TREATING TRAUMATIC BEREAVEMENT

Treating Traumatic Bereavement

A PRACTITIONER'S GUIDE

Laurie Anne Pearlman
Camille B. Wortman
Catherine A. Feuer
Christine H. Farber
Therese A. Rando

THE GUILFORD PRESS
New York   London

© 2014 The Guilford Press
A Division of Guilford Publications, Inc.
370 Seventh Avenue, Suite 1200, New York, NY 10001
www.guilford.com

Printed in Canada

This book is printed on acid-free paper.

Last digit is print number: 9   8   7   6   5   4

The authors have checked with sources believed to be reliable in their efforts to provide information
that is complete and generally in accord with the standards of practice that are accepted at the time of
publication. However, in view of the possibility of human error or changes in behavioral, mental health,
or medical sciences, neither the authors, nor the editors and publisher, nor any other party who has been
involved in the preparation or publication of this work warrants that the information contained herein
is in every respect accurate or complete, and they are not responsible for any errors or omissions or the
results obtained from the use of such information. Readers are encouraged to confirm the information
contained in this book with other sources.

Library of Congress Cataloging-in-Publication Data

Pearlman, Laurie A.
    Treating traumatic bereavement : a practitioner's guide / Laurie Anne Pearlman, Camille B. Wortman,
Catherine A. Feuer, Christine H. Farber, Therese A. Rando.
        pages cm
    Includes bibliographical references and index.
    ISBN 978-1-4625-1317-8 (pbk.)
    1. Bereavement—Psychological aspects.   2. Post-traumatic stress disorders—Treatment.
3. Sudden death—Psychological aspects.   4. Death—Psychological aspects.   5. Grief therapy.
I. Title.
    RC455.4.L67P43 2014
    616.85′21—dc23
                                                                    2013022787

*To those individuals who have endured
the sudden, traumatic death of a loved one
and to the therapists who commit to helping them*

About the Authors

Laurie Anne Pearlman, PhD, is a clinical psychologist and independent trauma consultant based in western Massachusetts. She is a member of the Complex Trauma Task Force of the International Society for Traumatic Stress Studies, a Fellow of Division 56 (Trauma Psychology) of the American Psychological Association (APA), and cofounder of the Traumatic Stress Institute/Center for Adult & Adolescent Psychotherapy. She has received awards for her clinical and scientific contributions from the International Society for Traumatic Stress Studies and the Connecticut Psychological Association, and for contributions to professional practice from APA Division 56.

Camille B. Wortman, PhD, is Professor of Psychology at Stony Brook University in New York. Her research focuses on how people react to the sudden, traumatic death of a loved one. She is a recipient of the Distinguished Scientific Award for an Early Career Contribution in Psychology from the APA, and a joint award from the APA Science Directorate and the National Science Foundation recognizing the achievements of women in science. She has authored four books and over 100 articles and book chapters.

Catherine A. Feuer, PhD, is a cognitive-behavioral psychologist in private practice in St. Louis, Missouri. Her clinical work, research, and publications are in the areas of anxiety disorders and posttraumatic stress disorder. She was formerly a postdoctoral fellow and Assistant Research Professor at the Center for Trauma Recovery at the University of Missouri, St. Louis. In her private practice, she treats trauma clients, including survivors of sudden, traumatic loss.

Christine H. Farber, PhD, is a clinical psychologist based in central Connecticut, where she practices psychological consultation informed by her interests in archetypal and humanistic psychology. She is Adjunct Professor at the University of Hartford's Graduate Institute in Professional Psychology and serves on the board of directors of the Connecticut Psychological Association, which has honored her with numerous awards.

Therese A. Rando, PhD, is Clinical Director of The Institute for the Study and Treatment of Loss in Warwick, Rhode Island, which provides psychotherapy, training, supervision, and consultation. She is a diplomate of the American Academy of Experts in Traumatic Stress (Board Certified Expert in Traumatic Stress and Board Certified in Bereavement Trauma). A recipient of numerous professional awards, she is the author of over 80 works, including *How to Go On Living When Someone You Love Dies*, *Treatment of Complicated Mourning*, and *Coping with the Sudden Death of Your Loved One: A Self-Help Handbook for Traumatic Bereavement*.

Preface

In writing this book, we came together with one goal: to improve the treatment available to people who have experienced the sudden, traumatic death of a loved one. Such deaths take many forms. In some cases, the death may have come about through the deliberate actions of another, as when a young woman is murdered by her ex-boyfriend. In other cases, the mourner may have contributed to the loved one's death, as when a father purchases a handgun that he neglects to lock up, which his teenage son then uses to commit suicide. In still other cases, the survivor experiences many profound losses in addition to the loved one's death, as when a tornado touches down in the neighborhood. To some degree, these survivors will face different issues: Some will live in fear that another loved one may be killed, some will struggle with guilt, and some will be exposed to bureaucracy at every turn as they try to rebuild what was lost. Despite these differences in how people experience the death, these losses share two common elements: Survivors of such losses can expect to experience painful feelings of grief as well as symptoms of trauma such as flashbacks, sleep disturbances, and problems with concentration. Treatment that focuses on only one of these elements is unlikely to be effective.

In this book we present a multifaceted therapy for these survivors. Our comprehensive treatment approach supports mourners in addressing both the trauma *and* grief associated with their losses. The treatment approach has three core components: building resources, processing trauma, and facilitating mourning. Briefly stated, the treatment will help traumatic bereavement clients develop the internal and external resources they need to process the traumatic dimensions of the death. The trauma processing, using cognitive-behavioral and exposure techniques, allows clients to address the trauma complicating their grief. Facilitating the processes of mourning enables clients to accommodate their loss. Through resource building, trauma processing, and the work of mourning in the context of a supportive relationship with their therapist, mourners are gradually able to adopt healthy new ways of moving forward in the world without the deceased.

WHO WE ARE AND HOW THIS BOOK CAME ABOUT

This book is the result of a long-term, stimulating collaboration among five psychologists who share a common aim: to help people with traumatic bereavement come to terms with what has happened and, ultimately, to lead more fulfilling lives. Some of us have sudden, traumatic losses in our personal backgrounds; all of us have encountered these survivors in our professional and personal lives. Their anguish and lack of treatment options motivated us to develop this approach.

On many occasions, we have had the opportunity to speak with survivors of traumatic loss who were disappointed in the treatment they received. Here are four examples:

1. About a year after losing her son in an accident, a woman began seeing a therapist. After 9 months of weekly treatment, the therapist told her, "You have a lot of trauma symptoms and I don't know how to treat those. We can either take a break, and I will attend some trauma workshops, or I can refer you to someone else."

2. A man whose son, a pedestrian, was killed by a drunk driver, struggled with flashbacks about what had happened that night. "My therapist advised me to stop dwelling on these thoughts, and to just put them out of my mind and try to think about something more pleasant. He implied that the problems that I had with these thoughts reflected a lack of willpower on my part."

3. A young man lost his brother, whom he had not seen in a year, in an airplane crash that he had witnessed while awaiting his arrival at a small airport. Two years later, still plagued by images of the crash, he entered therapy. After he told the therapist that he wanted to preserve some sense of connection to his older brother, the therapist told him that he had attachment problems and required intensive psychotherapy for what obviously were long-standing issues.

4. About 6 months after losing her husband in an industrial explosion, a woman made an appointment with the employee assistance person at her husband's workplace. She showed up at the appointment with her two daughters, ages 10 and 12. As she expressed it, "I told him a little bit about what happened to Robert and he literally went running out of the room. He said that he didn't have the training to help us. I thought he would send in someone else, but that didn't happen."

In addition to hearing from survivors, we have had countless conversations with therapists who had a strong desire to help traumatically bereaved clients, but who were uncertain or misguided about how to do so. In some cases, it appeared that therapists were unaware of the prevalence or the intensity of trauma symptoms. Similarly, many therapists seemed to be uninformed about the duration of these symptoms, not recognizing that following a traumatic death, debilitating symptoms of grief and trauma can last for several years.

As they learned more about traumatic bereavement, some therapists conveyed concerns that in the past, they may have responded inappropriately to bereaved clients' disclosures of traumatic experiences. Some expressed regret that they pathologized clients who displayed intense and prolonged trauma symptoms. For example, one therapist stated, "If I knew then what I know now, I would have been able to legitimize my client's responses to his loss. This would have made a big difference." Another therapist treated a woman whose daughter had been shot, told us that one of the most difficult aspects of the loss was what the client witnessed when she discovered her daughter's body. "I have to admit that I had great difficulty initiating discussion around this issue. When it did come up, I told myself that we should not focus on it too long or it might destabilize my client. I can now see that my client was avoiding this topic, and I was aiding and abetting her effort to do so." We have also reflected on our own difficulties in doing this work. Our personal reflections, heartbreaking stories from survivors about inadequate and incompetent treatment, and the suffering of our colleagues caused by regret or a sense of helplessness are what led to our collaboration and determination to create a treatment approach that would be accessible to therapists who wished to help the traumatically bereaved.

This treatment approach has truly been a co-creation, blending our different perspectives and backgrounds. Camille Wortman gathered and convened our group based on her vision of bringing together the accumulated wisdom in the fields of trauma and grief. We have spent hundreds of hours together sitting around a big worktable, participating in conference calls, writing and then editing each other's work, as well as sharing meals, laughter, and our own losses. After developing the approach, we pilot-tested it with clients at the Traumatic Stress Institute/Center for Adult and Adolescent Psychotherapy, formerly located in South Windsor, Connecticut (and now closed). Following the terrorist attacks of September 11, 2001, we were invited to teach our approach to psychotherapists from three universities in New York: Pace, Stony Brook, and Columbia. With each step, we have reshaped and refined the treatment approach. At many points along the way, individuals and groups who were interested in implementing our treatment program contacted us. Consequently, we decided to publish it as this book, which provides the background for this treatment approach, as well as the details of its implementation.

These chapters bring together cutting-edge work in the fields of trauma and loss. We draw from a wealth of clinical experience concerning ways to help clients build their resource base, process the traumatic elements of the death, and accommodate the loss and move forward with their lives. We address many specific issues that confront therapists who choose to work in the field of traumatic bereavement. Some of these problems concern the challenging matters and questions our clients bring to us. For example, a mourning parent may ask us why God allowed her child to die. Others stem from the nature of the work itself. For example, we offer support and guidance regarding how to help a reluctant client understand the value of recounting the murder of her child. We believe our approach represents the best integration and elaboration of the theory, research, and clinical wisdom that the fields of trauma and bereavement have to offer.

In collaborating on this book, we have made every effort to be mindful of the tension that often characterizes the relation between clinical research and practice (see, e.g., Bridging Work Group, 2005; Jordan, 2000; Neimeyer & Harris, 2011). Authors associated with the Bridging Work Group have emphasized that there is a gap between the interests, values, rewards, and work settings of bereavement researchers and those of practitioners. As the Bridging Work Group (2005) expressed it, "Many practitioners regard research as holding little relevance for their work, and many researchers believe that clinical practice has little to contribute to the scientific study of bereavement" (p. 93). The divergence in points of view was highlighted by the title of an early conference on improving communication between the two groups: "Therapists Are from Venus. Researchers Are from Mars" (Jordan, 2000).

The very composition of our team guards against the emphasis on theory or research over practice. Four of us are clinical psychologists who have had active psychotherapy and consultation practices focused on trauma (L. A. P., C. H. F., and C. A. F.) or bereavement and trauma (T. A. R.). The fifth (C. B. W.) is an academic psychologist who specializes in grief, and who serves as a legal consultant for survivors of sudden, traumatic death. As a group, we represent a variety of theoretical approaches, including cognitive-behavioral theory, psychodynamic theories, trauma theory, and humanistic psychology. Our broad experience base includes a wide range of clients and issues, which have informed and enriched the development of this approach. We considered each component of our treatment approach from multiple perspectives. Although all of us collaborated fully in developing the treatment approach, and each has contributed varying amounts of content to it in earlier iterations, Laurie Pearlman and Camille Wortman have played the primary role in writing the final version of the book. They contributed equally to this endeavor.

LANGUAGE

Authors must choose terms that convey their meanings as specifically as possible and terms that include all who might be part of the work. We have alternated use of the masculine and feminine pronouns. At times, we have addressed therapists as "you" and other times used "we" to acknowledge our own participation in this community. In describing those we are treating, we have alternated the term "survivor" with "mourner," "client," and "the bereaved."

We sometimes refer to the deceased as the "significant other." We chose this term in an effort to be as inclusive as possible when referring to the person who died. While many survivors will have had a positive attachment with their deceased family member or friend, others will have had highly ambivalent relationships or largely negative attachments for which terms such as "loved one" may seem inappropriate. Yet, in any of these cases, the connection will have been *significant*. In the text, we alternate among "loved one," "significant other," and "the deceased."

WHO MAY BENEFIT FROM THIS BOOK?

We wrote this book for psychotherapists and counselors who want to work more effectively with people who have experienced a sudden, traumatic death. In the past decade, there has been increasing interest in treating this population. There is growing awareness that traumatic bereavement may require treatment approaches that are unique to the specific challenges these survivors face. Many clinicians with a sincere interest in treating them have received little formal training in how to help. We have addressed this book to psychotherapists, with the implicit understanding that therapists also have had losses and may themselves be consumers of this type of treatment at some time.

For the most part, our target audience is psychotherapists who treat people with a variety of typical life problems such as divorce, job loss, and chronic stress. In all likelihood, these therapists have treated some clients with a "normal" or "typical" loss, such as the death of an elderly parent, but may not have treated many clients who experienced a traumatic loss. Our approach will show clinicians how to augment their skills to treat individuals experiencing traumatic bereavement.

Some therapists may have had the opportunity to treat a number of clients who have experienced a traumatic death. These therapists may feel that they would benefit from a treatment approach developed especially for this population, as well as treatment tools and resources that will help them to implement the approach.

We designed the treatment for clinicians representing a wide variety of experience levels and theoretical frameworks. We offer those with a particular orientation to therapy (e.g., cognitive-behavioral therapy) the opportunity to recognize the importance of including additional treatment components (e.g., building self capacities), and provide resources for doing so. We also describe ways to apply their particular orientation to this unique population—for example, how to change maladaptive thinking patterns in people who have experienced a loss of this kind.

Regardless of their level of experience or their theoretical orientation, many therapists rely on a grief or bereavement approach in treating the loss of a loved one. The basic idea is that clients must work through their grief by accomplishing certain tasks, such as accepting the loss. We demonstrate why such an approach, by itself, is insufficient to treat traumatic bereavement. The treatment approach described in this book assists clients in coping with trauma as well as grief.

We believe practicing psychotherapists working from a trauma, bereavement, or general background will find this book a useful overview of the problem and a source of ideas about treating clients. We hope it serves as a key reference for clinicians interested in traumatic bereavement. Scholars who may be looking for a clinical base for their study of sudden, traumatic death may also find the book informative. In addition, the book is useful as a teaching tool in graduate programs designed to train clinical practitioners. It is ideal for use in graduate courses in clinical psychology, social work, pastoral care, nursing, and related fields dealing with the treatment of traumatic bereavement. We also hope to inspire research on this approach to allow for its further development. Above all, we hope this book assists therapists in bringing relief to the thousands of survivors who are struggling with the ramifications of traumatic loss.

Acknowledgments

We would like to convey our heartfelt thanks to many people whose support in the process of writing this book was invaluable. Jim Nageotte, our acquisitions editor, provided guidance, encouragement, and wisdom at every step along the way. Our gratitude for all he has contributed to the book is beyond measure. Barbara Watkins, our developmental editor, provided incisive feedback and constructive suggestions. Her thoughtful analysis was instrumental in determining the structure of the book and shaping its content. Jane Keislar, editorial assistant, did an outstanding job of keeping track of loose ends. From the beginning, she stayed on top of the myriad details of this complex project, and thus kept us from losing our way. Marie Sprayberry, our copy editor, made many superb modifications to the text, thus greatly improving its clarity and readability. Laura Specht Patchkofsky, our production editor, kindly supported and guided us through the process of moving from a manuscript to a book. And last but not least, we want to acknowledge The Guilford Press for everything they have done to enhance the likelihood that our book would be successful. As indicated above, they have provided a team of outstanding professionals to work with us on the project. They have been very responsive to every issue we have raised. They have also been patient with us, allowing us to develop our ideas in our own way and at our own pace. Many of us have published books with other publishers, and we all agree that working with Guilford is as good as it gets.

Cherie Mahady, Camille Wortman's extraordinarily capable assistant, helped with a multitude of tasks, from finalizing the references to dealing with permissions. She did everything we needed when we needed it, and did it all with grace. Kathleen Albin, Jessica Latack, and Nicole Pitesa each read portions of the text. They provided invaluable suggestions, many of which appear in the book. We also want to thank Pamela Deiter-Sands and Dan Abrahamson for early support of the project that led to this work. To all of you, we express our profound thanks.

Each of us would like to make the following additional acknowledgments:

To Ervin—with gratitude for his intellect, compassion, love, and devotion, which nurture and sustain me. —L. A. P.

To Paul, the sustaining force in my life for nearly 50 years; and to Jeremy, Andrew, Katie, and Noah. Each of them has inspired me and brought me great joy. —C. B. W.

To my parents—Margaret and Michael—for all of their love, encouragement, and support; and to my children—James, Charlie, and Liam—for their love and enthusiasm. Thank you with all of my heart. —C. A. F.

To Lawrence, whose courage to allow an awareness of death and loss has deepened his capacity for both love and compassion. —C. H. F.

For laying the foundation, I gratefully acknowledge my parents, Thomas A. and Letitia G. Rando; for nurturing me along the way and enabling the meaning that makes it all possible, I am deeply indebted to Anthony, Elizabeth-Ann, Tommy, and B.B. —T. A. R.

Contents

> Downloadable versions of the reproducible handouts in this book, plus supplemental handouts and a sample 25-session treatment plan, are available at *www.guilford.com/pearlman-materials.*

PART I

FUNDAMENTALS OF TRAUMATIC BEREAVEMENT

CHAPTER 1

Sudden, Traumatic Death
and Traumatic Bereavement

One hot summer day when she was 6 years old, Emily discovered her father's lifeless body hanging in their garage. It was a grisly scene, replete with horrific sights and smells. Thereafter, Emily saw a succession of therapists. Each one addressed with her the psychological impact of dealing with her father's decision to take his own life, the resulting sense of abandonment that she experienced while growing up fatherless, and her grieving for all she had lost. Although she improved somewhat over the years, Emily continued to experience frequent nightmares, some emotional numbness, fear of intimacy, an exaggerated startle response, and increased agitation in hot, humid weather. Somehow, she felt unable to move on with her life.

It was fully 25 years before one therapist finally asked Emily, "Exactly what did you see when you found your father?" Finally someone had begun to tap into Emily's experience of the grotesque circumstances associated with her father's death, not solely the deprivations it had caused.

For many of us, the description above is disturbing to read. Like other survivors for whom this treatment is designed, Emily experienced the sudden, traumatic death of a significant other. In the instant she found her father dead, her life was fundamentally changed. She struggled on her own with trauma symptoms for 25 years, despite seeking help. As bereaved survivors attempt to pick up the shards of their lives and move forward, what lies ahead for them? If survivors want or need professional help, what sort of treatment would be most useful? This book addresses these questions.

Our goal is to provide a comprehensive treatment approach for therapists working with individuals who have experienced the sudden, traumatic death of a loved one. These mourners face the twin tasks of mourning the loss of their loved one and coping with the trauma that accompanied the death. Some therapists may not bring such a dual focus to their work with survivors of sudden, traumatic loss. Historically, the fields of *traumatology* (focusing on the study of traumatic events and their aftereffects) and *thanatology* (focusing on the study of dying, death, and bereavement) have existed relatively independently of one another, despite their conceptual, clinical, and often empirical relationship (Rando, 1997). This curious phenomenon has persisted despite the reality that most traumatic experiences include loss, and that most major losses have traumatic elements (see Rando, 2000).

This book presents a treatment approach designed to address both trauma and grief. In this chapter, we provide an overview of the psychological consequences of sudden, traumatic death, and broadly describe our integrated treatment approach for traumatic bereavement. Traumatic bereavement arises from an interaction between the circumstances of the death and other situational variables on the one hand, and aspects of the survivor (e.g., gender, attachment style, religious beliefs, personality) on the other, all within a particular social and cultural context.

Sudden, traumatic death is abrupt and occurs without warning. Although lack of anticipation alone can render a death traumatizing to a survivor, a death is more likely to be traumatic if it is untimely; if it involves violence or mutilation; if the survivor regards it as preventable; if the survivor believes that the loved one suffered; or if the survivor regards the death, or manner of death, as unfair and unjust. Other kinds of deaths likely to be regarded as traumatic include a death perceived as random (i.e., the loved one was in the wrong place at the wrong time); a death caused by a perpetrator with intent to harm; a situation where the survivor witnessed the death; a situation where the survivor is confronted with many deaths; and situations where the survivor's own life is threatened. Following a sudden, traumatic death, a survivor may experience *traumatic bereavement*, which is associated with enduring problematic reactions, including symptoms of trauma and grief. Causes of deaths most likely to precipitate traumatic bereavement include accidents, homicide, suicide, natural disasters, and war. In addition, acute natural events (e.g., a brain aneurysm) can have violent or traumatic elements.

TRAUMATIC DEATH PREVALENCE

According to the *National Vital Statistics Report* (Heron, 2012), the largest group of people who die between the ages of 1 and 44 do so as a result of a sudden, traumatic event. In most cases, a single traumatic death triggers a cascade of suffering and heartache, affecting the spouse or partner, parents, siblings, and children of the person who died. The tragedy may also affect extended family members, close friends, and coworkers.

Causes of traumatic deaths change over the lifespan. Accidents are by far the most common cause of death in all age groups younger than 44. For example, those in the 15–19 age group are approximately eight times more likely to die in an accident than to die from cancer, which is the leading cause of natural death in this group. Beginning at age 15, homicide and suicide emerge as prevalent causes of death. Among the 15–19, the 20–24, and the 25–34 age groups, suicide and homicide are among the top three causes of death, along with accidents. Those in the 15–19 age group are approximately six times more likely to die as a result of homicide or suicide than of cancer. Moreover, while deaths from accidents, homicide, and suicide become less prevalent after age 44, deaths resulting from sudden cardiovascular events become more prevalent.

These figures provide a conservative estimate of the prevalence of sudden, traumatic deaths. They do not include deaths from natural disasters, war, or terrorist attacks. They also do not include sudden deaths that result from heart attacks, strokes, or aneurysms.

PSYCHOLOGICAL CONSEQUENCES OF SUDDEN, TRAUMATIC DEATH

Following the sudden, traumatic loss of loved ones, survivors typically experience painful trauma symptoms (such as disturbing, intrusive thoughts), as well as grief symptoms (such as yearning for their loved ones). Because of the way the death occurred, the survivor is typically flooded with intense and painful affect. The deaths often completely overwhelm their defenses, leaving them unable to cope. As one survivor expressed it, "It was as though someone cut my insides out." In most cases, their symptoms are more intense and prolonged than those experienced by survivors of natural deaths.

If a death was sudden, was perceived as random, and occurred without warning, feelings of shock may be profound. A survivor may feel helpless, confused, and unable to grasp the implications of what has happened. Such deaths are also likely to evoke intense death anxiety, leading these bereaved person to fear her own death as well as that of surviving loved ones. As one father indicated following his wife's murder, "I was terrified that I would also be killed and that my children would be left with no parents."

Untimely deaths often cause distress because survivors feel their loved ones were cheated. If the loss was untimely or viewed as preventable, feelings of anger may be predominant. Most mourners in this situation find it difficult to live with the fact that their loved ones' deaths were unnecessary. Anger is also a common reaction to deaths that are regarded as unjust. Most survivors believe that perpetrators should be held accountable for what has happened. Particularly if a perpetrator intended harm or was cruel or callous, a survivor must confront the human capacity for malevolence. Deaths resulting from intentional acts of violence often trigger powerful feelings of generalized rage, as well as rage specifically directed toward the perpetrator.

A violent death typically results in mutilation of the loved one's body, such as when the deceased died in a fiery car crash or was shot at close range. In such cases, vivid images of the loved one's body are often seared into the survivor's mind. Such images typically emerge even in cases where the survivor did not witness the fatal incident. These disturbing images often return as intrusive thoughts or as parts of dreams or nightmares. In addition, the violence associated with the death and the mutilation of the body are likely to heighten the survivor's concern with what the loved one experienced during the final moments of her life.[1]

As we detail in later chapters, research has identified a set of core issues that survivors of sudden, traumatic death typically experience (Wortman, Pearlman, Feuer, Farber, & Rando, 2012). First, it is common for survivors to question their religious beliefs, or even to feel betrayed and turn against God. In such cases, religious faith can become a casualty of the death. Second, survivors are often preoccupied with whether their loved ones suffered at the time of their death. Third, most mourners are troubled by their inability to make sense of what has happened. Finally, survivors often struggle with feelings of guilt. This was the case for the parents of a young man named Greg, who was an honor student and a varsity athlete. When he turned 17, Greg began working evenings and weekends at a convenience store to save money for college. One evening at about 11:00 P.M., Greg and the manager were murdered during a botched holdup attempt. Greg's parents experienced intense guilt following his death. About 8 months before the tragedy, he had asked his parents whether he could take karate lessons. They said no, reasoning that his schedule was already overloaded. After the tragedy, they berated themselves for this decision, thinking that if he had taken the classes, he might have survived the assault. In Chapter 3, we discuss each of these core issues in more detail.

In attempting to understand why a traumatic death can evoke so many debilitating reactions, we must recognize that such a death typically provokes an existential crisis. The nature of the loss forces most mourners to question assumptions that they previously took for granted (see Bowlby, 1969; Marris, 1975; Parkes, 1971). These include beliefs that the world is meaningful

---

[1]To avoid awkward "he or she/his or her" constructions, we alternate throughout this book between feminine and masculine third-person singular pronouns.

and operates according to principles of fairness and justice, that one is safe and secure, that the world is benevolent, and that other people can generally be trusted (Janoff-Bulman, 1992).

The traumatic death of a loved one challenges these fundamental assumptions. Often the bereaved simply cannot absorb what has happened; the loss seems incomprehensible. It demonstrates that life is capricious and unpredictable. The dismantling of basic assumptions about the world may also invalidate much of the bereaved's past behavior. For example, two young parents did everything possible to protect their 3-year-old son, such as putting locks on their kitchen cabinets and buying the most highly rated car seat. Despite their precautions, the child was killed in a motor vehicle crash caused by an under-age driver who had been drinking. In addition to the loss itself, it was painful for his parents to recognize that they were unable to protect their child. Should the couple have other children, they are likely to experience intense and prolonged anxiety about the safety of those children.

It is generally well established that the presence of trauma symptoms interferes with the process of accommodating the loss (Rando, 1993, 2013). An important part of successful mourning involves recollecting the loved one and reviewing the relationship that was lost. Gradually, the mourner is able to put her life with the deceased into perspective, and to begin moving forward. When a person has suffered a traumatic loss, attempts to recollect the loved one are often associated with distressing memories or images, such as what happened during the loved one's death. These thoughts and images are so disturbing that in many cases, individuals try to avoid thinking about their loved one, making it far more difficult to process their loss. An additional burden is that survivors often become alarmed at the intensity of their trauma symptoms. As one man explained following the murder of his daughter, "I'm the kind of guy who would never even hurt a fly. But after her death, all I thought about was killing the man who did this to her. I kept thinking about all the ways I could kill him. I really thought I was going crazy."

Trauma symptoms are likely to undermine the resources survivors have available to deal with day-to-day living. Physiological hyperarousal and the resulting sleep and concentration difficulties, for example, can sap a mourner's energy and make it difficult to function well at work and at home. While coping resources are impaired as a result of the tragedy, the demands placed on the mourner often increase dramatically following the loss. For example, one woman whose husband died in an occupational accident experienced major difficulties with her surviving sons. Her 15-year-old quit the soccer team his deceased father had coached; the boy also became sullen and argumentative. Her 6-year-old started having nightmares on a frequent basis and began wetting the bed—something he had not done since he was toilet-trained.

Traumatic deaths are more likely than natural deaths to bring mourners into contact with situations that can be profoundly disturbing. For example, one couple rushed to the hospital to see their teenage daughter, who had been shot by her ex-boyfriend. Upon arriving, they were told that their daughter did not survive. The young woman's mother cried out, "I want to hold my baby." The nurse in charge informed her that her daughter's body was "evidence" for the case against the perpetrator, and that no contact or touch was permitted. Other issues that often emerge in regard to a traumatic death and exacerbate a survivor's distress include removal of the loved one from life support, insensitive death notification, identifying the body, a request for an autopsy (and the autopsy itself), lack of an intact body to bury, media attention, and criminal or civil trials. Most of these situations occur around the time of death. Consequently, survivors are forced to contend with them while in the throes of acute grief.

Many of the factors that can characterize traumatic deaths tend to occur together. A single mother lost her only child, a 10-year-old boy, when he was shot and killed in the home of a classmate. The gun, without adequate safety devices, was loaded at the time of the shooting. It was stored in a completely accessible, unlocked bedroom closet. The child's death was sudden and, at age 10, was untimely. It was regarded as preventable because if the gun had been stored properly, the accident would not have happened. A subsequent investigation revealed that her son did not touch the gun, but was accidentally killed while his classmate was playing with it. This led the mother to believe that her son's death was unfair. In most cases, the impact of these factors is cumulative: The more of them that are present, the more intense and prolonged the survivor's distress is likely to be.

PERSISTENT AND PERVASIVE EFFECTS OF TRAUMATIC DEATH

Back in the 1980s, one of us (Camille B. Wortman) was contacted by the Insurance Institute for Highway Safety, a private foundation. The foundation was interested in the long-term psychological effects of losing a spouse or child in a motor vehicle crash. A study was designed to investigate this issue. Interviews were conducted with people 4–7 years following the death of their spouse or child in a car accident. The researchers also interviewed control respondents who had not lost loved ones. The purpose of the study was to determine whether people continued to be affected by such losses years after they occurred. Would most respondents be functioning well, or would they still be struggling with the ramifications of the death?

The results provided compelling evidence that the traumatic death of a spouse or child poses long-term difficulties (Lehman, Wortman, & Williams, 1987). Comparisons between bereaved persons and controls revealed significant differences on several psychological symptoms, including depression as assessed on the SCL-90 scale (Derogatis, 1977). Following the loss, bereaved respondents also became anxious that something bad would happen to another family member; this anxiety did not arise among controls.

Bereaved individuals also reported a significantly lower quality of life than did control respondents, as assessed by the Bradburn Affect Balance Scale (Bradburn, 1969). This scale measures the extent to which respondents find their activities interesting and meaningful, experience feelings of pleasure and enjoyment, and feel proud about things they have done.

Whereas some bereaved couples reported that the death of a child had a pronounced negative impact on their marriage, others said that the death brought them closer together. As a group, however, the bereaved parents in this study tended to report more stress in their marriages and were significantly more likely to seek and obtain a divorce than controls. Bereaved parents were also significantly less likely than controls to be working for pay, and to be working at the same job that they held before the loss. When they did remain at the same job, they tended to have difficulty sustaining interest in and motivation for their work. Following the death, bereaved spouses and parents reported earning significantly less family income than controls. Bereaved parents were also significantly more likely to move. Many commented that their prior homes were an endless source of painful memories.

Bereaved spouses reported more difficulty in getting involved in leisure activities and in carrying out their housework. They also scored significantly higher on loneliness than did controls. Both groups also reported more conflict with relatives and friends than controls. For example, they were more likely than controls to indicate that these relationships made them feel hurt and disappointed. As we describe in more detail below, those who lost a spouse or child were more likely than controls to experience problems in their relationships with surviving children—for example, agreeing that they felt more "emotionally worn out." Moreover, in response to an open-ended question about the impact of their spouse's death on their surviving children, an overwhelming majority of respondents (73%) reported that their children had suffered negative effects. Forty-seven percent of responses were coded as "extremely negative effects," including depression, drug abuse, and suicide.

Negative effects were common even in cases where surviving children or siblings were quite young. Reports of withdrawal, obsessive behavior, and anger were typical. For instance, one mother spoke of her 5-year-old daughter's reaction to the loss of her father: "She stopped playing. She hasn't been the same since then. She doesn't show interest like she used to." Another mother described how her daughter was affected by the traumatic death of her older brother: "[My daughter] was very withdrawn for 1½ years. When her emotions finally came out, it was almost a disaster. She said she didn't love any of us any more because it would only hurt her."

The results revealed significant differences in mortality between bereaved and control respondents. By the time we started the study, more than 6% of those individuals who lost a spouse or child had died; none of the respondents in the control group had died. This is a very high mortality rate for such a young population (most of the respondents were in their early 40s).

The interview also included a number of questions to determine whether the bereaved were still dealing actively with their loss. Over 90% of those who had lost a spouse or child had experienced thoughts or memories of their loved one during the past month. Of those who had such thoughts, 56% of the bereaved spouses and 68% of the bereaved parents reported that these memories made them feel "hurt and pained," and none of the respondents were able to block unpleasant thoughts when they wanted to. Sixty percent of the bereaved spouses and 67% of the bereaved parents reported that during the past month they had had at least one conversation with a friend or family member about their loved one.

Despite the time that had elapsed since their loved ones' deaths, the data indicated that most respondents had not achieved a state of resolution regarding their loss. Nearly 50% of those who lost a spouse or a child stated that they had relived the accident or the events surrounding their loved one's death during the past month. Approximately 60% of the bereaved respondents reported having had thoughts during the past month that the accident was "unfair" or that they and their loved one had been cheated.

If a person is having difficulty coming to terms with the death of a spouse, child, or parent 4–7 years after it occurred, others might conclude that the person is coping poorly with the loss. What these data suggest is that lasting distress following the traumatic death of a family member is not a sign of individual coping failure. Rather, such distress is typical in response to this type of loss.

Since the motor vehicle study was conducted, a number of additional studies have corroborated these findings. For example, in an important study on the impact of losing a child through accident, suicide, or homicide, Murphy, Chung, and Johnson (2002) found that 5 years after the loss, a majority of mothers and fathers were experiencing significant mental distress. The percentage of mothers and fathers meeting formal criteria for posttraumatic stress disorder (PTSD) was still considerably higher than for women and men in the general population. Moreover, a majority of mothers (61%) and fathers (55%) continued to reexperience visual or mental imagery of their loved one's death (Murphy, Johnson, Chung, & Beaton, 2003). These and other studies have shown that following a traumatic death, it is common for a survivor to experience painful symptoms of trauma and grief for many years. Although feelings of distress may decline over time, there is some question about whether survivors of sudden, traumatic death ever recover fully. Thus we prefer to use the term *accommodation* to *recovery* when referring to the goal of the mourning processes. As one bereaved mother expressed it, "You don't get over it; you get used to it." In fact, traumatic bereavement can become chronic and debilitating. People may experience such profound and persistent changes as feelings of emptiness and alienation from others, a loss of meaning or purpose in life, and feelings of impending doom. Because friends, relatives, and even therapists are often not aware of the enduring impact of these losses, they may convey to the bereaved that they should be adjusting more quickly than they are. In fact, the bereaved themselves often mistakenly regard their continuing distress as a sign of personal inadequacy or coping failure.

THE NEED FOR INTEGRATED TREATMENT OF TRAUMATIC BEREAVEMENT

The description of Emily's traumatic experience at the beginning of this chapter illustrates the importance of addressing traumatic elements of the situation, in addition to those involving loss. Treatment must address integration of the trauma as well as accommodation to the loss. In Emily's case, the therapists she saw had focused on helping her to mourn—a task that seems like the natural thing to do, and that is in fact an important aspect of the treatment process. Yet, because they did not appreciate that she had been traumatized by what she experienced— overwhelmed by the terrible sights and smells, and helpless in the face of all the horror—a significant aspect of her experience remained unresolved. A survivor who is unable to address the traumatic aspects of a death continues to experience trauma symptoms, and these symptoms compromise the survivor's ability to mourn the loss fully. Therapy must address the two in combination. Without this dual and integrated focus, survivors may experience continuing emotional pain and distress.

Given the prevalence of sudden, traumatic deaths and the profound disruptions associated with traumatic bereavement, it is essential that effective treatment be available. In our experience, survivors frequently encounter difficulty in identifying treatment options that address their unique concerns and needs. As we describe in Chapter 7, several papers within the clinical literature have discussed the interaction of trauma and grief. For the most part, however, this work has not been integrated into a comprehensive treatment approach. The twin demands for healthy mourning and trauma integration, and the breadth and intensity of traumatic bereavement responses, call for a multifaceted approach.

AN OVERVIEW OF OUR TREATMENT APPROACH
FOR TRAUMATIC BEREAVEMENT

The goal of the treatment approach described in this book is to help an adult survivor address the traumatic stress associated with the death and the way it occurred, so that the survivor can process the grief surrounding her loss. The ultimate goal is to help clients reinvest in their lives in ways that are fulfilling to them. As shown in Table 1.1, this treatment is composed of three core components: (1) building a survivor's internal and interpersonal resources; (2) processing the traumatic death both cognitively and emotionally; and (3) moving through the processes of mourning. Psychoeducation in these areas is an important element, as are between-session independent activities assigned to clients. A supportive therapeutic relationship is essential as well. This treatment is based on theory as well as on empirically validated practices for treating grief and trauma. We have also drawn from years of clinical experience, and from a pilot study

TABLE 1.1. Components of the Treatment Approach

Resource building
- Self capacities
  - Inner connection
  - Self-worth
  - Affect management
    - Recognizing affect
    - Tolerating affect
    - Modulating affect
    - Integrating affect
- Coping skills
  - Breathing retraining
  - Self-care
- Social support
- Bereavement-specific strategies
- Meaning and spirituality
- Values and personal goal setting

Trauma processing
- Cognitive processing
  - Cognitive restructuring of cognitive schemas and related psychological needs disrupted by trauma
  - Identifying and challenging maladaptive automatic thoughts
  - Activity scheduling
- Emotional processing
  - Prolonged (*in vivo* and imaginal) exposure

Mourning
- *Recognize the loss*
- *React to the separation*
- *Recollect and reexperience the deceased and the relationship*
- *Relinquish the old attachments to the deceased and the old assumptive world*
- *Readjust to move adaptively into the new world without forgetting the old*
- *Reinvest*

Psychoeducation and independent activities

Therapeutic relationship

that tested the approach. We describe each of the treatment's components below and in more detail in Part IV, as well as in the client handouts in the Appendix. In addition, we have provided online supplementary handouts that, while not essential, may be useful to clients. These handouts are available at the website supplement for this book (*www.guilford.com/pearlman-materials*).

Resource Building

Clients who have experienced traumatic bereavement need to process the trauma and engage in active mourning. To build the foundation for those two tasks, this treatment approach first focuses on preparing survivors by developing six specific resources. These resources support clients in the therapy process and help them manage day-to-day life. They are woven throughout the treatment; clients are asked to engage regularly in some resource-building activity between sessions. We describe resource-building activities in Chapter 10.

Self Capacities

Self capacities are skills people use to regulate internal states. The three self capacities essential to internal stability are *inner connection* (internal bond with positive images and memories of loved ones or other positive attachment figures), *self-worth* (the ability to feel like a good enough person), and *affect management* (the ability to recognize, tolerate, modulate, and integrate strong feelings). These "feelings skills" are drawn from *constructivist self development theory* (CSDT; Pearlman, 1998) as well as attachment theory (Bowlby, 1969), and are discussed in more detail in Chapters 2 and 10.

Coping Skills

Coping strategies are actions people take to manage, tolerate, or reduce the demands of a stressful situation (Folkman, 2001; Lazarus & Folkman, 1984). We can empower our clients by helping them to examine the coping strategies they are using and by educating them about strategies that may be more effective. Two important coping strategies within our treatment approach are breathing retraining and self-care (i.e., adequate sleep, nutrition, and physical exercise).

Social Support

Emotional and instrumental support from family members, friends, neighbors, and coworkers can help to counter the isolation that survivors of traumatic bereavement may experience. The therapist encourages survivors to identify people who can help them when the treatment is challenging. For example, a support provider might accompany the client in exposure activities, such as visiting the deceased person's grave.

Bereavement-Specific Strategies

Bereavement-specific issues are events or occasions that evoke powerful memories or emotions ("subsequent temporary upsurges of grief"; Rando, 1993, 2013) related to the deceased or to her death. These situations often arise without warning and pose one of the greatest trials for the traumatically bereaved. Our treatment approach addresses these situations directly with clients, helping them to develop constructive strategies for anticipating these challenges whenever possible and coping with them when anticipation is not possible.

Meaning and Spirituality

A sudden, traumatic death can assault a survivor's sense that life is meaningful. An essential aspect of this treatment approach is to help the client create or recover a connection with something that makes her life feel worth living. This connection can serve as an inner resource to be called upon when needed for self-soothing.

Values and Personal Goal Setting

The purpose of *values* work with survivors of traumatic bereavement is to help them regain a sense of purpose and direction in their lives by identifying what matters to them most at this point. Values work helps people choose to move forward in meaningful directions and become engaged in activities they view as worthwhile. It can also propel movement forward in a client who seems to be stuck in the mourning process. For example, clients can be helped to realize that despite the loss, they have values that are important to them. These may include nurturing young people, learning new things, or maintaining a relationship with members of their extended family. Therapists can assist clients in developing goals that are consonant with their values. This should encourage involvement in activities that will help the client move forward.

Trauma Processing

When the client has adequate resources, trauma processing can begin. Cognitive-behavioral therapy (CBT) provides the empirically validated underpinning to trauma processing in our treatment approach (see Chapter 7 for a discussion of relevant research and Chapter 11 for a description of how to utilize these treatment elements). Another approach that is widely utilized for the treatment of trauma is eye movement desensitization and reprocessing, or EMDR.[2]

Although our treatment approach relies on techniques from CBT to process the loss, therapists trained in EMDR can use that technique for trauma processing (for a discussion of the use of EMDR to treat complicated mourning and traumatic stress, see Sprang, 2001).

Cognitive Processing

We utilize *cognitive processing therapy* (Resick & Schnicke, 1992, 1993; Resick et al., 2008) and cognitive techniques such as identifying, monitoring, and challenging problematic automatic thoughts; the downward arrow technique for identifying problematic beliefs; and the behavioral experiments of activity scheduling. These techniques help survivors change maladaptive cognitions that often emerge following sudden, traumatic deaths. Maladaptive cognitions (e.g., "I can't trust anyone") often present obstacles to the mourning process. Identifying and changing these cognitions can help the mourning process to proceed. CSDT (McCann & Pearlman, 1990b; Pearlman, 2001; Pearlman & Saakvitne, 1995) outlines five need areas that are the basis for core assumptions and beliefs about self and others within CPT (Resick & Schnicke, 1993). These trauma-sensitive need areas—safety, trust, control, esteem, and intimacy (Pearlman, 2003)—are the foundation for the cognitions targeted in this treatment approach.

Emotional Processing

Another aspect of the treatment relies on prolonged (imaginal and *in vivo*) exposures, drawn from *emotional processing theory* (Foa & Kozak, 1991; Foa & Rothbaum, 1998; Rachman, 1980). Exposure helps to counter the avoidance of people, places, and things that remind survivors of

---

[2]EMDR combines brief imaginal exposure to trauma material with therapist-induced rapid eye movements (or some other type of bilateral stimulation, such as finger tapping or auditory clicks). Investigators have begun to explore the application of EMDR to grief. The most recent edition of EMDR developer Francine Shapiro's book (Shapiro & Forrest, 2004) includes a chapter on grief (see also Solomon & Shapiro, 1997). Solomon and Rando (2007) have delineated how EMDR can be used within a comprehensive framework for the treatment of grief and mourning. They presented specific guidelines for using EMDR to facilitate the mourning process. According to Solomon and Rando, EMDR deserves more attention as a technique for processing the traumatic elements of a loss.

the traumatic aspects of the death and its aftermath. It also assists survivors by reducing the emotional intensity of traumatic memories and images. Imaginal exposure primarily takes the form of written assignments, the main one being written accounts of the death or of learning about the death. Clients are instructed to write an account of the death three times over the course of the treatment and are asked to read the account daily. For *in vivo* exposure, a therapist and client create a fear and avoidance hierarchy of avoided or anxiety-provoking situations. The survivor is then supported in moving through the list at his own pace, starting with the least distressing situation. *In vivo* exposure to situations is primarily carried out as an independent activity. Before initiating trauma processing via exposure, it is important to assess the adequacy of the client's coping resources. If this step is not taken, trauma processing may result in the retraumatization of the client. Therefore, building or strengthening a client's self capacities, in addition to assessing them along the way, is an essential element of this approach.

Mourning

There is a growing consensus that clients can be helped more effectively by treatments that focus on specific mourning processes, such as recognizing the permanence of the loss, rather than a sequence of discrete stages. In this treatment, we rely on the six "R" processes of mourning developed by Rando (1993, 2013) for conceptualizing healthy mourning. These "R" processes are as follows: *Recognize the loss; React to the separation; Recollect and reexperience the deceased and the relationship; Relinquish the old attachments to the deceased and the old assumptive world; Readjust to move adaptively into the new world without forgetting the old;* and *Reinvest*. Healthy mourning is the path to accommodating the many and varied losses that are typically associated with sudden, traumatic deaths. Among traumatically bereaved clients, the mourning process is often impeded by unprocessed trauma. Within this integrated treatment approach, a focus on the individual processes of mourning is interwoven with trauma processing.

Over the years, countless portrayals of the mourning process have appeared in the literature. Two of the most influential are Freud's (1917/1957) concept of *griefwork* and Bowlby's (1969, 1980) and Kübler-Ross's (1969) *stage models* of grief. In this book, we examine these models closely and consider their relevance to grief therapy as it is practiced today. In developing our treatment approach, we have drawn from approaches that have for the most part been developed after the griefwork and stages views, and often in reaction to their limitations. In addition to Rando's "R" processes, these theoretical developments include the *stress and coping* model (Lazarus & Folkman, 1984), which addresses individual differences in response to the death of a loved one, which stage models cannot; the *continuing-bonds* approach, which clarifies that it is not necessary to sever all or most ties to the deceased, and that in fact such ties can be beneficial (Klass, Silverman, & Nickman, 1996); research on *positive emotions* (Folkman, 1997a, 2001), which illustrates the surprising role these emotions can play in facilitating the mourning process and promoting healing; the *dual-process model* of bereavement (Stroebe & Schut, 1999; M. S. Stroebe, Schut, & Stroebe, 2005), which emphasizes that mourners must focus not only on painful aspects of the loss, but on feelings and behaviors that are restorative, and that provide a respite from intense distress; and the *meaning-making approach* developed by Neimeyer and his associates (e.g., Holland, Currier, & Neimeyer, 2006; Holland & Neimeyer, 2010; Neimeyer, 2001; Neimeyer & Sands, 2011; Shear, Boelen, & Neimeyer, 2011), who have demonstrated that a search for meaning is a fundamental part of the mourning process.

Psychoeducation, Worksheets, and Independent Activities

Psychoeducation—providing clients with information about their symptoms, adaptations, and recovery—is a critical aspect of this treatment. It takes place within virtually all sessions, and is reinforced by informational handouts. Other handouts for clients reinforce and expand upon in-session work; the worksheets and independent activities provided in these handouts support resource building, trauma processing, and mourning. Clients can also use these handouts to support their continuing progress after therapy ends. Purchasers of this book have permission to reproduce all of the handouts, which are located in the Appendix and online (*www.guilford.com/pearlman-materials*). The handouts that are essential to this treatment approach are in the Appendix and on the website. Additional, supplemental handouts are on the website only.

Therapeutic Relationship

We list the therapeutic relationship in Table 1.1 as a separate element of the treatment in order to highlight its importance. As in all trauma therapies, the presence of a compassionate guide on the journey is essential in working with survivors of traumatic death (see, e.g., Pearlman & Courtois, 2005; Pearlman & Saakvitne, 1995).

Treatment Structure

The treatment approach described in this book includes a rich array of material that can help traumatically bereaved clients within any theoretical framework, treatment length, or format (structured or unstructured). The therapist can plan the treatment in a variety of ways depending on a client's needs and resources, as well as on the therapist's and client's preferences. In Table 1.2, we list the session topics we have used in implementing the treatment. To provide a more comprehensive overview of our approach, we have expanded this list into a 25-session treatment plan, which is available on the book's supplemental website at *www.guilford.com/pearlman-materials*. The topics we include, and the way these topics are sequenced, are based on our experience with a series of pilot therapies.

The treatment can be tailored for clients who need only certain elements of the treatment or are only able to participate in a limited number of sessions. One can think of the approach as modular, and select all or any of the three core treatment components (resource building, trauma processing, and mourning) as needed for each client. The sample session format described in Chapter 9 (see Table 9.2) can be used to address any of these topics. In using this approach, it is important to integrate the treatment elements. We recommend that each session contain tasks from one or more of the three core treatment components, as well as psychoeducation about traumatic bereavement. These elements are interwoven over the treatment course, with each session having one or more specific topics as a focus.

Session Topics

People experiencing traumatic bereavement present with a vast array of symptoms, adaptations, and needs, and we would not expect that every therapy would address all of these topics. These topics (see Table 1.2) are sequenced as they would be to address a typical traumatically bereaved client. As we describe in Chapter 9, this approach can be adapted for cases in which the client

TABLE 1.2. Main Topics and Subtopics for the Treatment Approach

Session 1. Orientation
Orientation to the treatment
Discussion of sudden, traumatic death and traumatic bereavement (T, M)[a]

Session 2. Treatment Goals and Growth
Treatment goals and tools
Self-care (R)
Exploring the impact of the death (T, M)
Overview of the six "R" processes of mourning (M)

Session 3. *Recognize the Loss*; Feelings Skills (Self Capacities)
The first "R" process (M)
Breathing retraining (R)
Feelings skills (R)

Session 4. Automatic Thoughts
Introduction to the cognitive therapy model for change (T)
Identifying automatic thoughts (T)

Session 5. Automatic Thoughts (Continued)
Challenging automatic thoughts (T)

Session 6. *React to the Separation*; Exposure
The second "R" process (M)
First account of the death (T, M)

Session 7. Secondary Losses and Social Support
Secondary losses (M)
Building social support (R)
Second account of the death (T, M)

Session 8. Resource-Building Activities: Social Support and Values Work
Values work (R, M) and personal goal setting (R, M)
Third account of the death (T, M)

Session 9. Personal Goal Setting and Psychological Needs
Personal goal setting (Continued)
Psychological needs (T)
Foundation for ending therapy

Session 10. Obstacles to Accommodation
Obstacles to accommodation (T, M)

Session 11. Review of Previous Topics

Session 12. *Recollect and Reexperience the Deceased and the Relationship*
The third "R" process (M)
Positive and negative aspects of the relationship with the loved one (M)

Session 13. *Recollect and Reexperience the Deceased and the Relationship* (continued)
Review of the relationship with the loved one (M)

Session 14. *In Vivo* Exposure
Fear and avoidance hierarchy (T)
In vivo exposure activity (T)
Writing assignment: Relationship with the deceased (T, M)

Session 15. *In Vivo* Exposure and Guilt
Guilt, regret, and sudden, traumatic death (T, M)
In vivo exposure activity (T)

Session 16. *In Vivo* Exposure and Anger
Anger and sudden, traumatic death (T, M)
In vivo exposure activity (T)

Session 17. Transforming the Pain
Anger, regret, and guilt in sudden, traumatic death (T)
Letter to the deceased (T, M)
In vivo exposure activity (T, M)

Session 18. Bereavement Challenges
Bereavement-specific issues (M)
In vivo exposure activity (T)

Session 19. The Assumptive World; *Relinquish the Old Attachments to the Deceased and the Old Assumptive World*
Discussion of the assumptive world (M)
The fourth "R" process (M)

Session 20. *Readjust to Move Adaptively into the New World without Forgetting the Old*; Spirituality
The fifth "R" process (M)
Writing assignment: Meaning of the loss (T, M)
Spirituality (R, M)

Session 21. New Relationship with the Deceased; Termination
Writing assignment: Continuing the relationship with the deceased (M)
Ending therapy

Session 22. Self-Intimacy and Identity
Self-intimacy (R)
Identity (R)

Session 23. Other-Trust, Other-Intimacy; Social Support
Other-trust (R, M)
Other-intimacy (R, M)
Social support (R, M)
Writing assignment: Final impact statement (M)

Session 24. *Reinvest*; Termination
The sixth and last "R" process (M)
Termination

Session 25. Final Review and Termination

[a]We have designated subtopics in this table as promoting resource building (R), trauma processing (T), or mourning (M), as appropriate. Some subtopics contribute to addressing more than one of these components. Subtopics without those designations contribute to the development and flow of the treatment. Although the topics are presented according to the sample 25-session treatment plan on this book's website, therapists may select any topics and subtopics that are relevant to a client's treatment.

does not need all aspects of the treatment. However, some of these topics must be addressed before others. Most important, resource building must precede trauma processing, unless you determine the client has the necessary resources to commence with exposure work. In addition, the six "R" processes build upon one another, and the trauma-processing and resource-building work provides the foundation for movement through the six "Rs." Again, the sample session format described in Table 9.2 can be used to address any of these topics.

CLINICAL INTEGRATION

"Hi, Emily. I'm glad to see you back this week." Dr. Sandra Roberts had been working with Emily for just 2 weeks, and she had been unsure whether Emily would return. In their first session, Emily had mentioned being in therapy on several occasions throughout her life and feeling that these therapies had not helped her move through her grief. Why couldn't she just forget the terrible images and smells that intruded on her days and nights? Sandra was hoping Emily would feel optimistic about this new therapy, but she also understood that Emily might be reluctant to expect further change.

Emily launched right in. "You asked me last week what I saw and what I experienced when I found my father dead all of those years ago. You seemed interested in the details. I think about these details often, even now. But I have rarely talked about it. It just always seemed so taboo, and so gruesome, you know?"

Sandra nodded.

"I felt something like relief when you asked me that," said Emily. "I know there's fear there—fear about going into these details, but also relief."

"Well, as I said, I'm glad you're here, and I think you're brave for seeking help in the midst of your fear. Today I'd like to talk about what I think we can do together. I'd like to give you an overview of the treatment plan I have in mind. Does that sound OK to you?"

This time it was Emily who nodded. Sandra continued:

"As you know, at a very early age you experienced a traumatic death. You were left to deal with the loss of your father and the grief that resulted from his sudden absence. This is a lot for a little girl to deal with." Emily was listening attentively as Sandra spoke.

"Mixed in with that was the fact that the experience of finding your father hanging in the garage was traumatic. What I mean by that is that it probably evoked a reaction of shock and horror. It was a scene that was so unexpected—so far outside any framework of understanding that you may have had—that it probably felt pretty unreal. On the other hand, I imagine there was a way in which it was all too real. That is, the sights and smells and your own bodily sensations as you took this in were all in high focus."

Emily felt a wave in her stomach as Sandra described the scene as being "all too real." She became more fidgety in her seat and found that her voice cracked as she tried to speak. "I can remember it pretty vividly. I feel anxious hearing you talk about it—anxious in the way I described last week. Sometimes this anxiety comes up out of nowhere. Right now it feels connected to what you are describing."

"You seem very connected to your experience, and you're able to articulate it. That's great, and it will be helpful as we move forward. I think what you have experienced all these years is *traumatic bereavement*: symptoms, feelings, and a state of being resulting from a combination of loss and trauma, or from a death that was also traumatic in its circumstances. Does that make sense to you?"

"It does," said Emily.

"I think you've done a lot of grieving for your dad over the years, and you've probably done less work with the traumatic aspects of your experience of his death. If we can work on processing some of the trauma, we may find that the mourning work we do together is different from the work you've done in previous therapies. By also focusing on the traumatic aspects of your experience, the process of mourning your father may go deeper or beyond where you've been so far, and it may feel more complete. That's the idea of this treatment approach, and if you're on board, I will lead you through some exercises designed to process both your thoughts and feelings about the trauma. Along the way, we'll continue to move through the process of mourning your father in steps that I'll introduce during our sessions. My hope is that we will be able to assess where there might be obstacles along your path and to address these obstacles in a way that frees you up. At times, it will be difficult to do this work, but I'll make sure you have the resources and coping strategies to get through it." Sandra looked directly at Emily and asked, "Do we have a plan?"

"We have a plan," said Emily, and from there they launched into the therapy.

CONCLUDING REMARKS

As Emily's case illustrates, traumatic bereavement differs from the experience of losing a significant other to a death that stems from natural causes. Furthermore, as we have stated throughout this chapter, traumatic bereavement is more than the sum of loss and trauma. It is a unique phenomenon, marked by characteristics that include existential crisis, the taxing of an individual's resources, and pervasive and persistent symptoms and problematic adaptations.

Based on research with this population, relevant theoretical information, and our own clinical experiences, we have designed a treatment approach to address traumatic bereavement. Emily's therapist, Sandra, described this approach well: It focuses on assessing obstacles along the path of moving through mourning and addressing these obstacles by first shoring up resources, and then processing the trauma on both the cognitive and emotional levels. This treatment approach addresses the particular obstacles to mourning that a traumatic death presents.

We hope that the theoretical information in Parts I, II, and III paints a comprehensive picture of the experience of traumatic bereavement while pointing to treatment implications, which are then detailed in Parts IV and V. Our intention is to support you, our readers, in your work with traumatically bereaved clients, offering knowledge and tools that you can integrate with your own talents and style of psychotherapy.

CHAPTER 2

Theoretical Foundations

Eduardo's twin brother, Jorge, died in a motorcycle accident 2 years ago. He was shocked by the deadly accident, unable to grasp the reality of his brother's sudden death. They were only 23 years old; this couldn't be happening. Jorge had saved as much as he could from every job he ever had for that bike. It was brand new, and on the first day out, as he was merging onto the highway, the motorcycle malfunctioned, throwing him onto the dirt shoulder. Breaking his neck, he died instantly. Since that time, Eduardo had been struggling with an array of trauma symptoms, including sleep disturbance, concentration problems, and intrusive thoughts about what his brother suffered that day. In addition, he was experiencing powerful symptoms of grief, such as yearning for his brother and crying at the drop of a hat. His symptoms of grief and trauma were exacerbating one another. At work, crying spells interfered with his concentration on the job. Yearning for Jorge triggered traumatic images of his death and made it more difficult for Eduardo to sleep. He found himself avoiding reminders of their relationship, including childhood memories, even though another part of him wanted to recall fond memories and talk about his sibling and best friend. "When I think of Jorge, my mind always goes to how he died," Eduardo said.

Throughout this book, we use the terms *sudden, traumatic death* to refer to the death itself; *sudden, traumatic loss* to refer to a survivor's experience of the death; and *traumatic bereavement* to refer to the enduring problematic reactions that can result from the death. Traumatic bereavement is greater than the experience of trauma plus that of grief. As the case of Eduardo illustrates, people who lose a loved one suddenly and traumatically experience a more complex phenomenon. In this chapter, we lay out the theoretical foundations of our treatment approach—a synthesis of fundamental concepts, definitions, and language. This includes a discussion of loss, grief, and mourning; psychological trauma and trauma processing; and the intersection of loss and trauma, traumatic bereavement. In addressing these issues, our guiding criterion has been the utility of these concepts for clinicians and other treatment providers who must respond to the needs of traumatically bereaved clients.

LOSS

Loss is ubiquitous in human life. It is a central phenomenon in our existence. Virtually all change involves loss, and all individuals encounter loss repeatedly during their lifetimes.

A friend betrays your trust; a love affair ends; a child leaves for college; your sister develops a chronic illness; you move across the country; your car is stolen; your hearing diminishes; your partner dies. As these examples illustrate, a loss can be *physical*, referring to the loss of something tangible, or *psychosocial*, referring to a loss that is abstract or symbolic (Rando, 1993, 2013). A house that burns down, a watch that is stolen, and the death of a significant other are examples of physical losses. A shattered dream, such as being able to retire, is an example of a psychosocial loss. The death of a loved one necessarily involves psychosocial as well as physical losses. As an example, when a partner dies, the surviving partner may experience the loss of the other's physical presence (physical loss) as well as the loss of the other's roles in his life, such as lover, confidant, best friend, co-parent, or traveling companion (psychosocial losses).

It is important to distinguish between primary and secondary losses. A *primary* loss is the initial loss (in this case, the death), and a *secondary* loss is any loss that goes along with or develops as a consequence of the initial loss (Rando, 1993, 2013). Both primary and secondary losses can be either physical or psychosocial in nature. For instance, when the main breadwinner in a family dies, the family may have to relocate for economic reasons. The loss of the family home is a secondary physical loss; the loss of feeling connected to others in the community is a secondary psychosocial loss.

Some secondary losses refer to things a person no longer has as a result of the death. For example, if Jane's mother cares for her children during the day, her mother's death will result in the secondary loss of her day care provider. It is important to keep in mind, however, that secondary losses can also include the survivor's hopes and dreams for things that, as a result of the death, can never happen. Following her mother's death, for example, a young woman may mourn her inability to develop a good relationship with her mother while she was alive.

A special case of secondary symbolic, psychosocial losses is the shattering of assumptions, personal constructs, or schemas—known as *violation of the assumptive world*—which typically occurs in the aftermath of loss. For example, a woman whose husband is scheduled for surgery may believe that most surgeons are capable and can be trusted. If a surgeon makes an error that contributes to the husband's death, this may shatter her belief. Consequently, she may have great difficulty seeking the care of a physician, even when she is quite ill. If a doctor tells her that she or another close family member requires hospitalization, she is likely to experience intense anxiety. The shattering of one's assumptive world is particularly relevant to traumatic bereavement, and we address it in some depth in Chapter 3.

In some cases, secondary losses may be as important to deal with as primary losses, if not more so. This was clearly the case with Malcolm, who was 20 years old when his father died in a hunting accident. Malcolm was in college pursuing a degree in accounting at the time. His father's death forced Malcolm to drop out of school, in order to take over the family dry cleaning store that his father had owned and operated. This sacrifice was necessary to provide sufficient income for Malcolm's mother and two siblings. In addition to losing his father, Malcolm lost his vocation, his independence (he had to move back home), his day-to-day interactions with his close friends from college, and his role as a carefree young adult (he assumed his father's role in the family as eldest male and chief provider). Until Malcolm could identify and mourn these secondary losses, he would continue to struggle with the ramifications of his father's death.

The secondary losses that mourners experience following a traumatic death are determined in large part by the role relationship that was lost. Following the death of a spouse, the surviving spouse may struggle with a loss of identity, feeling as though a part of herself has died. She may also experience the loss of a caring presence day-to-day, the loss of her partner's participation in childrearing, and the destruction of her hopes and dreams for the future. When a child dies, parents must contend with the loss of their identity as parents, which is centered around caring for and nurturing the child. In many cases, they also lose a sense of meaning and purpose that was provided by the parental role. They can no longer enjoy or celebrate the child's milestones and accomplishments. In addition, a child often embodies the parents' hopes and dreams for the future; these are often shattered by the child's death.

The death of a parent is also associated with a unique set of secondary losses. These may include a lifelong emotionally supportive relationship, recognition and praise for accomplishments and achievements, guidance and advice at important crossroads, and a loving presence in the lives of grandchildren.

In most cases, mourners experience some secondary losses right away. For example, a widow may miss her husband's companionship immediately after his death. Yet it may take weeks, and perhaps months or even years, for survivors to become aware of the full range of secondary losses associated with the death. When tax season comes around, for example, a widow may recognize that she needs help with a task that her husband had previously handled. She may be confused about whom to contact for assistance.

GRIEF AND MOURNING

Grief and mourning resulting from a traumatic death are both qualitatively and quantitatively different from the grief and mourning that follow nontraumatic death. Although many people use the terms *grief* and *mourning* interchangeably, they are different. Understanding the difference is important to being able to help those suffering from traumatic bereavement. Technically, to say *grief and mourning* is redundant, since grief is the beginning part of mourning. However, they are separated in this book when it is necessary to pay specific attention to particular aspects of the initial period of mourning (i.e., grief), as distinguished from the subsequent action-oriented mourning processes occurring after that grief.

Grief

We use the term *grief* to refer to the psychological, behavioral, social, and physical reactions to the experience of loss (Rando, 1993, 2013). This definition has seven important clinical implications:

1. Grief is a natural and expectable reaction to an important loss.
2. People experience grief in virtually all realms of life.
3. Grief is expressed in a wide variety of ways. There is no right or wrong way to grieve.
4. Grief is not static, but changes continually over time.
5. Grief does not necessarily decrease in a linear fashion over time. For example, it may decrease for a while, then increase around the anniversary of the death.
6. Any important loss, not just death, can trigger grief.
7. The nature of a person's grief response depends on the person's unique perception of what she has lost, as well as on situational and personal factors (these factors are discussed in Chapters 5 and 6, respectively).

Although there is great variability in how people respond to the death of a loved one (Bonanno et al., 2002), there is general agreement about the grief symptoms most likely to accompany a loss. Survivors typically experience shock or numbness, symptoms of depression, and anxiety. Most people report an overwhelming sense of loss, as well as strong feelings of longing or yearning for the person who died. It is common for survivors to feel a profound sense of emptiness and to feel as though a part of them has died. They often speak of pain or heaviness in their chests. Bereaved individuals often lose interest in the world around them and feel hopeless about the future. Things that were once important do not seem to matter much any more. Fatigue, restlessness, irritability, anger, and guilt may also be present.

In the days, weeks, and months immediately following a death, responses such as disbelief, sadness, confusion, rage, and feeling overwhelmed are all common. Each of these reactions has behavioral, interpersonal, and physical correlates, such as withdrawal from social interaction, neglecting one's own self-care, and sleep difficulties. These natural responses to a significant loss reflect the experience of grief.

By itself, grief is insufficient for dealing effectively with loss, whether it is a natural death or one stemming from potentially traumatic circumstances. This is because, in order to cope successfully with loss, one must do more than merely react to it. This is where accommodation and the active processes of mourning come in. Thus grief is to mourning as infancy is to childhood: It's the beginning phase, but not the entire experience.

Accommodation and Mourning

Ultimately, in order to cope with loss in a healthy way, a person must accommodate it. To *accommodate* means to make room for something—to adapt or adjust. Accommodation is an active process. It involves reconciling differences in order to integrate one thing with another, for example, old ways of perceiving the world with new realities.

Because loss entails change, it demands accommodation. The death of a significant other is a major change and, as illustrated in our description of secondary losses, brings about numerous other changes as well. A major loss calls for multiple adjustments and a great deal of accommodation on the part of the survivor. When the death is traumatic, mourning will require a more extensive reorientation to life, due to the intensity and breadth of the adjustments required. Grief—merely reacting to the loss—will not accomplish this goal. It is a necessary but not a sufficient condition to do so. This is why the more active processes of mourning must be engaged.

Some have used the term *mourning* to refer to the cultural or public display of grief (Rando, 1993). As used in this book, however, *mourning* is the active process of coping with a death. This entails engaging in six processes, described below, that promote the personal readjustments and reorientations required to accommodate the loss of a significant other. These reorientations relate to the survivor's relationships with the deceased loved one, the self, and the external world (Rando, 1993, 2013).

Essentially, grieving is *reacting* to the personal experience of loss; mourning goes further and involves actively *dealing* with that loss. Whereas grieving involves experiencing and expressing one's reactions to the loss, mourning continues past that to serve the function of adaptation through accommodation. An understanding of this distinction allows a therapist to appreciate how much painful inner work remains after acute grieving subsides. The experience of grief helps people to recognize that their loss is real, and prepares them for the later changes they will need to undertake to accommodate the loss. It is therefore a significant entry into active mourning.

There is an important, if subtle, implication here that is crucial to effective work with survivors of loss. Many survivors will choose, consciously or unconsciously, to remain within the experience of grief and resist moving into mourning. In grief, they feel connected to the deceased. Some survivors may experience the pain of grief as an attachment to the deceased. The active accommodation of the loss in mourning can feel like resignation, accepting precisely that which one wishes to resist. It can feel tantamount to acknowledging that it is "OK" that the loved one is gone. Such acceptance can seem intolerable. Losing a significant other can leave anyone feeling powerless. Resisting acceptance—whether by remaining within grief or by not moving through mourning more fully—can give the illusion of control, even as it ultimately robs the survivor of true empowerment. Our treatment approach facilitates movement from grief into and through the active processes of mourning, resulting in accommodation of the traumatic loss.

An Overview of Mourning Processes

Knowledge of the processes of healthy mourning provides therapists with a powerful tool to assist clients in moving forward. Below, we provide a broad overview of how healthy mourning unfolds over time to permit accommodation of the loss. In our experience, most survivors' initial orientation toward mourning is one of avoidance. Over time, mourners typically enter a confrontation phase, in which they begin to deal with the reality of the loss and its implications. An accommodation phase usually follows, in which mourners are able to make a number of changes in how they view their situation, which helps them to move forward. These include their view of the loss, themselves, and the world, as well as their view of their relationship with the deceased. We list these categories of responses in Table 2.1. In describing these categories, we are not proposing that people go through an invariable sequence of responses. Without question, there is considerable variability in the process of mourning losses. However, there are common responses to major losses over time.

When mourning is not progressing toward accommodation, as is often the case in traumatic bereavement, the therapist's task is to assist the client in moving through these phases in an adaptive and healthy way. This involves successful completion of six specific processes, as described in Chapter 1 (the six "Rs"; Rando, 1993). A major component of this treatment entails facilitating these six processes. We introduce them briefly here and describe them in more detail in Chapter 12. Each "R" operates at a different point in the mourning process. For example, the first "R," *Recognize the loss,* is relevant to assisting the client in moving beyond avoidance, while the second "R," *React to the separation,* involves confronting the loss.

Below, we provide a brief description of the three broad categories of mourning and the "R" processes that characterize each.

Avoidance

Upon learning of a death, most mourners are overwhelmed. They are unable to comprehend what has happened. They typically feel a strong desire to resist acknowledging the death. Mourners may also experience denial, which can serve as emotional anesthesia as they begin to face the reality of the loss. At this time, many survivors require assistance with the first "R"

TABLE 2.1. The Six "R" Processes of Mourning in Relation to the Three Phases of Grief and Mourning*

Avoidance phase

1. *Recognize the loss*
   - Acknowledge the death
   - Understand the death

Confrontation phase

2. *React to the separation*
   - Experience the pain
   - Feel, identify, accept, and give some form of expression to all the psychological reactions to the loss
   - Identify and mourn secondary losses

3. *Recollect and reexperience the deceased and the relationship*
   - Review and remember realistically
   - Revive and reexperience the feelings

4. *Relinquish the old attachments to the deceased and the old assumptive world*

Accommodation phase

5. *Readjust to move adaptively into the new world without forgetting the old*
   - Revise the assumptive world
   - Develop a new relationship with the deceased
   - Adopt new ways of being in the world
   - Form a new identity

6. *Reinvest*

Note. From Rando (1993). Copyright 1993 by Therese A. Rando. Reprinted by permission.
*A slightly reworded, more layperson-friendly version of the same "R" processes appears in Handout 6, The Six "R" Processes of Mourning.

process, which is *Recognize the loss*. This is a crucial first step in the mourning process because if the loss is not recognized, there is nothing to mourn. When survivors come to treatment at this stage of mourning, the therapist's role is to help them to acknowledge the finality and permanence of the death.

Confrontation

Following acknowledgment of the death, most mourners enter into a painful interval where they confront the loss and gradually come to understand its impact. Three "R" processes come into play during this time. Most clients will require assistance with the second "R," *React to the separation*. It is important for therapists to assist their clients in experiencing and expressing the pain associated with the primary loss. To process this loss fully, they will also need help in identifying and mourning their secondary losses. The third "R" is *Recollect and reexperience the deceased and the relationship*. Therapists can aid clients in reviving and reexperiencing their feelings for their loved ones. The goal is for them to reach a point where they are able to remember the deceased and their relationship realistically, and then to reexperience the feelings associated with what they remember.

The fourth "R" process, which is also important during the confrontation phase, is *Relinquish the old attachments to the deceased and the old assumptive world*. A therapist's goal is to help a mourner let go of ties to the deceased that are problematic in light of the death. It is also important for clients to relinquish assumptions about the world that they held prior to the loss but that are not, in fact, true. As noted earlier, the sudden, traumatic death of a child may shatter a father's assumption that parents can protect their children.

Accommodation

Over time, most mourners come to understand the value of accommodating the loss, and become more receptive to interventions designed to facilitate that process. Still, it is not without struggle. The goal of the fifth process is to help the client *Readjust to move adaptively into the new world without forgetting the old*. The mourner learns to go on without the deceased, while finding ways to experience a healthy connection with her. For example, the mourner may become involved in a political cause that was important to the deceased. Other changes may involve adopting new ways of being in the world to compensate for the absence of the deceased (e.g., learning new skills).

Reinvest is the sixth and final "R" process. Here the mourner reinvests emotional energy once devoted to the relationship with the loved one in other people, projects, and so on. Ideally, this process of reinvestment will bring about fulfillment, gratification, or satisfaction.

In all of these "R" processes, the therapist works to enable the mourner to learn to live with the loss and its implications in a way that allows for a healthy and life-affirming future. In Chapter 12, we illustrate the role each of the six "Rs" plays as mourning progresses. We also provide guidance, suggestions, and examples of how therapists might utilize the "Rs" in clinical work with traumatically bereaved clients.

No book on grief treatment would be complete without emphasizing the profound role that culture plays in the mourning process. As Rosenblatt (2008) has described, culture defines and influences everyone's experience of grief, and also shapes (and sometimes limits) its expression.

Although a full account of the role culture plays in traumatic bereavement is beyond the scope of this book, we wish to raise two points. First, many studies on the reaction to traumatic loss have been conducted in other countries and with respondents from other cultures. This is the case, for example, for studies reviewed in Chapter 5 about the impact of war and disasters in Bosnia and Kosovo. Although such studies were not designed to address cultural differences, they elucidate the responses specific to each culture. This information could be useful to therapists working with people from cultures different from their own.

Second, the few studies that have focused on bereaved individuals from particular cultural groups in the United States have provided important information about the vulnerability of those groups. For example, McDevitt-Murphy, Neimeyer, Burke, Williams, and Lawson (2012) conducted a study among African Americans to examine the impact of losing family members to homicide over the previous 5 years. These losses took an enormous toll on the study respondents. The authors reported that nearly half of the sample screened positive for depression, complicated grief, PTSD, or anxiety, even though for most respondents it had been several years since the incidents occurred. The authors emphasized that this group would benefit from treatment tailored to their unique vulnerabilities. (In our judgment, the treatment approach described in this book has considerable relevance for this population.)

For those interested in learning more about culture and grief (in particular, information that has direct application to clinical practice), we recommend a book chapter by Klass and Chow (2011), which addresses, among other things, how culture "polices" the expression of grief; the book on African American grief written by Rosenblatt and Wallace (2005), which describes the ethnically specific challenges faced by African Americans, and also discusses cultural institutions of central importance to many African Americans, such as the Black church; and the book by Houben (2012), which provides a rich account of the values and traditions of Hispanic individuals, a cultural group increasingly seeking mental health treatment.

PSYCHOLOGICAL TRAUMA

A survivor who experiences the sudden death of a loved one as shocking or overwhelming is likely to suffer psychological trauma along with loss. We define *psychological trauma* as the experience of threat to life or to bodily or psychic integrity that overwhelms an individual's capacity to integrate the threat. In addition, the survivor feels as if she were going to die or disintegrate (Pearlman & Saakvitne, 1995). The events or experiences that give rise to psychological trauma following the sudden death of a loved one include aspects of the death and the context in which it occurs. As described in Chapter 1, survivors are particularly likely to experience deaths as traumatic if they are sudden, untimely, perceived as preventable, regarded as unjust, and/or viewed as resulting from an intentional act such as murder. Other important factors include whether the death involved violence or mutilation of the body, and whether a survivor believes that her loved one suffered during his final moments (see Chapter 5 for a comprehensive discussion of these characteristics). For example, upon witnessing the death of her partner in a motor vehicle crash, a woman may experience shock, terror, and helplessness. She may feel as if she is in a slow-motion horror movie from which she cannot escape. It is this *experience* (and not the crash or the death) that is the psychological trauma.

By definition, a traumatic experience often remains unassimilated within the survivor. Many people think of PTSD when psychological trauma is mentioned. Survivors who are unable to integrate overwhelming experiences may develop PTSD symptoms related to the event, such as intrusive thoughts or images or avoidance of reminders; negative changes in thoughts and mood; and changes in arousal and reactivity. Greater integration of the experience leads to symptom reduction.

Whereas PTSD is the diagnosis most commonly associated with the experience of trauma, or traumatic bereavement, it is certainly not the only one. Nor do these PTSD symptoms constitute a comprehensive description of psychological trauma. Survivors of sudden, traumatic loss can exhibit a broad range of problematic responses. Major depression, generalized anxiety disorder, panic disorder, acute stress disorder, substance abuse, and dissociative disorders are examples of other disorders that can be associated with traumatic stress (see, e.g., Kristensen, Weisaerth, & Heir, 2012). In some instances, problematic reactions to traumatic events and experiences may not fit any diagnostic category at all.

Another way of understanding problematic responses to potentially traumatic events focuses on the self rather than on symptoms. CSDT (McCann & Pearlman, 1990b; Pearlman, 2001; Pearlman & Saakvitne, 1995), mentioned in Chapter 1, elucidates both the domains of the self most vulnerable to traumatic experience and the process by which these vulnerabilities are activated. It gives clinicians a tool for understanding their clients' unique experiences of traumatic bereavement, and thus provides the link among survivors' experiences, their symptoms, and their specific treatment needs. Events in and of themselves do not lead directly to specific psychological responses. Every individual experiences and processes those events, attributes meaning to them, and integrates them into existing frameworks (or is unable to do so). With its focus on the self, the CSDT framework augments and enhances understandings offered by diagnostic categories. In addition, CSDT offers a framework for potential therapeutic intervention that grows out of its delineation of the domains of self most likely to be disrupted by traumatic bereavement. With its focus on early development and attachment, CSDT suggests the importance of a developmental perspective on how a person is affected by traumatic experiences. Finally, the theory emphasizes a relational orientation in any treatment designed to address traumatic attachment experiences, including traumatic loss.

Disrupted Domains of the Self

CSDT describes five domains of the self that are most vulnerable to disruption through severe attachment losses, including sudden, traumatic death (see Table 2.2). An individual who experiences the sudden, traumatic death of a loved one may suffer injury or disruption to particular domains of self—for example, the need for safety, the ability to use sound judgment, or the capacity to tolerate strong feelings.

Trauma symptoms are the more visible signs of those invisible domains of self that have been disrupted. Examples of symptoms and, in parentheses, the corresponding disrupted domains, include the following: a decreased ability to tolerate strong feelings of anger, and a related feeling of anxiety because the emerging anger would be unacceptable (self capacity/

TABLE 2.2. CSDT: Domains of the Self Affected by Traumatic Life Experiences

Frame of reference: Frameworks for understanding life
- *Identity:* Perceptions and experience of self
- *Worldview:* Life philosophy, notions of causality, moral principles
- *Spirituality:* Awareness of intangible aspects of experience; meaning and hope

Self capacities: Abilities that allow for navigation of the intrapersonal or inner world
- *Inner connection with benign others:* Internalized positive experience of others
- *Self-worth:* Sense of one's value
- *Affect tolerance:* Ability to experience, tolerate, manage, and integrate strong feelings

Ego resources: Abilities that allow for navigation of the interpersonal world (e.g., judgment, boundary management, foreseeing consequences)

Psychological needs and related cognitive schemas: Motivating factors and related beliefs
- *Safety:* Oneself (self-safety) and loved ones (other-safety) are generally safe and secure
- *Trust:* One can trust one's own perceptions and judgment (self-trust) and most other people can be trusted (other-trust)
- *Esteem:* Oneself (self-esteem) and others (other-esteem) are worthy of respect
- *Intimacy:* One can be aware of one's thoughts and feelings (self-intimacy) and experience deep connection with others (other-intimacy)
- *Control:* One can manage one's behavior (self-control) and can be effective in the world (other-control)

Body and brain: Physiological and somatic effects

Note. The social and cultural context—including traditions, mores, and norms—shapes the survivor's and others' responses to potentially traumatic events. From Saakvitne, Pearlman, and the Staff of the Traumatic Stress Institute (1996). Copyright 1996 by the Traumatic Stress Institute/Center for Adult & Adolescent Psychotherapy LLC.

affect management); a sense that the world is meaningless, leading to withdrawal from one's spiritual community (frame of reference/spirituality); difficulty believing that loved ones are safe, resulting in fears about their whereabouts (psychological needs/safety); and questioning one's judgment, resulting in difficulty with decision making (ego resources). Individuals experiencing traumatic bereavement often present with such symptoms when they come for treatment. The symptom picture of traumatic bereavement is discussed in detail in Chapter 3. The domains of self relevant to this treatment approach, based in CSDT, are discussed below.

Self Capacities

Self capacities are inner abilities that allow individuals to manage their psychological world and regulate their internal states. The three self capacities within CSDT are internalizing benign others (those who care for a person), maintaining positive self-worth, and regulating emotion. A person who can practice these skills effectively is better equipped to manage the internal states that mark traumatic bereavement, and therefore to process the experience of the loss. In other words, in order to process a traumatic loss effectively, a survivor needs to be able to experience intense feelings, memories, and sensations over time, without avoiding or dissociating from them. The survivor needs to remain connected to her experience. For these reasons, the above-named self capacities lay the groundwork for processing the traumatic loss within this treatment approach. Because a traumatic event can disrupt the very capacities needed for healing and recovery, effective treatment must attend to the strengthening of those capacities.

Effective treatment must take into account a person's developmental history as well. There is clear evidence that vulnerability to potentially traumatic experiences is shaped by a person's attachment history—particularly attachment experiences that occur during the first years of life, when the brain is developing most rapidly (Allen, 2013). Healthy attachment interactions provide the foundation for the skills to tolerate, modulate, and integrate feeling states and emotional experiences (Bowlby, 1969, 1988; McCann & Pearlman, 1990b; Schore, 1994; see Chapter 10 for a more detailed discussion). A person's developmental history is therefore relevant to his capacity to manage the inner experiences that mark traumatic bereavement. If a person did not have positive attachment experiences while growing up, then effective treatment requires attention to the development of these capacities. Treatment with a person who evidenced well-developed capacities before the traumatic death will still need to attend to buttressing those capacities, which may have been diminished by the traumatic death. Again, because such capacities are crucial to managing traumatic bereavement, an assessment of developmental history is essential, as is an assessment of post-loss capacities, regardless of developmental history. We discuss such assessment in Chapter 8.

Ego Resources

Ego resources are the basis for those skills that support a survivor as she negotiates external demands and her interpersonal world. In the aftermath of traumatic death, such tasks can be extremely taxing, rendering these skills indispensable. Being able to trust one's judgment when deciding when to return to work after a loss, setting appropriate boundaries in order to get increased rest and engage in more self-care, and assessing available avenues of social support are examples of ego resources that treatment can address to help a person move through traumatic bereavement. As is the case with self capacities, though, a traumatic death can compromise these skills at a time when they are most needed. Moreover, such skills often work hand in hand with self capacities. When a survivor's internal experience feels intense and out of control, it is more difficult to call upon resources that were once available but now seem out of reach.

Some traumatic bereavement symptoms are expressions of disrupted ego resources. Understanding this can help clinicians to empathize with clients and to intervene effectively. For example, a mourning, traumatized mother reports almost falling asleep at the wheel while driving her children to school. Rather than interpreting this as "self-destructive behavior," we can instead recognize that she needs help with accessing good judgment and asking for help from others. Like *self capacities, ego resources* are a domain of the self affected by traumatic bereavement. They form a background for understanding survivors' behaviors and are therefore a significant foundation of our treatment approach. The treatment addresses strengthening ego resources in its attention to developing coping skills, social support, bereavement-specific strategies, and values and goal setting, as discussed in Chapter 10.

Psychological Needs, Schemas, and Automatic Thoughts

We all have physical and *psychological needs* that must be met as we move through life. These needs motivate our behavior, and their fulfillment influences our well-being. The following five psychological needs are particularly sensitive to the effects of traumatic events, including traumatic loss: safety, trust, esteem, intimacy, and control (Pearlman, 2003). We experience each of these needs in relation to ourselves and to others. For example, we generally need to believe that both we and those we care about are safe in the world in order to move through our day-to-day lives unencumbered by anxiety. When these needs are for the most part fulfilled, we tend to take them for granted and pay little attention to them. When they are disrupted, they can take the form of automatic thoughts, which may contribute to an array of symptoms.

Cognitive and cognitive-behavioral theorists, drawing upon information-processing theory, suggest that we gather interrelated information in the form of *schemas*, or belief systems. Our schemas guide our attention, expectations, interpretations, and storage and retrieval of memories (Janoff-Bulman, 1992), as well as our social interactions (Pearlman, 2003). Distress can occur when people encounter information that is incongruent with a schema or when conflicting needs give rise to problematic schemas (e.g., the need for connection or intimacy can conflict with the need for control). As mentioned earlier, traumatic bereavement symptoms that stem from disrupted schemas will often reflect one of the five psychological need areas listed above. A father may view the death of his child as incongruent with the schema that good parents should be able to protect their children (reflecting needs for other-safety and other-control). In this case, an event has occurred that is schema-discrepant. The bereaved father may extrapolate from this discrepancy and decide that his poor parenting was the cause of the child's death. This belief is likely to result in self-blame, as well as intense anxiety about the safety of his other children.

Our schemas present themselves in our daily lives in the form of automatic thoughts. "My keys are hanging by the door" is an example of a benign automatic thought that occurs, mostly outside of awareness, for the woman who always leaves her keys on the same hook when she enters her home. Automatic thoughts often help us move through the world efficiently. We can also have automatic thoughts that reflect harmful, negative, or disrupted schemas. These may also occur without our awareness and can have a powerful impact on our moods, behavior, or physical sensations. Automatic thoughts in the wake of a sudden, traumatic death range from the existential ("I asked God to protect him, and He did not") to the everyday ("I will never be able to maintain the house without her").

An understanding of trauma-sensitive psychological needs is important for a comprehensive framework of traumatic bereavement. Problematic schemas can interfere with trauma processing and accommodation to loss. Cognitive therapy techniques, including those we draw upon in this treatment approach, help people to recognize these thoughts, to name the schemas underlying them, and then to challenge the thoughts that are associated with psychological distress (Lichtenthal, 2012). By listening to clients' language and narrative of events for disruptions within the five need areas outlined above, therapists can hone in on maladaptive beliefs common to traumatic experience that may be interfering with clients' progress. Clients can learn to do this for themselves as well. By identifying and challenging their automatic thoughts, they can remove some of the obstacles that are preventing them from accepting and processing the traumatic loss and from moving forward in their lives. Clients can also benefit, therefore, from knowing these categories of needs as they listen for their own problematic automatic thoughts. Handout 23, Psychological Needs (in the Appendix and online at *www.guilford.com/pearlman-materials*), describes each of the five needs in detail and is useful for therapists and clients alike. In Chapter 11, we provide detailed information about identifying and challenging automatic thoughts.

Frame of Reference and Assumptive World

As human beings, we all hold assumptions and beliefs pertaining to "big-picture" issues, such as how we define ourselves, why things happen in the way they do, and whether something like a higher power exists. We may believe that there is a meaningful trajectory to our lives, or not. We may assume that things happen for a reason, or not. We may believe that there is reason to hope for something we desire, or not. We may define ourselves according to certain roles, accomplishments, or ways of being. Taken together, our assumptions and beliefs constitute what CSDT refers to as our *frame of reference*. Frame of reference includes a person's identity, worldview, and sense of spirituality.

Like psychological needs, a person's frame of reference is articulated as a set of schemas and expressed in automatic thoughts. The schemas can be helpful or maladaptive, accurate or exaggerated, explicit or implicit. And as is the case with psychological needs, traumatic experiences usually violate aspects of a survivor's frame of reference. In fact, disrupted meaning and loss of hope are hallmarks of psychological trauma (Pearlman & Caringi, 2009).

Following the traumatic death of her husband, for example, a woman may feel unanchored in her identity as wife, partner, companion, and co-parent. When the traumatic death of a loved one shatters such roles and their associated meanings, the psychological and relational foundations of a person's life can be demolished—and, as we have mentioned in Chapter 1, a survivor may experience an existential crisis. So much of what the survivor assumed to be true about the world can be turned on its head, and this can happen in an instant. Traumatic death can evoke a violation or shattering of a person's *assumptive world* (Janoff-Bulman, 1992), or everything a person holds to be true about her self and the world. Awareness of this process is essential to a comprehensive understanding of traumatic bereavement.

Theoretically, the concepts of frame of reference and assumptive world overlap. For our purposes, we use these concepts interchangeably throughout the text. The delineation of frame of reference as including identity, worldview, and spirituality can help a therapist listen for particularly sensitive aspects of a person's *assumptive world* in any given therapy. Empathic attunement to a client's existential crisis is itself a therapeutic stance. Appreciating the specifics of such a crisis for any given individual also allows a therapist to address the last three "R" processes in an effective manner, and to address the work of reestablishing goals and values in the wake of the loss.

Brain and Body

At any given time, no matter what else is going on in our lives, our bodies are our vehicles for navigating the world. Our bodies are fundamental aspects of ourselves; some would say that we are our bodies. Any comprehensive understanding of the traumatized self must therefore include the body. In delineating domains of the self most vulnerable to traumatic experience, CSDT calls attention to the body. As a theory of trauma treatment, CSDT suggests intervention targeting the physiological effects of traumatic bereavement, with particular attention to affect regulation.

We have drawn upon research findings about the neurobiological correlates of the psychological experience of extreme stress and PTSD. This research informs our understanding of the experience of the body in traumatic bereavement (Bremner, 2006; Bremner et al., 1995, 1999, 2003; Heim & Nemeroff, 2009; Shin, Rauch, & Pitman, 2006; van der Kolk, 2006). Much of this research has been conducted with individuals diagnosed with PTSD and/or with survivors of childhood abuse or neglect. We include this information because, in our judgment, survivors of traumatic bereavement often suffer from physiological dysregulation.

Describing the clinical implications of clinical neuroscientific research, van der Kolk (2006) suggests that clients with PTSD "lose their way in the world" (p. 280) because of their diminished capacity to be engaged in the present. Trauma therapy, he concluded, ought to facilitate self-awareness and self-regulation, helping clients to regain their capacity to respond more fully in the present moment. The emphasis on building and strengthening self capacities within our treatment approach may effect greater self-awareness and emotional regulation among traumatically bereaved clients. Ideally, this will address the possibility of overactivated, hyperaroused, and/or sensitized central nervous systems. Within our treatment approach, breathing retaining and drawing on an internalized benign other are examples of interventions that can help clients to regulate their emotions.

Engaging mourners in active coping behaviors, goal setting, and narration of the traumatic death (all elements of this treatment approach) may have the effect of stimulating cortical activity. (Such activity may be diminished in trauma survivors, potentially resulting in impaired judgment or difficulty with goal setting, for example.) These strategies also offer clients experiences of empowerment and mastery. Furthermore, because survivors often experience their symptoms viscerally, clinicians can strengthen the therapeutic alliance by understanding the physiological processes underlying their clients' symptoms and articulating this understanding to clients as appropriate.[1]

---

[1]We refer readers who are interested in a deeper understanding of the psychobiology of trauma to the following excellent resources: *Being a Brain-Wise Therapist* (Badenoch, 2008), *In an Unspoken Voice* (Levine, 2010), *The Polyvagal Theory* (Porges, 2011), *The Body Remembers* (Rothschild, 2000), and *Healing Trauma* (Siegel & Solomon, 2003).

Symptoms as Adaptations

CSDT establishes an approach to symptoms that respects their adaptive qualities. Throughout the text, we sometimes describe the manifestations of traumatic bereavement as adaptations rather than as symptoms. This term is intended to emphasize that the visible signs of disrupted domains of the self represent survivors' best efforts toward managing or adapting to overwhelming internal states. The term *adaptations* conveys the positive implication that survivors are doing the best they can under the circumstances. *Symptoms* conveys pathology, which can lead to victim blaming or failure to appreciate survivors' strengths. Of course, adaptations may result in negative consequences, even as they represent attempts to cope. For example, a mother struggling with painful and intense affect following the death of her child may begin overusing alcohol to help dull the pain. While creating problems, this response is an understandable attempt to manage agonizing feelings.

Understanding the varied expressions of traumatic bereavement as adaptations to an overwhelming event and the corresponding internal states that the person has been unable to integrate reduces the likelihood of pathologizing common and natural responses to unexpected terrible events. For example, one bereaved wife talked with her therapist about seeing her deceased husband every night and having conversations with him. It would be most useful for the therapist to create a shared understanding of this experience as an adaptation to the loss. In this case, the survivor's intense longing for her husband's companionship might have led to her envisioning that she was conversing with him. Identifying this perception as a hallucination and treating it with antipsychotic medication would be counterproductive. Not only might this be a misunderstanding of a particular adaptation, but it could block an opening for exploring this client's particular experience of adapting to the inner emptiness left in the wake of the loss. This treatment approach understands symptoms as adaptations and supports healthy, adaptive coping strategies.

Processing Psychological Trauma

As noted in Chapter 1, our treatment approach draws heavily on cognitive processing theories and CBT. These models combine cognitive techniques with behavioral applications. One goal of our integrated approach is to assist clients in addressing those posttraumatic stress and post-loss symptoms that most interfere with the tasks of mourning. CBT techniques assist in (1) locating the disruptions to particular domains of the self as described above, because such disruptions often show up in a person's automatic thoughts; (2) addressing avoidance of trauma material, including emotional and other internal responses to the traumatic death; and (3) implementing and practicing adaptive behaviors that support a survivor's movement forward in his life.

Our use of CBT techniques within the treatment approach is based in the notion that a person's mood, thoughts, and behaviors all affect one another (Beck, Rush, Shaw, & Emery, 1979), as described by the model shown in Figure 2.1. The multidirectional arrows in the figure signify that the cycle can begin anywhere in the loop, and that addressing one aspect of the loop (e.g., thoughts) can affect the other aspects (e.g., mood). Cognitive-behavioral theories focus on mechanisms of change in thoughts (cognitions) and behaviors. Some theories also address related physical sensations.

Processing the trauma entails addressing the disruptive and distressing elements of the thought–mood–behavior loop as they are manifested for a particular client. Leading a client

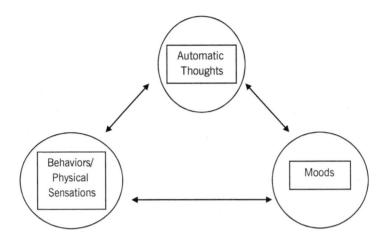

FIGURE 2.1. The cognitive model. Based on Beck, Rush, Shaw, and Emery (1979).

through this process requires that the therapist understand something about how the various elements relate to one another for the client. For example, a man whose spouse died may believe he failed his partner. This belief may make it impossible for him to move forward with meeting new people and dating, which may reinforce his belief that he is an inadequate person.

One important aspect of CBT that is relevant for this treatment approach involves *avoidance behaviors* and how these relate to disrupted schemas. For instance, the painful consequence of touching a hot stove makes us likely to avoid touching hot stoves in the future. This type of learning, *conditioning*, plays an important role in some traumatic experiences. An event as significant as a sudden, traumatic death can condition a survivor to avoid anything related to the painful feelings associated with the loss. Our brains naturally create quick associations, and an emotional reaction prompts us to avoid potentially painful situations.

Behavioral conditioning can occur over time with repeated "trials" of learning. A person who has experienced traumatic bereavement may have learned from successive trials, or real-life experiences, that expressing emotion about the loss to others will result in a painful, awkward silence. The survivor therefore begins to withdraw and to avoid talking to people about the death. People can learn other associations in a single instance when a sufficiently powerful emotion accompanies the trial. For example, a survivor may become very distressed at the sight of planes because his loved one died in a plane crash. Survivors often avoid internal, emotionally painful states as well, thereby preventing them from experiencing their feelings and from emotionally processing the loss. Of course, avoidance of external and internal stimuli usually go hand in hand.

We can begin to see the dilemma. Traumatically bereaved clients often attempt to avoid feeling their emotions about the death and the way it happened. They avoid thoughts that evoke emotion, as well as people, places, and things that remind them of the loss. Although this avoidance may temporarily ease their pain, the longer-term consequences contribute to the experience of being "stuck" in their grief and mourning, unable to move through the "R" processes described earlier. It may be particularly difficult, for example, to *Recollect and reexperience the deceased and the relationship* when doing so brings up painful affect or traumatic memories. Survivors may successfully suppress emotions in the short term, but these emotions may later surface unexpectedly. Such behavioral patterns tend to reinforce maladaptive schemas. Withdrawal from life means that bereaved survivors do not have experiences that might challenge their maladaptive schemas. And disengagement from emotions means that they miss the opportunity to mourn in healthy ways. Disengagement from others further eclipses opportunities to receive much-needed social support. Chapter 11 details the specific use of CBT techniques for processing the traumatic loss on both a cognitive and an emotional level.

A RELATIONAL TREATMENT APPROACH

Understanding personal development in the context of an attachment paradigm allows us to appreciate that individuals develop within relationships, can suffer injuries within relationships, and can heal within relationships as well. The loss of a significant other will call a person's attachment system into play (see, e.g., Fraley & Shaver, 1999; Parkes, 2001). The survivor's attachment paradigms (or *internal working models*; Bowlby, 1988) and experiences will mediate responses to traumatic loss, which in turn will affect those paradigms. This may be particularly true in the case of a sudden, traumatic death; the survivor does not have an opportunity to say goodbye. Sensitivity to the therapeutic relationship, including its eventual end, is an important element within this treatment approach.

The sudden death of loved ones can reinforce survivors' beliefs that relationships will likely end traumatically, placing them at greater risk of a poor outcome. Yet, without relationships, the essence of human experience is diminished. In addition to whatever therapists do or say, their predictable, compassionate presence serves as a balm to painful attachment losses from the past. Thus, in this treatment approach, we regard a therapist's commitment to respectful connection with a client as an intervention of significance.

INTEGRATION IN THE TRAUMATIC BEREAVEMENT TREATMENT APPROACH

There are two key aspects to the role of integration in our treatment approach: integrating mourning and trauma resolution, and integrating theory and practice. First, *integration* refers to the fact that a survivor of a traumatic death must deal with the dual tasks of mourning the loss and resolving trauma—tasks that both overlap and interfere with one another. In creating an effective treatment for individuals grappling with both loss and trauma, we have recognized the importance of integrating trauma resolution into the work of facilitating adaptive mourning. We have further recognized that it is essential to help clients build and access the resources needed to engage successfully in such processing work. Research has affirmed the importance of developing self capacities, or the ability to regulate one's emotions, before providing too much emotional challenge (e.g., Cloitre, Koenen, Cohen, & Han, 2002; Korn & Leeds, 2002; see Chapter 7 for a discussion of this research). This recognition is also the basis for the widely utilized phase-oriented treatment for psychological trauma, which recommends building an internal foundation for the challenging work of processing memories of traumatic experiences. Various clinical approaches to addressing psychological trauma reflect this model (Allen, 2001; Briere, 1996a, 1996b; Cloitre, Cohen, & Koenen, 2006; Korn & Leeds, 2002; Linehan, 1993; McCann & Pearlman, 1990b; Saakvitne, Gamble, Pearlman, & Lev, 2000).

Throughout our treatment approach, the development of self capacities supports the necessary regulation of arousal. This, in turn, assists with the processing of traumatic imagery and memories (Cloitre et al., 2006; Korn & Leeds, 2002; McCann & Pearlman, 1990b; Pearlman, 1998), which further facilitates mourning. In addition to the development and strengthening of self capacities, the treatment approach emphasizes attention to those ego resources that promote effective coping in the world. Clients are guided to practice a variety of activities and strategies, which are generally referred to as *resource building*. These strategies help them to access and utilize their ego resources and to engage with the world in adaptive ways.

The treatment approach integrates three core components, described in Chapter 1: the development and strengthening of self capacities (McCann & Pearlman, 1990b; Pearlman & Saakvitne, 1995) and other resources necessary for the effective, safe engagement with traumatic bereavement material; trauma processing, largely accomplished through CBT interventions and exposure to traumatic bereavement material (Foa & Rothbaum, 1998); and the tasks and trajectory of mourning based on Rando's work, as described earlier in this chapter (Rando, 1993). Supported by an empathic therapeutic relationship and a client's own commitment to healing, practically carried out through independent activities, these three core components work together to facilitate moving forward with life in fulfilling ways.

The treatment approach also integrates theory with practice. We realized early that we could not create a one-size-fits-all treatment for this population. Rather, we offer an approach that includes a flexible trajectory, necessary tasks and interventions, and topics likely to require attention. In order for therapists to utilize this approach well, and to target particular clients' needs, a comprehensive understanding of mourning, the traumatized self, traumatic bereavement, and CBT techniques is required. Thus our use of *integration* to describe this treatment approach refers to the fact that foundational theoretical concepts inform the implementation of the therapeutic approach, and that therapists need to be familiar with these concepts in order to utilize the treatment effectively. Of particular relevance is a firm understanding of the domains of self most vulnerable to disruption by a traumatic loss. Such an understanding affords therapists a means of assessing the self capacities necessary for trauma processing, a framework for identifying problematic adaptations and existential injuries, and a means of connecting visible symptoms with a client's inner experience.

One potentially useful way of conceptualizing a traumatic bereavement therapy is to think about it as a journey through the "R" processes. In collaboration with the client, the therapist assesses supports for this journey and works to develop those resources as needed. Also in collaboration with the client, the therapist assesses obstacles to the journey. Some of these obstacles will be related to disruptions to domains of the self resulting from the traumatic loss. It is useful to think of responses to these disruptions as adaptations and to ask whether a particular adaptation is helping a client to accommodate his particular loss, or not. In other words, is this adaptation assisting a client through his journey? If not, how might the client adapt in a different way? This treatment approach is designed to help therapists and clients answer this question together.

Two people may endure the death of a loved one that looks similar, yet may have two very different sets of reactions. In a community tragedy such as a terrorist attack, some individuals may struggle most with the sudden, unexpected violation of their community. Others may focus on the lack of preparedness demonstrated by their community agencies. Some may withdraw from loved ones, while others cling desperately to family and friends. Some may struggle with self-trust needs, while others are challenged more by other-safety needs. Each of these responses has different treatment implications in terms of the types of resources that must be developed and the specific nature of interventions used. In this chapter, we have laid out the theoretical concepts that inform the approach. In Parts II and III, we describe living with traumatic bereavement as well as risk factors before moving into the specific interventions of the treatment approach in Parts IV and V.

CLINICAL INTEGRATION

Pauline walked into the break room after her session with Eduardo. She was glad to see her clinical supervisor, Erin, sitting there with a cup of coffee.

"Do you mind if I join you?" she asked Erin.

"Of course not. Have a seat. How's it going?"

"Well, I think," remarked Pauline, noticing the tone of doubt in her own voice. "I just met with that new client I've been seeing—the one whose twin died in a motorcycle accident a couple of years ago."

Erin nodded. "You're using that new traumatic bereavement approach with him, right?"

"Yeah. It's been useful to think about the therapy in this way. It's helped me not to minimize the traumatic aspects of his experience, not to focus solely on the loss."

"That's interesting," said Erin. "I imagine the traumatic aspects of a sudden death might be overwhelming—not just to him, but to you, too. What are you doing differently as a result of being mindful of the trauma?"

"I'm not sure," said Pauline. "We've only met three times so far. Eduardo seems to be really stuck on how unfair the experience was, and is. He's pretty young. Prior to this, he had never experienced any sort of tragedy or major loss. His life was going well, and he believed life was fair—that people get what they deserve. Eduardo also thought the world of his brother. His death shook him to his core, in large part because he believed Jorge, maybe more than anyone, deserved a good life. Eduardo hasn't been able to reconcile this."

"Don't you think such a death would shake anyone to his core?" Erin wondered aloud.

"Well, yes and no. Eduardo has had lots of trauma symptoms, as well as those of grief. Jorge was his best friend, and he misses him terribly. He feels empty without his twin, and yet he cannot remember the times they had together in any way that brings him comfort. He just imagines Jorge lying on the roadside, dead. Two years later, he is still experiencing disturbing imagery and a predominant feeling of emptiness. I'm now thinking his attachment to the idea that life should be fair gets in the way of processing all of this. Does that make any sense?"

"Yes," said Erin. "Can you say any more about his attachment to fairness?"

"It's as though Eduardo needs this to be true—that life is fair. There's this impasse within his psyche, and for as long as it's there, I don't think he'll be able to move forward with his life. Eduardo lost not only his brother, but also his whole frame of reference, and assumptions about how the world works. It feels to me like his very identity is built upon this idea of fairness."

"That belief or frame of reference sounds like a good focus for your work with him," Erin said.

"Yes, I think you're right," Pauline answered.

CONCLUDING REMARKS

Throughout this chapter, we have laid out foundational and theoretical information related to the phenomenon of traumatic bereavement. Rando's (1993) work describes mourning as an active process that ideally promotes the personal adjustments necessary for a person to accommodate his loss. When a death is traumatic, as Jorge's death was for Eduardo, a survivor's abilities to make such adjustments and accommodate the reality of the loss can be compromised in specific ways. CSDT, based in attachment theory, points to those aspects of the self that are most vulnerable to disruption by traumatic experience, including a traumatic death. In doing so, CSDT provides a framework for possible targets of intervention.

Cognitive-behavioral theories further inform the various mechanisms of intervention that we discuss more completely in Part IV. We believe that a survivor needs to confront, rather than avoid, the death and its circumstances; work to accommodate the new reality; and work through the obstacles to doing so that are often related to maladaptive schemas or beliefs. The working-through process as described in this book fosters the awareness and confrontation of these beliefs.

Pauline understood that Eduardo needed help addressing obstacles to mourning his brother's death—obstacles that were related to both the traumatic nature of Jorge's death and the resulting trauma symptoms, as well as Eduardo's own belief system. Her foundational understanding of the phenomenon of traumatic bereavement allowed her to listen for those obstacles, or places where Eduardo was stuck in his mourning of Jorge. Her ultimate goal was to assist Eduardo in moving through his mourning, so that he could reinvest in his life without the physical presence of his twin. We hope that the information provided throughout this book will assist you, our readers, as you work with clients to develop adaptations that best assist them with their tasks of mourning.

PART II

LIVING WITH
TRAUMATIC BEREAVEMENT

CHAPTER 3

Psychological Dimensions

James lost Raphael, his partner of 7 years, when Raphael died in a manufacturing accident. Upon learning of the accident, James rushed to the plant, where he saw the aftermath. Images of blood, broken machinery, his partner's body, and Raphael's coworkers, who were themselves in shock, were etched into his mind. In the months following the accident, James spent a lot of time trying to find out what happened and who was to blame. He spoke with employees who had witnessed the incident, as well as the manager in charge, but found no one who could explain it. Given the nature of Raphael's death, James also found himself preoccupied with the question of how much his partner had suffered and with his own associated feelings of powerlessness. These disturbing thoughts interfered with his sleep. When he did manage to fall asleep, it was a restless experience, marked by nightmares revolving around themes of Raphael's death. He wanted the intrusive imagery, the loneliness, and the pining to stop.

The monumental impact of Raphael's death on James is striking. "It is as though the wrath of God has been unleashed on me," he said. Similarly, a man who lost his son said, "Even if someone had dropped an atom bomb in the middle of our community, we could not have been more affected" (Dyregrov, Nordanger, & Dyregrov, 2003, pp. 149, 151). Survivors often experience a traumatic death as a wound to their fundamental sense of self; the injuries are deep and far-reaching.

The material presented in this chapter and the next three offers a comprehensive description of traumatic bereavement, in order to give clinicians a framework of possibilities for working with traumatically bereaved clients. This chapter and the next present the phenomenology of traumatic bereavement, describing what it feels like to the survivor. This chapter describes common psychological responses to sudden, traumatic death, which often complicate the mourning process. We link the common symptoms or adaptations to their source: the violation of the assumptive world, which includes disruptions in underlying psychological needs and frame of reference.

SYMPTOMS AND ADAPTATIONS

As we have discussed in Chapter 2, many symptoms of traumatic bereavement are *adaptations* to this extraordinary event and the inner experiences it evokes. Many strategies that start out as adaptive eventually become problematic, prolonging distress and pain. For example, initially avoiding painful feelings can help clients get through the day, and can keep them from becoming completely overwhelmed. If it continues over time, however, such avoidance can become an obstacle to moving through the mourning process.

Table 3.1 provides a comprehensive list of symptoms that survivors of sudden, traumatic death may experience. We include this list to illustrate the wide range of ways in which traumatic bereavement manifests itself. Many of the symptoms fit into multiple categories. Readers will recognize some of these symptoms as hallmarks of grief, and others as those of trauma. However, they cease to be easily separable within the experience of traumatic bereavement. They are all expectable responses to sudden, traumatic death, and one of our important tasks as clinicians is to normalize them as appropriate for our clients. We encourage therapists to consider each client's particular constellation of symptoms as that person's experience of, and adaptation to, traumatic death.

SHATTERING OF THE ASSUMPTIVE WORLD

Survivors of traumatic death must contend with the shattering of their most basic beliefs and understandings about the world. This is termed *violation of the assumptive world* (Janoff-Bulman, 1992). This disruption in beliefs is one process that gives rise to the symptoms of traumatic bereavement outlined in Table 3.1 on pages 42–43. When the survivor can no longer trust her perceptions of the world, of other people, or of herself, a multitude of problematic adaptations can result.

As described in Chapters 1 and 2, CSDT (Pearlman, 2001; Pearlman & Saakvitne, 1995; Saakvitne et al., 2000) outlines five psychological need areas that are particularly vulnerable to assault from a traumatic experience: safety, trust, control, esteem, and intimacy (Pearlman, 2003). Within each need area, people hold beliefs related to self and others (e.g., self-esteem, or valuing oneself, and other-esteem, or valuing others). The experience of a traumatic loss is likely to influence assumptions, beliefs, or internal working models (Bowlby, 1988) related to these five need areas. We refer therapists who want to provide clients with more information about these needs to Handout 23, Psychological Needs.

In addition, traumatic experiences usually violate survivors' *frame of reference*, or big-picture ways of understanding themselves and the world. These include identity, worldviews, and spirituality (particularly meaning and hope). After the traumatic death of his wife, for instance, a man may feel that his roles as husband, partner, companion, and co-parent have been shattered. The loss of these roles and their associated meanings can shatter the psychological and relational foundations of his life.

Listening for these need-related themes in a client's statements reflects empathic attunement and helps the client to feel understood. When the therapist accurately identifies critical needs—for example, control or intimacy—the therapeutic relationship grows stronger, the therapist knows how to guide the work, and the therapy moves forward more effectively.

Sudden, traumatic deaths are likely to evoke intense fears that something else bad is going to happen. A survivor may feel that danger is lurking everywhere, and that there is no way to protect loved ones from harm (other-safety). As one bereaved mother expressed it, "You're always waiting for this other shoe to drop" (quoted in Finkbeiner, 1996, p. 81). From this place of fear, individuals understandably may become rigid, overprotective, and avoidant in their attempts to defend against another traumatic loss (other-control). Of course, in some instances, the client not only feels unsafe but also is actually at increased risk of harm. An example would be a case of homicide in which the perpetrator is still at large and/or has threatened other family members.

The events that bring about traumatic death frequently undermine a survivor's ability to trust. Problems with trust are particularly likely in those situations where the life of the deceased was in the hands of another person. As noted above, survivors of medical malpractice typically have great difficulty trusting doctors or other health care professionals in the future (other-trust). Deaths that occur when a child is at school or with a babysitter are also likely to damage the survivors' assumptions about trusting others. Losses of this sort also lead survivors to question their own judgment (self-trust). For example, a man who lost his infant son because the doctor failed to diagnose and treat pneumonia blamed himself for choosing that particular doctor.

Moreover, traumatic deaths affect survivors' desires to be close to others (other-intimacy)— even members of the immediate family. As one father stated following the death of his son in a motor vehicle crash, "I just couldn't get that involved with my other son after the first one died." Individuals often have a difficult time with self-intimacy (being aware of and familiar with their own internal states) as well; they may deny their feelings and needs in an effort to avoid the associated pain.

In some cases, the death shatters the client's assumptions about the deceased. Information that was previously unknown may surface following the death. For example, parents may learn for the first time that their child was involved in destructive or illegal activities. This may shatter their assumptions that she was a well-adjusted person who used good judgment. Deaths of this sort can leave parents with the painful realization that they did not really know their own child.

In addition, survivors of a traumatic death may develop new beliefs that can generalize in ways that promote or prolong painful affect (Pearlman, 2003). For example, Arthur allowed his teenage daughter to go out with a young man whom he did not know very well. While driving, the young man was speeding and failed to negotiate a turn. Arthur's daughter was killed instantly when the car struck a tree. Consequently, Arthur developed a belief that "I must monitor my children's behavior at all times in order to keep them safe." He became a harsh disciplinarian with his son, restricting his activities, controlling his choice of friends, and imposing a strict curfew. As a result, his son became extremely angry and resentful. He avoided his father as much as he could, and lied to his parents about his social activities and relationships. Their previously warm and loving relationship was transformed into one characterized by conflict and mistrust. Such disruptions contribute to prolonged suffering, as they often separate survivors from their loved ones at a time when they have a deep need for connection and support.

In addition to the disruption of an assumptive world, a survivor may experience the stirring of long-held beliefs that were problematic even before the significant other's death. For example, throughout her childhood, Joan's father had told her that she was "no good." When her son committed suicide, the belief that she was no good (self-esteem) emerged as a significant element of her grief.

The shattering of their worldviews has profound implications for how survivors think about and process the loss. In most cases, survivors will try to make sense of what has happened, but may be unable to do so. They may have trouble reconciling the death with their religious views, and may feel betrayed or let down by God (other-trust, worldview). Many survivors are preoccupied with thoughts about causality and responsibility (self-trust, worldview) and accountability

TABLE 3.1. Common Responses to the Sudden Death of a Loved One

Psychological	Physical	Behavioral	Social
Emotions	Trembling, shaking, "jumpiness"	Searching behavior to recover the lost loved one	Lack of engagement with other people or usual activities due to preoccupation with the loved one and the loss
Anxiety, fear	Muscle tension, aches, soreness	Being "on guard" with heightened awareness of surroundings, hypervigilance	Decreased interest, motivation, initiative, direction, and energy for relationships
Shock, emotional numbness	Stomach upset, nausea	Social withdrawal or isolation	Boredom
Separation pain, sadness, sorrow, anguish	Grinding teeth, clenching jaw	Disorganized activity, erratic behavior	Being critical of others, showing anger or irritation with others
Yearning, pining, longing	Tiring easily	Increased intake of medicine and/or psychoactive substances (such as drugs, alcohol, caffeine, nicotine)	Loss of or changes in usual patterns of social interaction
Helplessness, powerlessness, feeling out of control	Exhaustion	Distractibility	Feeling alienated, detached, or estranged from others
Anger, hostility, irritability, impatience	Headaches	Crying or tearfulness	Jealousy of others without loss
Guilt, self-reproach, regret	Heart palpitations	Diminished self-care	Dependence on others, clinginess, and avoidance of being alone
Depression, hopelessness, despair	Shallow and rapid breathing	Decreased effectiveness and productivity in personal, social, or work situations	
Loss of pleasure or enjoyment of formerly enjoyed activities	Shortness of breath	Avoidance of/clinging to people, places, or things that are reminders of the loved one, the death, or associated events	
Decreased interest, motivation, initiative	Numbness, tingling sensations	Self-destructive, impulsive, addictive, immoderate, or compulsive behaviors (e.g., gambling, indiscriminate sexual activity, overworking, overeating, excessive shopping/spending money, overexercising, fast driving)	
Fear of going crazy	The sensation of being smothered	Hiding grief for fearing of driving others away	
Feeling violated or mutilated	Dizziness		
Vulnerability, insecurity, inability to feel safe	Dry mouth		
Loneliness	Sweating		
Shame	Cold, clammy hands		
Abandonment	Hot flashes or chills		
Relief	Chest pain, pressure, or discomfort		
Thoughts	Diarrhea or other abdominal distress		
Disbelief	Frequent urination		
Denial	Tightness in the throat, difficulty swallowing		
	Heightened arousal		
	Agitation		

Confusion, bewilderment

Disorganization, distractibility

Preoccupation with the loved one and/or the death

Inability to remember aspects of events surrounding the death

Impaired concentration, comprehension, mental functioning, memory, problem solving, and decision making

Reexperiencing aspects of events surrounding the death; intrusive thoughts and images; dreams, nightmares, flashbacks

Increased or decreased spirituality; confusion about spiritual beliefs

Shattered assumptive world—changes in the way one thinks about oneself, the world, others, life in general

Meaninglessness, senselessness

Disillusionment

Lowered self-esteem, feelings of inadequacy

Negative thinking, pessimism

Perceptions

Feelings of unreality, depersonalization, dissociation

Paranormal experiences pertaining to the loved one (such as hearing or seeing the person or having a sense of his presence)

Development of a perceptual set for the deceased

Startling easily

Difficulty falling or staying asleep

Physiological reactivity upon exposure to reminders of the death

Appetite disturbance leading to weight loss or gain; food doesn't taste right and is difficult to eat

Feeling as if there is a "lump" in the throat

Tendency to sigh

Feelings of emptiness

Reduced immune response

Constellation of vague, diffuse physical complaints

Hair loss

Irritability, outbursts of anger

Sighing

Changes in sexual activity level

Note. From Rando (2014). *Coping with the sudden death of your loved one: A self-help handbook for traumatic bereavement.* Copyright by Therese A. Rando. Adapted by permission.

43

(other-trust, worldview). It is also common for mourners to be tormented by feelings of guilt and questions of whether and how much the deceased may have suffered. We discuss these issues in more detail below. Each adds to the challenges of accommodating the death and moving constructively into the future.

Core Issues Created by Violated Assumptions

Difficulty Accepting the Loss

As noted above, it is common for survivors of sudden, traumatic deaths to experience difficulty accepting that their loved one is actually dead. As Rando (1993) has explained, many people state that they accept the death, but it is clear from their remarks that they do not fully comprehend the finality of the loss and all of its ramifications. Consequently, it is difficult for the mourning process to commence. In the study by Lehman and colleagues (1987), described in Chapter 1, the respondents were interviewed 4–7 years after losing a spouse or child in a motor vehicle crash. Nearly 40% of the bereaved spouses and parents indicated that they sometimes felt the death was not real and that they would wake up and it would not be true. In addition, 32% of the bereaved spouses and 41% of the bereaved parents indicated that, even though they realized it was not possible, they sometimes imagined that their spouse or child was coming back.

In cases where the deceased's body is not recovered, such as in an airplane crash or a terrorist attack, it may be particularly difficult for the survivor to accept the death. Even when the body is present, problems accepting the death may make it hard to part with the loved one's possessions. In addition, these problems may make it difficult to deal with tangible reminders that the loved one is gone, such as the gravesite. "When I visit my child's grave, it confronts me with her death in a way that is almost too painful to bear," said one mother.

Grappling with Meaning

Most survivors of traumatic loss report that at some point, they attempted to make sense of, or find meaning in, their loved ones' deaths. According to Davis (2001), the search for meaning may take many forms, such as finding emotional meaning (e.g., believing that one's loved one is with God and is no longer suffering); developing new goals or a new purpose; experiencing transformative personal growth; or finding benefits or redeeming features in the loss.

However, available evidence does not support the belief that, over time, most survivors are able to make sense of what has happened and move forward with their lives (see Wortman & Boerner, 2007, for a review). In our experience, survivors frequently comment that now that their loved ones have died, life holds no meaning. For example, parents are likely to view the death of a child as a violation of the natural order. As one father indicated, "You're not supposed to bury your children" (Rosof, 1994, p. 17). Survivors of traumatic death typically make statements like these: "Tomorrow comes and tomorrow comes," and "I don't care what happens to me" (quoted in Finkbeiner, 1996, p. 191). In the Lehman and colleagues (1987) study described previously, the majority of the respondents (68% of bereaved spouses and 59% of bereaved parents) said that they had not made any sense of, or found any meaning in, the deaths 4–7 years afterward. In addition, 85% of spouses and 91% of parents had asked the question, "Why me?" or "Why my spouse/child?" Of these people, 60% of the bereaved spouses and parents said they were unable to answer the question.

Cleiren (1993) found that 14 months after the loss, 74% of those who had lost a loved one in a motor vehicle crash could not find meaning in what had happened. Murphy, Johnson, and Lohan (2003b) obtained similar findings in a study that focused on parents who had lost a child as a result of homicide, suicide, or a fatal accident. They found that 43% of the respondents had not found any meaning in their child's death by the end of the 5-year study. In the case of homicide, 66% of respondents were unable to find meaning. Evidence is clear that survivors are more likely to have difficulty finding meaning after a sudden, traumatic loss than after a loss stemming from natural causes (see Neimeyer & Sands, 2011, for a review).

These and other studies have demonstrated that the mourning process is especially painful for people who search for meaning but do not find it (Davis, Wortman, Lehman, & Silver, 2000). For example, Lehman and colleagues' study (1987) reported that of the respondents who were unable to find meaning in the loss, 73% of the bereaved spouses and 81% of the bereaved parents reported that it was painful for them not to have found meaning in the loss. Moreover, among those who seek meaning, the inability to find it is a significant predictor of poor post-loss adjustment in the majority of these studies. Neimeyer (2001) has suggested that sudden, traumatic losses impair the ability to create meaning, and that this may be the mechanism through which traumatic loss can bring about intense and prolonged distress.

Questioning One's Faith

Among practitioners and laypeople alike, it is believed commonly that a deep religious or spiritual commitment may facilitate coping with loss. Park and Halifax (2011) have noted that for many individuals, "religion or spirituality underlies their general approach to life and forms the system of meaning through which they experience and understand the world" (p. 358). Religious or spiritual beliefs may mitigate threats to meaning, since most faiths have doctrines that explicitly address the meaning of death. Such beliefs may help people make sense of the traumatic loss by providing a framework for incorporating negative events (Pargament & Park, 1995; Park & Cohen, 1993). For example, a religious doctrine may emphasize that a traumatic incident was the will of God (see, e.g., Dull & Skokan, 1995). Specific tenets of a faith, such as the belief that the loved one is in a better place or that the mourner will be reunited with the loved one someday, may also reduce the likelihood of an existential crisis.

Whereas some people may find solace in their religious beliefs, it is also common for survivors of traumatic loss to question faith-related beliefs, and sometimes to abandon them altogether. A woman who had lost her son in an accident several years previously found that the loss triggered a powerful and long-lasting crisis of faith. Although she had been actively involved in her church before the loss, her views toward God shifted dramatically following her son's death: "If there is a God, [He is] not a loving God and I want nothing to do with him. . . . If He has no control over our lives, why bother to pray to Him? . . . the hell with you, God" (quoted in Finkbeiner, 1996, pp. 167–168).

Wilson and Moran (1998) maintain that following a major traumatic experience, "God is viewed as absent from a situation which demanded divine concern, divine protection, and divine assistance. The God in whom one once believed no longer deserves devotion. Consequently . . . in these situations, faith becomes impossible" (p. 173). Like many of a person's fundamental beliefs, those related to spiritual and/or religious practices may be subject to abandonment, renegotiation, or recreation. The task for clinicians working within this treatment approach is to help clients develop a perspective on these issues that contributes to their healing.

Preoccupation with Causality, Responsibility, and Blame

In the wake of a traumatic death, it is common for a mourner to become preoccupied with the question of why the loved one died and who should be held accountable for the death. Typically, this preoccupation represents the mourner's attempt to rework his worldview and to regain a sense of order, control, and justice in the world following the destruction of his basic assumptions.

Particularly after deaths that are unexpected or perceived to be preventable, survivors often experience a need to learn everything about what happened. They may obtain copies of police reports, autopsies, and other documents in order to gain as much information as possible. Many survivors feel conflicted about reading such documents, since they recognize that the information often includes traumatic content and that it may confirm the death, which they still have not fully accepted. In fact, many survivors find that the information included in the documents is more disturbing than they anticipated. One woman, whose husband died in an explosion at his job site, was determined to review the autopsy report so she could understand more about how her husband died and whether he had suffered. "His bosses told me that he died instantly, but how can they know?" she said. The report provided no definitive information about how long he lived once the accident had occurred. However, it did reveal that his injuries were far more extensive than she had been led to believe. Even in cases where mourners are not exposed to traumatic content, these documents are rarely definitive. In some cases, they are inconsistent with information about the tragedy from other sources, such as eyewitness testimony. In other cases, the information may be incomplete. Consequently, such documents often raise more questions than they answer, adding to the mourners' distress.

In cases where deaths were caused by identifiable individuals, it is common for survivors to experience a desire for retribution. Following a homicide, for example, mourners are often determined to ensure that the legal system holds the perpetrator accountable for what happened. As we discuss below, it is natural for survivors to believe that the person who brought about the loved one's death should receive punishment commensurate with the heinous act. In our experience, negative feelings toward the perpetrator are likely to intensify if he fails to show remorse for his actions. This perspective is supported by observations from the South African Truth and Reconciliation Commission, which revealed that when perpetrators confessed their guilt without remorse, the bereaved were left feeling insulted, angry, and dissatisfied with the process (Payne, 2008; Weiner, 2006).

Survivors are especially likely to struggle with the need for accountability, as well as a desire for revenge, in cases involving homicide. As Rando (1993) has indicated, these mourners typically experience anger that knows no bounds, as well as accompanying thoughts of retaliation and revenge. They may develop elaborate fantasies regarding ways to hurt, degrade, or even torture a perpetrator. As one mourner indicated, "I want him to experience the terror and physical pain that my daughter experienced." Most mourners are very frightened by the emergence of such feelings.

In therapy, clients may be reluctant to bring up these strong feelings and revenge fantasies, fearing that their clinician may be repelled or judgmental. These survivors are typically not aware that such thoughts are normal following this type of loss. Feeling angry can also be very empowering for survivors, and may represent a preferable alternative to the vulnerability and despair that may underlie the anger.

Feelings of Guilt

Many survivors of traumatic death experience powerful and disturbing feelings of guilt. Guilt feelings frequently emerge in cases where they would appear to be completely unwarranted. For example, one woman relocated her family from Denver to Chicago because she had an excellent job offer there. After they had been living in Chicago for about a year, her 13-year-old son was struck and killed while riding his bicycle. "Johnny did not want to move to Chicago, but my husband and I thought it would be best for the family," she said. "If we had not moved, he would still be alive."

Evidence from the motor vehicle study discussed earlier indicates that it is extremely common for survivors to experience self-blame and guilt even when they are not at fault (Davis, 2001). For example, many of the respondents lost a loved one when another motorist, either speeding or drunk, collided with the car occupied by their loved one. Not one of the respondents reported thinking, "If only the other guy wasn't drunk," or "If only the other guy had driven more carefully." Virtually all of the respondents offered explanations for what happened that implicated their own behavior—for example, "If I had taken my son to the ballgame that night, rather than letting him drive with a friend, it would not have happened."

Most parents have deep feelings of responsibility for the safety of their children, and these feelings are readily transformed into guilt after a child's traumatic death. As Rosof (1994) has put it, "Your job as a parent was to protect your child, and you could not" (p. 15). In attempting to understand what happened and why, survivors often question themselves mercilessly about things they did, as well as things they believe they should have done but didn't. Self-blame serves the purpose of shoring up the belief that there is some controllability in the universe and that what happens is not completely random (Janoff-Bulman, 1992). Rosof has emphasized that, despite the anguish that typically accompanies feelings of guilt, it is easier for survivors to find themselves guilty of some sin of omission or commission than to acknowledge how helpless they truly are.

In our experience, feelings of guilt are particularly pronounced after a suicide (see Chapter 5). It is common for survivors to experience intense anguish because they did not recognize the depth of their loved one's distress, or because they could not prevent what happened. However, feelings of guilt are prevalent among survivors of other kinds of sudden death as well. A college student whose father dies in a crash when driving drunk may feel guilty for not confronting him about his alcohol use. A mother whose infant dies as a result of sudden infant death syndrome (SIDS) may feel guilty because she was not watching the baby closely enough. A woman whose husband dies of a heart attack may experience guilt because she did not encourage him to alter his diet or to get more exercise.

Guilt often causes survivors of sudden, traumatic loss to scrutinize their behavior during the days and weeks before the death. It is common for them to focus on any sign of conflict and exaggerate the role this may have played in the death. For example, shortly before his mother left for work, a teenage boy had an argument with her about attending a party at his friend's house. When his mother was killed in an accident on the way to work, he could not help feeling that she was distracted by the argument and therefore less attentive to road conditions.

In addition to their own feelings of guilt, survivors often worry that those in their social network will blame them for the tragedy. Indeed, it is common for friends and acquaintances to make remarks insinuating that a survivor is to blame, even when such an assessment is unwarranted (see Rudestam, 1987). In our experience, such remarks are particularly likely be made after the death of a child. For instance, an elderly driver struck and killed a 12-year-old boy who had run into the street to retrieve a baseball. A neighbor berated the boy's mother because she did not have a fence around her yard. While such direct and unwarranted blaming of survivors is prevalent, it is even more common for people to deliver such remarks in more subtle form, which can make them more difficult to refute. A friend of this same woman asked her, "Where were you when your son was killed?"

Sometimes survivors' beliefs about others' judgments may be projections of their own feelings of guilt or shame. Survivors' sense that others are judging or criticizing their behavior typically leads them to withdraw from social contact. Social withdrawal can contribute to feelings of isolation and estrangement, which make it difficult for the healing process to begin.

Litz and colleagues (2009) have used the term *moral injury* to refer to the state that military service members can experience after "[p]erpetrating, failing to prevent, bearing witness to, or learning about acts that transgress deeply held moral beliefs and expectations" (p. 700). Although these occurrences are expected parts of the combat experience, they can nonetheless lead to social withdrawal, self-harming behaviors, reexperiencing (in the form of painful recall), helplessness, hopelessness, and enduring changes in beliefs about oneself and others, among other difficulties. The concept of moral injury is relevant to service members who may seek treatment for trauma- or bereavement-related challenges, and it may also be relevant to others who similarly struggle with moral aspects of the deaths of their loved ones.

Preoccupation with the Deceased's Suffering

Most survivors of sudden, traumatic deaths are preoccupied with questions about whether and how much their loved ones suffered. Many agonize about what their loved ones experienced during the final moments of life. Did they know they were going to die? Did they see it coming? Did they experience intense fear or terror? Ruminations about suffering appear to be most prevalent following deaths that are violent or mutilating, or that involve homicide. As one father expressed it, "I have nightmares about how my son struggled with his killer." Such ruminations are also prevalent in cases where the death was not instantaneous. Concerns about the deceased's suffering can tap into a person's other-control needs.

In 95% of violent deaths, loved ones are not with the deceased at the time of death (Rynearson, 1987, 2001). Hence the vast majority of survivors struggle with questions about exactly how their loved ones died. Furthermore, many survivors of traumatic deaths are deeply troubled that their significant others died alone. They are distraught that there was no one available to comfort their loved one in his final moments of life. "I wish I could have been there to hold his hand, stroke his face, and tell him how much I loved him," said one woman whose husband died in a motor vehicle crash.

CLINICAL INTEGRATION

James's sister, Pamela, had been worried about him for some time. She decided to talk to him about her concerns. "I know you had a bad experience with that therapist a year ago, but maybe someone else would be more understanding and could actually help you. I'm worried that I'm going to lose my brother forever."

Pamela was referring to his extreme withdrawal since Raphael's death 2 years earlier. James no longer socialized with friends; he had stopped going to the gym; he didn't spend time with his nieces and nephews as he used to; and, as far as his sister knew, he had quit playing guitar. Pamela not only missed her brother, but was deeply concerned for his health and well-being. As she and James spoke, he saw the look of concern on her face and considered what she had said. Still, he couldn't seem to get past the question the first therapist asked him almost a year ago: "Have you been able to find a silver lining in your experience of losing Raphael?"

The memory made him want to scream. "Silver lining?!" he thought. "There is no silver lining here! My life is over! My love is lost forever."

Although he had felt initially supported by that therapist, James never returned after she asked that question. He found it deeply offensive and took it as proof that the therapist couldn't understand what he was going through. What the therapist didn't fully understand, and what James himself found difficult to acknowledge, was that he was struggling with the utter meaninglessness of Raphael's death. After a year-long investigation of the accident and of working conditions at the manufacturing plant, no liability was apparent. There was no one to blame and no way to make sense of what had happened that dreadful day. Neither did James have a way of making sense of the death from a broader perspective. For James, there was no spiritual belief, no world-view, and no actual experience that imbued Raphael's death and his own loss with any meaning at all. If he were to give therapy another try, he would need the next therapist to understand this. He needed a therapist who could tolerate the radical uncertainty that now defined his existence. If he couldn't make sense of Raphael's death in some way, how could he continue with his own life? This was the question that James now needed some help exploring.

CONCLUDING REMARKS

Throughout this chapter, we have described traumatic bereavement as an extraordinary experience marked by disintegration of worldviews, depletion of resources, and disruption of basic psychological needs. Survivor clients need clinicians to convey understanding of and respect for their symptoms and struggles. Sound, ethical clinical practice requires that we know something in general about our clients' condition while remaining open to learning from them about their particular experience. In other words, we should not leave it to the clients to teach us what we need to know about traumatic bereavement; neither should we assume that we know how the clients experience traumatic bereavement in the context of their lives.

James's first therapist made a mistake by asking about a possible "silver lining." We can characterize the question as a mistake because in this case, James was struggling with a sense of meaninglessness that was just the opposite of what his therapist wondered about. James's experience can help us appreciate that knowing something about the role and nature of blame attribution, guilt, rage, and spiritual loss will be helpful in working with traumatic bereavement clients. At the same time, we can best help our clients if we also remain open to learning whether and in what ways these aspects of traumatic bereavement manifest themselves for each individual client.

CHAPTER 4

Domains of Life Affected

Kyle's younger brother, Jeff, died in a plane crash on his way to visit friends in the Midwest. At the time of the incident, both Kyle and Jeff were college students and were extremely close. Now that Kyle has returned to college following Jeff's death, he feels numb and as if nothing matters any more. Thoughts about Jeff's accident go through his mind, and he finds it difficult to sleep. Concentration problems plague him, particularly in his math and science courses, and Kyle is terrified that he will lose his scholarship and disappoint his parents.

Kyle is also worried about his parents. Before Jeff's death, Kyle looked forward to visits home during the school year—enjoying his mother's great cooking, shooting hoops in the backyard with Jeff and his dad, and watching sporting events as a family. Since Jeff's death, he instead has felt sadness and despair as soon as he enters his parents' home. His father is more withdrawn. It seems as though his mother's vitality has drained away. Her boundless energy was one of the things he admired most about her. Now she appears to be a shell of her former self. Cold cuts from the deli or pizza delivery have replaced family dinners. His friends at school have expressed sympathy, but they also tend to keep their distance because they don't know what to say. For Kyle, Jeff's death has changed everything. No matter where he turns, he confronts the painful consequences of what happened.

A sudden, traumatic death can impinge on virtually every aspect of a mourner's life. A comprehensive understanding of the domains of life it affects, including possible legal involvement, is crucial to successful treatment. As illustrated above, disruptions in these domains bring about additional assaults on mourners and their capacity to integrate and accommodate their losses. In this chapter, we describe the sorts of difficulties that survivors may encounter in the various domains of their lives.

Survivors of traumatic loss seek solace in a variety of places, including interactions with others or involvement in work, leisure activities, and faith communities. For a variety of reasons, their quests for comfort and support are often unsuccessful. Indeed, in many cases, survivors continue to accumulate painful and alienating experiences.

Survivors of natural deaths may also have trouble in many of the domains we discuss below. In most cases, however, survivors of traumatic deaths encounter situations that are more problematic. For example, upon returning to work, a woman whose husband killed himself is more likely to experience stigma and greater social discomfort than is a woman whose husband died of cancer. Following the death of a spouse by suicide or homicide, intrusive thoughts and concentration problems are common and can interfere with the survivor's ability to meet responsibilities at work and at home. Such problems are less prevalent following a natural loss. In fact, survivors of natural deaths rarely encounter some of the problems that bring about great distress for survivors of traumatic deaths. For example, these survivors are more likely to question their religious faith. They may also experience anguish at the hands of the criminal justice system. For example, the system may bring them into contact with a perpetrator who shows no remorse, or who receives a suspended sentence. Encounters of this sort give rise to further complications of mourning, beyond those the survivors have already sustained.

INTERPERSONAL RELATIONSHIPS

The Nuclear Family

In considering how a nuclear family may be affected by traumatic loss, it is important to keep three factors in mind. First, the particular stressors associated with any role (e.g., work) are likely to be more intense and prolonged following a traumatic death than one that has occurred through natural causes (Rando, 2013; Wortman & Boerner, 2011). Second, reactions to a given loss are importantly influenced by the role relationship each family member had with the deceased—for example, whether one has lost a spouse or a child. People viewing the loss through the lens of one role may have difficulty understanding aspects of the loss associated with other roles. Finally, within a particular family, there are typically dramatic differences in whether and how individuals express their grief and cope with their loss. Each of these factors is likely to contribute to family members' distress and can undermine relationships that were previously close and rewarding.

Unlike those who lose their loved ones through natural causes, survivors of sudden, traumatic deaths have no time to make a transition into the new roles required of them. If a woman experiences the traumatic death of her partner, she may suddenly have to take on responsibilities for unfamiliar roles, such as handling the family finances. In fact, she is likely to be confronted with a host of financial matters almost immediately after the death. These include issues pertaining to Social Security benefits, life insurance, and estate taxes, among others. These may exceed her abilities, particularly while she is in the throes of acute grief. In contrast, if a person loses his spouse to cancer, he will have weeks or months to prepare for taking over such tasks. Moreover, this process is most likely to proceed with input from the spouse.

Consider a case in which a man is killed in a helicopter crash, leaving behind a wife and an adolescent son. The son may be devastated because he can no longer turn to his father for support or advice. In addition, he may deeply miss his father's involvement and encouragement regarding his music activities. He may be troubled by the fact that, although his parents always attended his concerts together, his mother has rarely attended performances since his father's death. Over time, he may resent his mother's apparent lack of interest in him; he may sometimes feel that, in effect, he has lost both parents.

In many cases, one family member may be unaware of the issues that are most troubling to another. For instance, the mother in the example above may assume that her son understands that she will become more engaged in his activities as soon as she is able. She may also assume that her son is aware that she is struggling with complex issues surrounding her husband's estate that she must handle now.

It is difficult to correct such erroneous assumptions because most survivors try not to say or do things that will upset other family members. This adolescent boy may believe that if he talks candidly with his mother about how upset and disappointed he has been, she may become even more distraught. It is also unlikely that his mother will talk with her son about the enormous pressure she is experiencing in regard to financial issues. Yet it may be beneficial for him to have a better understanding of the burdens she is carrying, as this may lead him to judge her behavior toward him less harshly. In addition, open discussion about their respective losses may help each facilitate the other's mourning by diminishing their sense of isolation.

Survivors may also mourn differently because they have distinct styles of emotional expression. Whereas some mourners may benefit from discussing their feelings about the person who died, such discussions may increase others' distress. Mourners within the same nuclear family may also differ in their views regarding the value of displaying feelings. A bereaved parent may conceal his feelings in order to be strong for his partner. Similarly, parents may feel that it is inappropriate to express feelings of grief and distress in front of their children. They may feel that in the face of this tragedy, children need to believe that their parents are strong and capable. Finally, regardless of their attitudes about emotional expression, mourners are likely to differ in their ability to regulate and control the emotional distress they are experiencing. Such divergent responses can complicate the mourning process within the nuclear family and between immediate and extended family members.

Most people report a dramatic change in the atmosphere at home. As one mother explained following the death of her teenage son, "He would always walk through the door laughing and joking, often with some of his friends. Now all I hear is silence, and it kills me." Family members may also become more irritable and tense following the loss—a common result of the disrupted ability to manage strong feelings or express grief or anger directly. One man who lost his daughter stated, "The anger and frustration from what happened to our daughter seem to spill over into my relationship with my wife. We are far more irritable with each other now."

Some family members may interpret others' different approaches to mourning as indicating something negative. For example, a wife may fail to understand why her husband shows no emotion following his sister's death. She may question whether he really loved his sister. In addition, as family members struggle with their own anguish, there may be a contagion of negative affect that can intensify each person's grief. After a relatively good day at work, for example, one husband plummeted into despair when he returned home to find his wife sobbing.

In most cases, the home and yard contain many reminders of the loved one. Such reminders can intensify the pain of the loss. For example, one man had helped his wife plant daffodils along the side of their home the fall before she died. The next spring, when the flowers bloomed, he became distressed that she was not there to see them.

Marriage or Primary Partnership

Following the death of a child, members of a couple are sometimes able to pull together and provide some measure of support for one another, reflecting other-trust and other-intimacy. In fact, a mourning parent may feel that the partner is the only person who truly understands who and what was lost, and the couple may develop a closer relationship as a result of what happened. The notion that divorce after the death of a child is almost inevitable has been shown to be a myth (Murphy, Johnson, & Lohan, 2003a)—one that puts an unnecessary additional burden on bereaved parents. It is true, however, that divorce becomes more likely following the death of a child. Evidence suggests that the death of a child places strain on even the best partnerships. As discussed in Chapter 1, parents who had lost a child in a motor vehicle crash 4–7 years previously were more likely to divorce than parents who had not lost a child (Lehman et al., 1987).

As described above, a potential source of discord may be that the members of a couple have different mourning styles. For example, one partner may feel a powerful need to talk about what happened or about their child. The other partner may prefer to keep feelings inside. One partner's discussions about the loss may intensify the other's torment. As one husband explained it, "When my wife talks about what happened the day our daughter died, I know she is only trying to make sense out of it. But it literally makes me nauseated, and I have to leave the room." If one partner gives cues that he doesn't want to hear about the other's feelings, the other partner is likely to feel disappointed and hurt. Such feelings can diminish communication between partners and change the tenor of everyday tasks they previously enjoyed, such as preparing dinner or gardening together. As a result of living with these dynamics, it is common for each member of the couple to feel estranged from the other. According to Mehren (1997), spouses often report that they feel "shut out," and are at a loss as to how to establish the closeness they enjoyed previously.

It is common for partners to have difficulties negotiating their sexual relationship following the death of a child. Either person may experience a lack of interest in sexual intimacy after the loss. For example, one may feel that it is wrong to experience pleasure in light of what has happened. In some cases, however, the desire for intimacy may increase following the death of a child. As one man explained after the death of his only child, "Sexual intimacy helped me feel close to the only other person who meant anything to me." In cases where partners differ in their desires for intimacy, tension can arise. When both members of the couple lose interest in sex, their sex life may become yet another casualty of their child's death. (For more on the impact of child loss on sex and other aspects of a couple's relationship, see Rando, 1986, 1993.)

A couple may also have difficulty coping with other losses, such as the death of a parent, sibling, or close friend. If the loss affects one partner more deeply, the other may have a difficult time understanding what the first one is feeling. This is particularly likely to occur when one member of a couple loses a parent. People typically believe that the death of a parent should not cause an adult a great deal of distress. Hence, one partner often reacts with irritation when the bereaved partner appears distraught about such a loss. The bereaved spouse may feel unsupported by the partner, and both are likely to report a decrease in marital quality (Umberson, 2003).

For a same-sex couple, the loss of a loved one may pose an additional set of challenges in coping. For example, the surviving member of the couple may feel unwelcome at her partner's funeral. If sexual orientation has alienated the survivor from her extended family, she may also lack that potential source of social support.

Parenting

The death of either a partner or child leaves a surviving parent with a number of specific problems. Some problems in parenting are unique to people who have lost their partners. For instance, Marlene, the mother of four young children, lost her husband in an airplane crash. Prior to his death, Jon had participated fully in parenting and household activities. In addition to his role as primary breadwinner, Jon had assumed responsibility for paying the bills, planning for the family's long-term financial needs, and maintaining the house and car. The two of them shared driving the four children to different schools and attending their activities. Jon's death thrust Marlene abruptly into single parenthood.

Other difficulties are experienced both by survivors who have lost a partner and by those who have lost a child. When a person is in deep mourning as a result of such a loss, it is hard to be emotionally available to surviving family members. In many cases, it is challenging for bereaved parents to provide physical care for their children. Like many others, Marlene had difficulty with sleep after her husband's death. She would typically fall asleep around 4:00 A.M. She was often unable to get up at 7:00 A.M. to get her children ready for school. She was afraid to take sleep medication because she wanted to be sure she would hear the children if they cried out in the night.

Marlene felt that her children would benefit from continuing the family activities that they had enjoyed before Jon's death. Prior to the loss, they went skiing every other weekend during the winter, and took regular trips to the beach in the summer. However, she recognized that without her husband's income, these pastimes were not affordable. In fact, the financial constraints resulting from a loved one's death can prove devastating, and can greatly increase the distress associated with the loss itself. In Marlene's case, an immediate consequence of her husband's death was that she lost health insurance for herself and the children. This was particularly stressful in Marlene's case because one of her sons had a congenital birth defect that required regular treatment.

About 6 months after her husband died, Marlene recognized that she and the children could no longer afford to live in the family home. Clearly, such a loss has profound ramifications for all family members. In addition to everything else, Marlene had to get the house ready to sell and find a real estate agent. She also had to locate a suitable new home and deal with such issues as mortgage rates and closing costs. The children were faced with the loss of their many friends from the neighborhood. They also had to adjust to a new school.

In addition, it can also be difficult for surviving parents to enforce consistent discipline. Because of symptoms such as depression, lack of motivation, fatigue, and inability to concentrate, bereaved parents are sometimes lax in maintaining structure, boundaries, and routines for their children. At other times, chronic feelings of anger and frustration may result in frequent arguments. Children may find that sometimes the surviving parent does not notice indiscretions, while at other times she responds harshly.

Alternatively, a parent may realize that the child is having a difficult time, and provide gifts as a way of comforting him. Members of the extended family may also provide an excessive number of gifts. These diverse responses to the child, which often bear little relationship to his behavior, can lead to confusion and insecurity.

It is also common for parents to become overprotective following a traumatic death because their safety needs—for themselves and others—are likely to be affected by the sudden death. Survivors typically live in fear that something bad will happen to other family members. As one bereaved woman stated, "When my daughter was late coming home, and I could not reach her on her cell phone, I became hysterical." Parents often place many new restrictions on the behavior of their children. A 9-year-old girl who lost her brother complained, "I used to be allowed to go to sleepovers at my friends' houses, but now I'm not. I'm the only kid who's not allowed to go." Parents are likely to question teenagers relentlessly about where they are going and what they are doing. Such behavioral restrictions and increased scrutiny often contribute to feelings of animosity and resentment. These responses can also interfere with the development of autonomy in adolescents and young adults, which typically evolves in response to consistent guidance and age-appropriate regulation by parents.

Some bereaved survivors express deep concern about how children of the same gender as the deceased parent will fare without a role model to assist with gender role socialization. One man who lost his wife in an industrial accident was concerned about raising his two young daughters alone. "She used to take them shopping for clothes and talk to them about their feelings about boys," he said. Such concerns may also adversely affect the surviving parent's feelings of self-esteem, self-trust, and adequacy to parent alone.

Parents may be unaware that young children express their grief differently from adults. Very young children may simply be unable to comprehend the permanence and irreversibility of death or the concept of an afterlife. One grandmother who had lost her adult daughter was taken aback when her 4-year-old grandson asked at the funeral, "When is Mommy going to wake up?" She added, "He thinks heaven is an actual place you can visit, like McDonald's, and says we should go to heaven and pick Lucy up."

Young children are also likely to exhibit aggression, anxiety, and regressive behavior—evidence of setbacks in affect tolerance. Bedwetting is common following the traumatic loss of a parent or sibling. Unfortunately, many parents are unaware of the link between the loss and such regressive behaviors and consequently may react punitively to the child. Other common symptoms are stomachaches, headaches, difficulty tolerating separation from the surviving parent or other loved ones, and acting in ways that test (or may be designed, even if unconsciously, to elicit) limits.

Many times, teenage children become more rebellious and uncooperative around the house. They may perform more poorly at school and experience an increase in problematic behaviors. One of Marlene's sons began cutting classes and bullying classmates. Parents might have difficulty determining to what extent certain changes stem from the loss, and to what extent they stem from the fact that the child is now an adolescent. Such behavior can be particularly difficult for the surviving spouse if the deceased spouse handled discipline prior to the death. In any case, the surviving parent must now manage these challenging behaviors without the benefit of consulting with the partner.

Children often go out of their way to be "good" so as not to upset or disappoint the surviving parent. When parents are unable to function, surviving children may be forced into a caregiving role. In these cases, it becomes more difficult for such children to separate from the parent and become independent.

Parents often struggle with what to tell their children about the death, and about how to respond to a child's questions or comments. For example, the driver of a moving van was talking on his cell phone when he plowed into a car that was stopped at a red light. The 32-year-old driver of the car was killed on impact. The trucker received minimal punishment for this crime. As his wife stated, "Our 8-year-old son, Bobby, asked me why the trucker is not in jail and why he is still driving a truck. What am I supposed to tell him?" In another case, a 10-year-old boy whose father was killed by a drunk driver announced to his mother, "When I grow up, I'm going to kill the man who killed my daddy."

The Extended Family

Following a traumatic death, an adult survivor typically expects to receive emotional support from parents, siblings, and other relatives, particularly if they enjoyed good relationships prior to the loss. Sometimes this expectation is fulfilled, and mourners are able to establish a nurturing relationship with one or more family members. However, many bereaved survivors encounter unexpected problems in their relationships with members of their extended families.

One problem frequently mentioned by mourners is extended family members' refusal to acknowledge and talk about the deceased. As one mother expressed it, "They act as though my daughter never existed. This really hurts." Some family members avoid mentioning the deceased for fear of upsetting surviving members of the nuclear family, whereas others do so because they worry that they themselves will become emotionally overwrought if they bring up the topic. Still others simply feel at a loss for the "right" thing to say.

Whereas failure to acknowledge the deceased can be problematic, intense and repeated displays of distress can be equally difficult for survivors. As one woman indicated after the death of her daughter, "I used to enjoy going over to my mother's. But now all she does is cry about Cassie. I wish she would support me, but instead I feel that I have to take care of her."

Following the death of a spouse or partner, it is common for conflict to develop between the survivor and her in-laws. In-laws may begin to offer unsolicited advice about many topics, including how the surviving parent should raise the children and handle investments. Such behavior may reflect the in-laws' desire for control stimulated by the loss of their child. Of course, concern for the young family may also motivate such comments. Advice is most helpful when tempered by attunement to the young family's expressed needs and responses to advice.

Conflict may also emerge regarding particular possessions of the deceased. In the case of a natural death, the dying person has the opportunity to decide how to distribute his possessions. Following a sudden, traumatic death, however, family members must sort this out for them-selves. For instance, a man who killed himself had an extensive coin collection. His parents believed that they should have the collection, while his wife wanted to keep it to pass down to their children. In such disputes, each party may be looking for ongoing connection with the deceased.

Because of the aforementioned difficulties, the tenor of family gatherings may change. When attending a family gathering, both immediate and extended family members may feel as though they must "walk on eggshells" to avoid upsetting anyone. If survivors do lose their composure on such occasions, they may not receive much sympathy. One woman who had lost an infant son was attending her sister's baby shower. Although she worked hard to maintain her composure, her eyes welled up with tears a few times. After the shower, she overheard her mother say, "It's too bad Peggy can't be happy for Susan, instead of just focusing on herself and her own loss."

Finally, the fact that all family members are bereaved may affect the degree of support any family member can offer to another. When Jon was killed, Marlene naturally turned to his par-ents, who lived nearby, for help with the children. However, Jon's father was so deeply affected that he was unable to assist Marlene and required substantial support from his wife, who then was less available to support Marlene and the children.

STRUCTURES OF DAILY LIFE

Following sudden, traumatic deaths, most people will need to attend to their obligations and the basic requirements of daily life. These demands may include such tasks as maintaining the household, paying the bills, and bringing home a paycheck. It can be excruciatingly difficult to engage with such tasks when it feels as though one's world has been ripped apart. These burdens can also compromise people's ability to participate in therapy. Alternatively, a survivor may appear to become excessively involved in daily activities, to avoid facing the painful affect associated with the loss. One husband and wife found themselves at odds shortly after the death of their adult son in military combat. Almost immediately after their son's death, the wife threw herself into dismantling his condominium to prepare it for sale. Although her husband wanted to spend some time reviewing their son's art collection, she insisted on selling it, even though they did not need the money. In either case, clinicians and clients together must explore the psychological needs the clients' behavior is serving, and whether it is in fact adaptive for healthy mourning and accommodation.

Work

For many survivors of traumatic deaths, work is a means of maintaining a routine, structuring their time, and feeling competent. They hope that their jobs will help them focus their attention away from the loss, and perhaps fill the emptiness they feel. In many cases, mourners are fortunate to have supportive coworkers. Nonetheless, it is typical for survivors to have experiences at work that add to their distress. Particularly in the first several months after the loss, mourners may have difficulty keeping their emotions under control. They may become tearful when they encounter a reminder of the loss, such as a customer who has the same name as the deceased. They may also feel self-conscious around others. As one woman indicated, "I felt that my presence was making people uncomfortable. They kept some distance from me, probably because they did not know what to say or do."

Upon returning to work, many survivors face serious difficulties with concentration and memory. These common symptoms of traumatic bereavement can dramatically reduce a mourner's ability to function at work. If he is experiencing intrusive imagery, concentration difficulties may be even more pronounced. One survivor said, "My boss keeps asking me for the sales projections for next year. But how can I finish them when I keep seeing images of the accident?" These problems manifest themselves in different ways, depending on the nature of the job. Those who work in sales may be unable to remember the names of their customers or what products they need. Those who work in management or service fields may find it extraordinarily difficult to listen to the work-related problems of their clients or their subordinates. People who work with heavy machinery may be concerned that a lapse in concentration will result in an injury for themselves or someone else.

The deficits in motivation that often accompany traumatic bereavement can also erode survivors' ability to perform well at work. Many people report that because of the death, they no longer find their job as satisfying or interesting as they once did, and that they have to force themselves to perform tasks that they completed easily before the loss. In many cases, previously held plans or goals for professional advancement no longer seem possible. As one mourner indicated following the death of her sister, "I was planning to start taking classes toward my master's degree this summer. But at this point, there is no way I can handle work and school."

Physiological changes—including hyperarousal, an increase in headaches or stomachaches, and sleep difficulties—can also lead to lowered productivity. A reduced sense of physical well-being can make work feel more onerous.

Because of the problems described above, most mourners show a dramatic decline in work attendance. In addition to such factors as sleep disturbance and a decrease in motivation to complete the work, the ability to go to work on significant dates may affect attendance. Common impediments to work attendance include the anniversary of the death or the birthday of the person who died; the necessity of dealing with children who are ill (particularly if a survivor is a single parent); and the decision to be present in the courtroom if a (criminal, civil, or both) case is being tried. Dealing with these factors can also affect performance in many ways, such as enhancing the likelihood that a survivor will make errors, or will fall behind schedule by taking more time to complete job-related tasks. Survivors of sudden, traumatic deaths may experience a great deal of anxiety about their work performance. As one woman indicated, "I was always worried that I would let down my coworkers or my boss." Another man said, "Before my mother's death, I gave 150% at work. Now I can only give around 50%."

The factors that contribute to absences at work are also likely to result in tardiness. As one employee expressed it following the death of his partner, "For the last 16 years, I was only late on one occasion. Since Bob's death, I have been late about three times a week." In addition to anxiety, it is common for survivors to feel embarrassed or ashamed about their absences and tardiness. Moreover, many mourners have indicated that after the first month or so following the loss, their coworkers do not show much sympathy for their situation. "My boss told me flat out that she thought I was taking advantage of Jessie's death by missing so many days and coming in late all the time," said one mother who had lost her daughter.

In many cases, survivors also report difficulty with the day-to-day banter of colleagues. It is hard for some mourners to endure coworkers' comments about their families. One father lost his son shortly before the son was scheduled to begin college. When he heard a coworker mention that he was planning to take his daughter to college, the bereaved father suddenly started sobbing. Another survivor who lost his wife had difficulty showing sympathy for a colleague who complained that his wife was out of town for a week. Because of their discomfort with such conversations, many survivors minimize their contact with coworkers. As one mourner stated, "I used to eat in the lunch room, but now I eat at my desk."

Leisure and Recreation

For most people, recreational activities are enjoyable pastimes, providing relaxation and replenishment. After a traumatic death, however, it is often difficult for survivors to participate in leisure activities that they enjoyed with the deceased. One father said, "As my son was growing up, I taught him everything I know about fishing. We went fishing together on countless occasions and always had a great time. Since his death, I have no interest in fishing whatsoever. My friends have invited me to go, but I have declined. It would be too painful to be out there without him."

Vacations also present challenges to those who have experienced a traumatic death. Family members often struggle with whether they should return to a regular vacation spot or try a new destination. If they return to a destination they have enjoyed in the past, the trip is likely to trigger bittersweet memories. If they choose a new destination for a vacation, they may experience profound sadness that their loved one is not present to enjoy the trip. One couple lost their toddler when his condition was misdiagnosed in the emergency room and he did not receive the appropriate treatment. The following year, they took their surviving children to Disney World. It was painful for them to encounter Mickey Mouse, who had always been their toddler's favorite character.

These feelings are likely to emerge not only around vacations, but also around a host of activities family members enjoyed before the tragedy. Camping trips, sporting events, and religious and school functions are but a few examples. As one widow explained, "Every year we went to the annual charity ball at my workplace, and it was always a lot of fun. I have no desire to go by myself."

Following a traumatic death, it may also be difficult for survivors to enjoy television and movies as much as they did before the loss. Many mourners find it hard to relax while watching TV or films because they never know when they will encounter vivid reminders of their loss. For example, a couple who lost a blond toddler may find it difficult to witness the endless series of blond toddlers who appear in diaper and cereal commercials. Sometimes, out of a need to guard against the potential confrontation with such reminders, mourners remain in a constant state of hypervigilance. At other times, they may elect to quit watching TV altogether so as to avoid exposure to these cues. One man whose twin sister was shot in a robbery said, "I can hardly watch anything any more. Shootings occur all the time on TV and in the movies. I can't even watch the evening news." Even if the media do not expose survivors to images that evoke their loved ones' deaths, newspapers and magazines frequently carry stories that exacerbate survivors' distress. For example, a woman whose daughter was killed in a gun accident may find it painful to encounter an article about a recent mass shooting or about the easy availability of guns. In addition, watching TV or movies can bring about discomfort if mourners feel guilty when they enjoy these pastimes or momentarily forget about their loved ones.

In most cases, the distress associated with watching movies or TV is exacerbated when a mourner is in a social situation. In one case, a man was at the home of friends, and they were watching an action movie together. Near the end of the movie, there was a violent explosion. This man's father had died in an explosion the previous year while working on a pipeline. "The movie ended and they asked me if I wanted coffee and cake, and I was sitting there crying," he said. "Witnessing that explosion brought everything back."

Spiritual or Religious Community

As we have discussed earlier, the traumatic death of a spouse/partner or child can evoke a crisis of faith. Feelings of disillusionment may undermine survivors' motivation to participate in their faith-related activities or communities. Without their faith communities, survivors lose an important source of support and comfort.

Among those who continue to attend religious or spiritually oriented services, this experience may change dramatically after the loss. One woman who had gone to church with her husband for many years found it jarring to attend alone. Often the music played can stimulate great emotion, as can certain parts of the service. One Catholic widower remarked, "I cry when I hear the hymns at Mass, and I really lose it when I have to give others the Sign of Peace." A place of worship can also trigger disturbing memories if the funeral service took place there. As one woman indicated, "Whenever I go to the synagogue, I think about my son's funeral." Survivors also report feeling self-conscious in religious institutions, since these communities are defined in part by concern for others. "I found it hard when people asked me how I was doing," said one mother who lost a child. "I knew they wanted me to say I was doing OK, or that I was doing better. But that would have been a lie."

In some religious communities, survivors may also become the recipients of support attempts that are based on an assumption of God's omnipotence. As one father expressed it, "If one more person tells me that God needed my son more than I did, I'm going to throw up." Survivors are commonly told that what happened was God's will, that it was for the best, that their loved ones are in a better place, and that they will see their family members in the next life. Many people find such comments offensive. In addition, common responses to a traumatic death (e.g., questioning God's will) may elicit disapproval from members of a mourner's congregation, who may view such responses as blasphemy or demonstrating a lack of faith.

In some cases, members of a congregation may regard a mourner's decision to enter treatment as reflecting a lack of faith. As a result of these kinds of responses, it is common for survivors to distance themselves from their religious communities. Some change churches or temples so that they can practice their religious faith without constant scrutiny; others quit attending religious services altogether. As one former churchgoer stated, "Following my son's death, I began to question religious beliefs that I had held all of my life. I could not understand why God would allow my son to die. I thought attending church would be comforting, but every few minutes there was a reference to God's omnipotence or God's goodness."

THE LEGAL SYSTEM

If the death of a loved one was caused by another person, the perpetrator may be prosecuted criminally for causing the loved one's death. The death may have come about through murder, manslaughter, or criminally negligent homicide. In such cases, the local, state, or federal government, which seeks to determine the perpetrator's guilt or innocence and impose an appropriate sentence, may initiate legal action.

Individuals may also become involved with the legal system if they decide to file a civil suit, or a wrongful-death suit, on behalf of their deceased loved one. The most common causes of wrongful deaths include motor vehicle accidents, medical malpractice, use of defective products, and construction accidents. Unlike criminal trials, which are initiated by the government, civil suits are initiated by the loved one's surviving family members. In a criminal case, the penalty imposed is a sanction, such as a fine or imprisonment. In a civil case, a monetary judgment is entered against the perpetrator. In some cases, the perpetrator may be prosecuted in both a criminal action and a civil action.

In either a criminal or a civil case, survivors are typically motivated by a desire for justice. They want to see the perpetrator held accountable for what has happened. At the onset of a trial, survivors may be optimistic about receiving an acknowledgment from the legal system that what happened to their significant other was wrong. Many mourners have a fervent wish that as a result of the legal proceedings, what happened to their loved one will be less likely to happen to someone else. Consciously or not, they may also believe that they will experience some relief or healing if the perpetrator is found guilty.

People commonly hold beliefs and assumptions related to justice and fairness within their worldviews, and a traumatic death can deeply disrupt these beliefs. It is common for family members of individuals who have been murdered to express dissatisfaction with the legal system. In one study, dissatisfaction with the criminal justice system was highly correlated with respondents' ratings of anxiety and depression (Amick-McMullan, Kilpatrick, Veronen, & Smith, 1989).

It is most unfortunate that what begins as a search for justice or healing often ends in disillusionment and heartbreak. Disillusionment may stem from going through the legal process, facing an unfavorable outcome, or both. Parties can experience a number of delays during the judicial process, for which most people are ill prepared. Postponements, continuances, and appeals can prolong a legal battle for several years. In one case, a woman witnessed her husband being struck and killed while he was on the shoulder of the highway changing a tire. The perpetrator's blood alcohol level was three times the legal limit. She felt strongly that the perpetrator should be held accountable for this crime. Each time the matter was scheduled to be heard in criminal court, she took a day off work and drove to the courthouse, which was 50 miles away. The case was continued six times over a 2-year period. Many defense attorneys are motivated to continue such cases because it is a way to keep their clients out of prison. Such practices can be heart-wrenching and infuriating for survivors.

If a case does go to trial, survivors may experience considerable anxiety about the prospect of testifying in front of the judge and jury. Many bereaved survivors cannot imagine expressing their innermost thoughts and feelings in such a public forum. It can feel as though they are the ones on trial, and that they must prove how much they are suffering. In most cases, they are also fearful about what they will be asked during cross-examination. One mother was terrified that she would be questioned about how often she visited her son's grave. One aspect of the judiciary process that can be upsetting to survivors is that the defense attorney may attempt to shift blame from the perpetrator to the survivors or to the deceased. For example, a man was struck and killed while he was attempting to assist a distressed motorist on the side of the highway. In court, the defense attorney argued that he should have recognized the danger of stopping to assist another motorist.

It is also common for the alleged perpetrator's attorneys to scrutinize every aspect of the survivor's past. A single parent who lost her only son in a motor vehicle crash was shocked when the defense attorney unearthed her traffic violations from 15 years earlier, and when he berated her in front of the jury for accepting food stamps when her son was young. Defense attorneys are often intent on obtaining information about the plaintiff's behavior that will weaken the case. In one case where a woman's husband died because of medical malpractice, the defendants hired private investigators to determine whether she had begun dating again. She frequently saw them lurking outside her home and was frightened and intimidated by these tactics.

During legal proceedings, survivors often encounter information about their loved one or the manner of death that is shocking and disturbing. One woman was pushing her baby in a stroller when a drunk driver drove onto the sidewalk, hitting the stroller and killing the baby. The woman was horrified when she entered the courtroom and saw the mangled stroller, which the defense attorney planned to use as an exhibit. Another woman learned in the courtroom for the first time that when her brother's accident occurred, his body was dragged along the pavement for 200 yards.

Yet another troubling aspect of the judicial proceedings is that they bring survivors into contact with the perpetrator, usually for the first time. For most survivors, this encounter evokes powerful and unsettling emotions. As noted above, it is common for survivors to harbor seething rage toward the perpetrator. They hope that the perpetrator will recognize the magnitude of the loss she caused and show some remorse. In our experience, this almost never happens. One man whose mother was shot in a holdup attempt said, "He acted so nonchalant, as if he did not have a care in the world. He even smiled on some occasions. I was so angry, I could have killed him with my bare hands."

It is typical for survivors to feel that what happened to them and their significant others was profoundly unfair. They often believe that they have received a life sentence of pain and loss. It is rare for perpetrators to receive sentences that mourners view as commensurate with their crimes, especially in cases of vehicular homicide. In one case, a couple lost their teenage daughter when her car was struck by a vehicle traveling over 150 mph. The driver was returning from a bachelor party and was legally drunk. Her parents were infuriated that the perpetrator was not sentenced to any jail time; he was not fined; and, in fact, he didn't even get a traffic ticket. In those cases where the perpetrator receives a minimal sentence or no sentence, the survivors may feel that the value of the loved one's life was not acknowledged or recognized. As one father expressed it, "It was as if they said, 'Your daughter was killed, so what!'" Similarly, such an outcome can leave the survivors feeling as though their own pain and suffering do not matter.

In our experience, many bereaved individuals harbor a strong wish to convey what they have been through to the perpetrator. Since the 1990s, survivors have been able to make statements regarding the emotional suffering they have experienced as a result of their loved one's death. Such a statement is called a *victim impact statement*, and is used at sentencing. This information can be provided orally, in writing, or both. In our experience, the vast majority of bereaved people who have given such statements consider them to be meaningful and worthwhile.

SOCIAL SUPPORT

Social support is generally regarded as one of the most important resources for dealing with stressful life experiences. As we discuss in Chapter 10, supportive interactions with others help people to feel loved, cared for, valued, and understood. A survivor who is engaged in any of the domains described above, such as being at work or attending church, has the potential for receiving support. Unfortunately, available research indicates that survivors of traumatic loss rarely receive effective support. Studies on social support among the bereaved suggest three reasons why support may not be forthcoming. The first, which we have touched on above, has to do with the impact of a death on the support providers to whom a mourner has typically turned in the past. The second stems from survivors' strong inclination to withdraw from others after the tragedy, thereby cutting themselves off from interactions that are potentially healing. The third set of reasons results from the social ineptitude of those in the social environment, leading them to offer support that is ineffective or even harmful. We discuss each of these reasons below.

Impact of the Death on Potential Supporters

It can be especially hard on a survivor if the person who died was his major source of social support. This often occurs in the case of spousal loss, particularly for men. Many heterosexual men in our culture rely almost entirely on their wives for support and have few close friendships outside the marital bond. In addition to removing a major source of support, the traumatic death can render other potential supporters less effective, since the tragedy may also affect them, as discussed previously in the section "Interpersonal Relationships."

Mourners' Tendency to Withdraw

Studies have shown that people who have experienced the traumatic death of a loved one often choose to avoid or minimize contact with others. Research indicates that it is common for survivors to withdraw from others. In a study of how older adults coped with the death of their adult child, Malkinson and Bar-Tur (1999) noted that many of these parents inhabit "an emotional territory that is inaccessible and isolated, by building a fence between themselves and others" (p. 414). Dyregrov and colleagues (2003) assessed parents of children who had died as a result of SIDS, an accident, or suicide, an average of 1½ years after the deaths. Approximately 50% expressed agreement with the statement "I withdraw from others." Self-isolation was by far the most important factor associated with health problems, PTSD symptoms, and complicated grief in all three samples.

Survivors may withdraw for several reasons. Some mourners may feel too helpless, confused, or depleted to initiate social contact. As one woman expressed it following the suicide of her son, "When you experience such a disaster, you are not capable of asking for anything. You are completely lost" (quoted in Dyregrov, 2002, p. 656). These feelings may also make it difficult for survivors to respond to social overtures from others. Some people do not like to go out, especially at first, because they feel self-conscious. As one person indicated after the loss of her child, "I felt that everyone was looking at me and trying to figure out how I was doing." A woman who lost her spouse felt that she did not "fit in" with her former couple friends. As she expressed it, "I feel like a fifth wheel." In addition, she found it painful to realize that at the end of the evening, she would be going home alone. Some avoid socializing because they are afraid that they will make others uncomfortable, or that they will be "wet blankets" and ruin the gathering for others. Still others prefer to stay at home because they never know when they will encounter a reminder of their loss that will trigger distress. For example, a widower whose spouse loved lasagna became visibly upset when he went to a dinner where the host served lasagna.

In addition, mourners often have difficulty engaging in the types of interactions that typically occur at social gatherings. After experiencing a traumatic death, a mourner may find almost any subject trivial and meaningless. In our experience, mourners have particular difficulty with people who complain about relatively insignificant issues. For example, a woman whose husband died in an accident may become annoyed when her colleague complains because someone dented his car in the parking lot.

Parents who have lost a child may find it heartbreaking to hear others discussing their children's activities, accomplishments, or plans. Bereaved parents may also have difficulty when exposed to parents who are critical of their children. "At work today," one bereaved parent indicated, "I had to listen to my supervisor go on and on about how upset he was that his son didn't make the basketball team." For all of these reasons, survivors of traumatic deaths often feel more comfortable at home.

Others' Social Ineptitude

Research indicates that in many cases, survivors perceive remarks that people intend to be supportive as disappointing or hurtful. Dyregrov (2003–2004) conducted a study of the support difficulties encountered by parents who lost a child to SIDS, suicide, or an accident. She used the term *social ineptitude* to describe the responses that the bereaved often received from members of their social network. Problematic responses fell into three main categories. The first was anticipated support that failed to appear—for example, when people who were close friends prior to the loss did not contact a survivor after a death. The second category was avoidance of the bereaved (e.g., friends or acquaintances crossing the street or looking the other way when they caught sight of a bereaved person). As one mother stated after the traumatic death of her daughter, "I felt like I had the plague." Rando (1993) has noted that among those who have lost a loved one, bereaved parents are the most stigmatized and avoided because "their loss represents the worst fears of others" (p. 624).

The third category of social ineptitude Dyregrov identified was offering advice or support that recipients viewed as unhelpful. These included attempts to block discussions about the loss or displays of feelings (e.g., "You need to be strong for your children"), minimizing the problem (e.g., "At least he's not a vegetable"), invoking a religious or philosophical perspective (e.g., "She's a flower in God's garden"), giving advice (e.g., "You should not be going out to the cemetery every day"), and identifying with feelings (e.g., "I know how you feel—I lost my second cousin"). One might expect unhelpful remarks to be more prevalent among strangers or casual acquaintances than among the survivors' relatives or close friends. However, this does not appear to be the case (Lehman, Ellard, & Wortman, 1986). In one study, the bereaved consistently rated family members as less helpful than friends (Marwit & Carusa, 1998).

Survivors have reported that they experience such responses as deeply wounding. They leave the bereaved feeling that no one understands what they are experiencing. Such comments also contribute to survivors' discomfort at social gatherings. The bereaved typically find it helpful when others convey a supportive presence (e.g., "I'm here for you"); when they express concern (e.g., "I care what happens to you"); or when they offer tangible assistance, such as help with errands or meals. Most survivors also value interactions in which they can talk about the loss if they choose to do so (Lehman et al., 1986; Marwit & Carusa, 1998).

Some survivors elect to stay at home to avoid the difficult questions that others may direct toward them. People in a survivor's social network may ask insensitive questions about such matters as how the death occurred (e.g., "How fast was your husband driving?"), about financial issues (e.g., "How are you going to spend the insurance money?"), or about the loved one's possessions (e.g., "What are you going to do with his tools?") (Wortman, Battle, & Lemkau, 1997). Such questions or remarks can contribute to the survivor's tendency to withdraw from others.

CLINICAL INTEGRATION

It's been about 9 months since Kyle lost his brother, Jeff, to a plane crash. Now in his senior year of college, Kyle has been working with a psychotherapist, Xiu, in the counseling center on campus. During their ninth meeting, the following conversation takes place.

XIU: Hi, Kyle. How did you do with your independent activities this past week?

KYLE: Um, you know how we talked about bringing a friend home with me for the long weekend? Jeff and I both used to do that a lot. Our friends loved coming to our home when we had some time off at school because we have a comfortable house and our dad's a big sports fan and a really good cook. My friends always loved my mom, too, and she's an even better cook. When you're used to eating college cafeteria food and pizza, two chefs in the family is a big deal.

XIU: (smiling) Yes. And I know that going home is one of the things you've missed since Jeff's death.

KYLE: Yeah. I wasn't sure if Al would be able to have a good time because my parents aren't like they used to be. It took all the nerve I had, but I finally asked Al if he wanted to come home with me because his family lives too far for a weekend visit and he had nowhere to go. I thought that a sad house was better than staying in the dorm alone.

XIU: You were concerned about Al's feelings?

KYLE: Yeah, I guess so. He's one of the guys who know about what happened and all, so that made it a little easier. I called my girlfriend before I talked with Al; she really helped me get up the nerve to ask him.

XIU: That's great, Kyle. Do you see how calling Trish was an example of calling on social support and building those resources we've been talking about?

KYLE: Yeah, I guess so. For the most part, it's easier to rely on her, but I'm afraid of overwhelming her and pushing her away.

XIU: OK—I'm going to jot that down: Your fear of overwhelming Trish. It's something we may want to go back to and examine more closely. For now, can you tell me what happened when you talked with Al?

KYLE: Well, he was really cool about it and all. He's been to my house before, and so he was looking forward to it. But the next day I changed my mind. I canceled the trip. I disappointed Al and myself, and maybe even my parents.

XIU: OK. Let's go back a few steps and maybe learn something about the blocks you've been talking about. Do you remember how you felt, or what was going on inside of you, right after Al said he would come home with you for the weekend?

KYLE: I wanted to feel proud of myself; I thought I might, but I didn't. Instead, I felt that pit in my stomach that I always feel.

XIU: Always? That's a strong word. Do you always feel the pit? Did you feel it after talking with Trish?

KYLE: No, not always, and not after my call to Trish.

XIU: OK. So you did feel the pit after talking with Al. Are you aware of any thoughts you were having at the time?

KYLE: I'm not sure.

XIU: That's OK. What is your best guess about what you may have been thinking?

KYLE: I think I started imagining me and Al shooting hoops in the driveway. What if my mom was looking out the window while we played?

XIU: What if? What do you imagine would happen?

KYLE: (choking up) It's . . . it's like I'd be hurting her. She would see Al and me and think of Jeff and me, and . . . well, you know?

XIU: I think I do know, but I want to make sure I understand. What's the "and"? You said she would think of you and Jeff and—?

KYLE: Um. And she would think it's wrong if I was having a good time. (Xiu remains silent for a few moments, allowing space for Kyle to be with his inner experience. Kyle looks up at Xiu, then quickly looks away.)

XIU: Kyle, what did you notice just then? What was happening inside?

KYLE: I just felt sad, but also some relief. Well, that's not the right word. It's like I was aware of how heavy everything is, and somehow I felt lighter or something; I don't really know.

XIU: Sometimes when we can give a name or some expression to an inner experience, it does feel lighter. As though a small piece of the burden is lifting.

KYLE: (softly) Yeah.

XIU: You've said some important things today, Kyle. You were worried about Al having a good time. You didn't want to disappoint him. You were worried about being a burden to Trish. And you were concerned with possibly hurting your mom, and worried about disappointing her—not wanting to disappoint her. Not wanting to disappoint her with your happiness! That's all quite a burden, isn't it?

KYLE: Yeah, I guess it is.

XIU: And the part about disappointing or hurting your mom with your happiness, that's quite a dilemma: "If I'm happy, then I'll hurt Mom." It's especially a dilemma now, as you're trying to get through the last semester of your senior year, when there are a lot of opportunities for some happiness, or just a bit of fun.

Xiu again allows some silent space between words. He then asks, "What about Kyle?" Kyle's posture changes on hearing this question. He sits up straighter, indicating some interest in this question. He is vaguely aware that this issue is a theme they have touched on before, and on some level, he is grateful to have someone asking, "What about you?"

CONCLUDING REMARKS

When working with this treatment approach, we can address the domains of life affected by the traumatic death in various ways. We will want to assess which domains of life have been most disrupted or are most problematic as a result of the client's loss. For Kyle, the dynamics within his nuclear family, his relationships with friends, and his ability to experience pleasure and leisure have all been dramatically affected by Jeff's death. As Xiu has demonstrated in his work with Kyle, we also want to explore the client's inner experience in relation to these situations. What are his reactions? What is he telling himself about the situation? Which psychological needs are being activated? How are the client's self capacities being tapped or challenged? Furthermore, are these elements of inner experience helping or hurting him in his ability to cope, adapt, and move forward, both in general and within specific domains of his life? Finally, we'll want to explore how best to assist clients in adapting to and accommodating the changes they now face. In other words, we want to help clients develop healthy adaptations—those that support rather than inhibit the evolution of their mourning. Xiu again demonstrated how this can be done through examining Kyle's inner experience and helping him to confront difficult situations and practice coping strategies.

PART III

RISK FACTORS
AND RELATED EVIDENCE

CHAPTER 5

Event-Related Factors

Just as she did most other afternoons, Suzanne, a single mother, walked into her house at about 4:00 P.M., threw her bag and keys on the credenza, and called out to let her teenage daughter know she was home from work. Unlike other afternoons, there was an eerie silence in the house; once she entered the kitchen, Suzanne felt a chill throughout her body. She hadn't heard her daughter answer in her usual fashion. Suzanne would later describe this as "a feeling deep down in my bones that something was wrong." Suzanne doesn't remember the rest of that afternoon in any detail. She knows that she became more frantic when she entered her daughter's empty room and then began searching the house for clues to her whereabouts. They had spoken just hours before, as they did every afternoon, to confirm that her daughter would be home. Suzanne remembers that Sarah's voice had sounded strange, but she had chalked that up to adolescent moodiness. Suzanne also remembers her own horrific screams—although at the time she experienced them as though they were coming from someone else—when she descended to the basement to find Sarah dead. An empty prescription bottle of oxycodone lay next to her.

In this chapter, we continue a comprehensive description of traumatic bereavement. We focus on two sets of factors that influence how individuals experience and express traumatic grief: the characteristics of the death, and the type or mode of death. These dimensions are referred to as *risk factors*, since they typically affect the survivor's risk of a poor outcome. Each mode of death (e.g., accident, homicide) incorporates one or more of the characteristics of deaths (e.g., violence, randomness) described below.

Awareness of risk factors can provide a framework for understanding each client's thoughts, beliefs, emotions, behaviors, and vulnerabilities. Such information is invaluable in identifying specific issues that clients who have endured a particular type of loss often face. Following the violent death of a child, for example, it is common for the surviving parent(s) to struggle with intrusive thoughts about the unfairness of the death. Such images are usually less common following other kinds of losses, such as a spouse's fatal heart attack. Therapists who have a keen understanding of these issues will be in a better position to validate their clients' feelings, enhancing the likelihood that clients will feel heard and understood.

CHARACTERISTICS OF THE DEATH

In Chapter 1, we defined a *sudden, traumatic death* as one resulting from a precipitating event that is abrupt and occurs without warning. In this chapter, we discuss many characteristics of a death that, when present either individually or in combination, are likely to add to the impact of suddenness and lack of anticipation, and to precipitate traumatic bereavement in a survivor. There is empirical support for some of these elements, such as violence. Other factors, such as multiple deaths, have yet to be investigated systematically. In such cases, our discussion is based primarily on clinical observations—our own and those of other treatment providers. In discussing these elements, our goal is to elucidate the specific ways they can traumatize the mourner. Such knowledge can be indispensable to therapists in developing a treatment plan tailored to their clients' unique concerns.

Evidence suggests that the impact of the risk factors discussed below is cumulative. However, the intensity of a mourner's response to any specific risk factor depends on his subjective assessment or cognitive appraisal of the situation. Sometimes one factor (e.g., how much the loved one suffered just prior to death) brings more distress than others. This is why the therapist must focus not only on the array of event-related factors that are present in the situation, but on the client's unique responses to particular factors.

In exploring the impact of characteristics of the death, it becomes clear that some characteristics overlap with others. For example, unnatural deaths are usually violent. We have elected to discuss each characteristic individually, despite the overlap. This enables us to paint a more complete picture of the potential ramifications of the different kinds of death.

Unnaturalness

An unnatural death is markedly different from natural dying and typically prompts more extreme responses in a mourner (Rynearson & Geoffrey, 1999). In almost all cases, violent deaths are unnatural. The more unnatural the death, the more difficult it is for the survivor to integrate it into his inner life. There is a lack of any comfort that could be taken if this were a death that was anticipated and regarded as an appropriate exit from life. As Rynearson (1987) noted, "the peaceful dying of someone ringed by nurturing relatives is categorically distinct from the brutal dying of someone who is stabbed repeatedly by an assaultive thief or someone who is hit in a crosswalk by a drunk driver, or someone who is partially decapitated by a self-inflicted gunshot wound" (p. 78). The more unnatural or grotesque the specific circumstances of the death (such as a dismembered body), the more it breaches the survivor's sensibilities, and the more it interferes with healthy mourning (Rynearson, Schut, & Stroebe, 2013). In addition, mourners are more likely to view an unnatural death (e.g., one resulting from suicide or an accident) as "a senseless and wasteful loss of life" than a natural death (e.g., one resulting from illness) (Bailley, Kral, & Dunham, 1999, p. 267).

Violence

A large majority of sudden, traumatic deaths involve at least some violence. Mutilation or destruction often accompanies deaths involving violence. They are particularly traumatic because of the feelings they typically engender in the survivors: shock, horror, helplessness, vulnerability, anxiety, violation, and victimization (Rando, 1993). In most cases, such reactions lead to significant physiological hyperarousal, anger, guilt, and self-blame. Violent deaths rupture mourners' senses of invulnerability, security, predictability, and control, viciously violating their assumptive worlds (described in Chapter 3). In addition, they tend to undermine the mourner's ability to think or speak about the experience coherently. This, in turn, makes it far more difficult to process the loss and come to terms with what has happened (Currier, Holland, & Neimeyer, 2006). Consequently, there is a high risk of mental health problems following the violent death of a loved one (see Hibberd, Elwood, & Galovski, 2010, for a review; see also Rynearson & Salloum, 2011).

In most cases, violent deaths bring about posttraumatic stress symptoms (Green et al., 2005; Rynearson, 1987, 2001). Clients typically experience traumatic imagery that can be overwhelming and unresponsive to treatment. Of course, violent deaths result not only in intense and prolonged trauma symptoms, but in grief symptoms as well (see, e.g., Kaltman & Bonanno, 2003; Zisook, Chentsova-Dutton, & Schuchter, 1998). Kaltman and Bonanno (2003) found that, in contrast to people whose spouses died of natural causes, those who experienced the violent death of their spouse manifested significantly more PTSD symptoms during the 2-year duration of the study. Those who lost their spouse through natural means showed a decline in depressive symptoms over time, whereas those who lost their loved one through a violent means showed no drop in depressive symptoms over the course of the study (see Currier et al., 2006, for similar findings).

In some cases, a survivor may have harbored aggressive thoughts or fantasies toward a deceased person prior to the death. For example, upon learning that her husband is having an affair, his wife may have recurrent fantasies about harm befalling him. If so, his actual death may bring about feelings of guilt (Raphael, 1983), perhaps more so if the death is violent. Similarly, Raphael (1983) has asserted that violent deaths evoke primitive destructive fantasies and reawaken basic death anxiety and fears of annihilation, leaving survivors with these additional stresses to master. Horowitz (1997) maintains that in some cases, violent deaths evoke a powerful desire for retaliation. As we have noted earlier, survivors often imagine killing or torturing the perpetrator, and feelings of guilt sometimes follow these thoughts. Moreover, such deaths inevitably conjure up images of whether and how the deceased may have suffered. These images add enormously to the mourner's distress.

As noted in Chapter 3, in 95% of violent deaths from suicides or homicides, the persons die alone, in the absence of loved ones (Rynearson, 2005; Rynearson & Salloum, 2011). Survivors of such a death are at risk for being stuck in what Rynearson terms the *reenactment story* of the death. According to Rynearson (2005), survivors piece together this story from the media and from police and witness descriptions. It is common for survivors to replay this reenactment repeatedly in their minds.

Physical or Emotional Suffering before Death

Sometimes there is evidence that a loved one suffered, as when witnesses at the scene heard screams of anguish prior to the loved one's death, or when the medical examiner provides evidence that the death was not instantaneous. In other cases, a mourner may strongly suspect that a loved one suffered because of the way the death occurred. Regardless of how the events leading up to traumatic deaths unfolded, most survivors are concerned that their loved ones may have suffered. Thoughts about suffering are distressing because of the mourners' helplessness in the face of what happened (a challenge to schemas about control), the anger and guilt that result from the helplessness, and the associated imagery. As noted above, it is common for mourners to have elaborate and detailed thoughts about their loved ones' final moments, focusing on such things as whether they died in a state of fear or terror, experienced physical pain, or called out for the mourner as they were dying. As noted previously, some survivors become trapped in a repetitive cycle of imagining the suffering and death of their loved ones. Others may avoid thinking about the death to such an extent that the third "R" process of mourning (*Recollect and reexperience the deceased and the relationship*) does not take place.

Human-Induced Events

Although few comparative studies exist, available evidence suggests that it is more traumatic for people to contend with a human-induced tragedy than a natural one, such as an earthquake or tsunami. An exception to this occurs when humans cause a "natural" event, as was the case when poorly constructed levees gave way during Hurricane Katrina in 2005. The lack of an adequate response to an emergency or disaster, as with Hurricane Katrina, can also contribute to its psychological effects. A truly natural event usually brings forth relatively less anger and fewer violations of the survivors' assumptive world, although there still can be challenges, such as being left without a specific target for blame and anger (Rando, 2013). Two types of human-caused deaths create particular difficulty for survivors: those that survivors regard as preventable, and those that they view as intentional. Each of these types of deaths poses unique issues for the mourners.

Deaths Regarded as Preventable

Once a mourner receives information about a death, she may conclude that it occurred because of the negligence or carelessness of someone else. For example, there may be evidence that the pilot of a small plane was talking to co-workers and not paying attention, resulting in a fatal crash. Or a doctor may breach the standard of care by failing to prescribe needed antibiotics to a young boy who visits his office, resulting in seizures that prove fatal. Mourners are likely to view such deaths as senseless and unnecessary—in other words, as preventable. The fact that a mourner perceives a death as avoidable can cause him to ruminate about how someone, including himself, could have prevented it. For most survivors, such deaths raise issues of responsibility and accountability. They also affect the survivors' ability to trust and depend on others. For example, a man whose partner dies because of medical malpractice may want the physician to be held accountable for what she did. He may be devastated to learn that she will not be penalized and will still be allowed to practice medicine. It is typical for survivors to experience profound anger that such deaths occur, as well as feelings of anger and bitterness at the persons perceived to be responsible (Kristensen et al., 2012). It is also common for mourners to struggle with the injustice and unfairness of what has happened.

Complications following the loss may be greater in those cases where the behavior of the person(s) perceived as having caused it is more imprudent and/or unreasonable. In one case, a pedestrian was killed by teens who were joyriding in a parent's car. If the accident had occurred because an elderly woman temporarily lost control of her car, traveling just far enough onto the shoulder of the road to kill the deceased, fewer complications might have ensued for the survivors. The death of a loved one may also be more difficult to process in those cases where the perpetrator's negligence occurred on a regular basis and/or resulted in financial gain. This might occur in a death brought about by a trucking accident. If the trucking company routinely cut costs by hiring unqualified and inexperienced drivers, survivors may have great difficulty coming to terms with the loss.

In some cases, the deceased's own behavior contributes in some way to her death. For example, a teenager may sneak out of the house to take a ride with her boyfriend, and then die when he loses control of the car. In such cases, her parents' feelings of intense anger toward their daughter, as well as feelings of guilt, are likely to add to their distress because they view the accident as preventable. The perceived preventability of the death has violated their control schemas.

Deaths Caused by a Perpetrator with Intent to Harm

As noted above, psychological symptoms are particularly severe and long-lasting when the cause of death is of human design and conscious intention, as opposed to being a natural event or an accident. Homicide and suicide are examples of such deaths, and each type presents mourners with more potentially traumatizing elements than preventability alone. In addition to violating the mourners' assumptions about predictability, safety, and control, such elements are likely to undermine their trust in other people (Janoff-Bulman, 1988). In many such cases, the mourners view such deaths as evidence for the existence of evil forces in the world. According to Janoff-Bulman, an exaggerated sense of powerlessness and helplessness, along with a sense of "losing" a loved one to another human being, can elicit humiliation, shame, and a loss of self-respect. Outrage at the audacity of someone who takes a loved one's life can also be difficult to manage. We discuss homicide and suicide in more detail below.

Randomness

In some cases, survivors believe that their loved one died because she was in the wrong place at the wrong time. For example, Gretchen was scheduled to fly back to her home town following a business meeting in another city. The meeting ended early, so she was able to book an earlier flight. She was killed when the plane crashed. It was agonizing for her husband and parents to recognize that if she had taken a different flight, she would still be alive. Random events are frightening because they are uncontrollable; individuals cannot protect themselves from such events. For this reason, survivors sometimes assume blame for random events. It is easier for mourners to cope with such an event by taking responsibility for it, believing that they are in control of their lives, than to contend with the fact that they had no control. In such situations, the assumption of blame and of the consequent guilt is the price one pays to maintain the needed perception that the world is controllable. For example, Gretchen's husband might assume responsibility for her death because he had asked her to get home as soon as she could.

A related set of dynamics operates in a phenomenon called *blaming the victim* (Ryan, 1976). Here a survivor attempts to remove the event from the realm of a random occurrence by identifying what the deceased should have done or not done so that the event would not have taken place. Beliefs that contribute to victim blaming can be held not only by a survivor, but by acquaintances, friends, and family members of the deceased. For example, people may assert that "If she hadn't gone out alone at night, she wouldn't have been raped and murdered," or "If he'd worn his seat belt, he would not have been killed in the car crash." They derive some illusions of predictability and control by claiming that if they act differently than the deceased did (e.g., not going out alone at night), then they can avoid future tragedy (e.g., not being raped and murdered). Victim blaming by others can complicate the survivor's loving attachment to the deceased, creating ambivalence and guilt in the survivor, who does not want to hold blame toward the deceased loved one.

Multiple Deaths

We use the term *multiple deaths* to refer to cases where two or more loved ones die in the same event. Such deaths may stem from a natural or human-induced disaster, from a motor vehicle crash, from a murder–suicide scenario, or in cases of mass violence (such as a shooting episode in a public setting). In most cases, multiple deaths create a state of *bereavement overload* (Kastenbaum, 1969; Rando, 1993, 2013), and are consequently more difficult to handle than the death of a single loved one or even two sequential deaths. The process of mourning for one person often compromises the process of mourning for a second person. A vicious cycle often exists wherein the survivor is unable to mourn the death of Person A in the best way because of the emotions, unfinished business, and remaining reactions connected with Persons B and C. Each of these deaths, in turn, cannot be mourned adequately because of the incomplete mourning and stress associated with the death of Person A.

Situations involving multiple deaths raise a number of challenges. Multiple deaths are often associated with such a deluge of pain that a survivor is unable to function. Multiple deaths can also engender *psychic numbing* (Lifton, 1976), which can interfere with engagement in mourning processes. The mourner may also experience survivor guilt because she did not die. She may come to believe that her continued existence has been purchased at the cost of the loved ones who died. In addition, multiple deaths may have an adverse effect on the mourner's social support system. In many cases, one or more persons to whom the mourner would ordinarily turn for support have also been killed. Others in the social support network may also be incapacitated by grief and trauma symptoms, and thus may be less available. For all of these reasons, multiple deaths are likely to interfere with the six "R" processes of mourning. Such processes as facing the pain, mourning secondary losses, and relinquishing attachments are far more difficult when the survivor is mourning the deaths of two or more people.

Multiple deaths can also be complicated for survivors who lost only one loved one, but also acquaintances, neighbors, or other community members. This instance includes shootings in public settings such as schools (as in Newtown, Connecticut, in 2012) and movie theaters (as in Aurora, Colorado, also in 2012). In such a case, a whole community will be affected. An individual mourner's private grief becomes part of a larger narrative. Such events also tend to attract major media attention, including anniversary commemorations. Although mourners may experience additional support in such cases, they alternatively may find that their mourning is taken over by the community, which may choose ways to mourn or commemorate the deceased that do not meet any individual mourner's needs or style.

Threat to One's Own Life; Confrontation with the Deaths of Others

In some cases, a mourner's own life is threatened during the incident in which a loved one dies. For example, a couple may be involved in a car crash in which the husband dies, while the wife sustains serious injuries but survives. A scenario of this kind faces the survivor with a host of coping challenges. These often include watching the loved one suffer and die, and then struggling with subsequent gruesome images of the scene of the accident. If the loved one dies instantly, the survivor may feel heartsick that she was unable to tell him that she loved him and to say goodbye. The survivor may also experience guilt that she was not able to take some action that would have prevented the accident. In such situations where there was a threat to survival, the more the survivor experienced this life threat and thought she was going to die in the situation, the more emotional reactions, traumatic stress symptoms, and potential long-term problems she may have.

Being present at the scene of the loved one's death has the potential to bring the survivor into contact with the deaths of many people. One's presence at the scene typically results in a highly aversive sensory bombardment in terms of sights, smells, sounds, and kinesthetic feelings. Examples of such situations include air crashes, natural disasters, and war (Rando, 1993). Common responses include shock, horror, terror, helplessness, anxiety, and fear. Such factors as the sheer number of dead bodies encountered, as well as the extent of damage or mutilation to the loved one's body, can increase the horror of the situation. These stimuli can evoke overwhelming traumatic stress responses, including hyperarousal, numbness, intrusive images, flashbacks, avoidance, and extreme vulnerability.

As Kristensen, Weisaeth, and Heir (2009) have noted, those who are directly exposed to a disaster and experience a threat to their own lives are far more likely to develop PTSD than those who are not directly exposed to the disaster. This will be the case for those who survive shootings in schools and other community gathering places. Such survivors may need to review and reexperience the event in their thoughts, as well as to defend against it by avoiding it or shutting it out. Clearly, such personal confrontations with death, which raise the deepest questions about the meaning and value of one's life, can have a profound impact on the process of coping with the death of an important other (Rando, 1993).

According to Rynearson (2010), approximately 5% of violent deaths are witnessed by survivors. This may occur in a variety of different situations. For example, those who are present at the scene of a mass shooting at a school or movie theater may witness others' deaths. Or, following a motor vehicle crash, the driver may witness the passenger's death (or vice versa) while they are waiting for help to arrive. Evidence suggests that witnessing the death results in a significant increase in PTSD symptoms (see Kristensen et al., 2012, for a review). For example, Brent and colleagues (1992) found that survivors who witnessed the suicides of their loved ones or found the bodies had more PTSD symptoms than those who did not.

Untimeliness

When a young person dies, we typically feel that he has not had the opportunity for the kind of fulfillment in life to which he was entitled. It is a death "out of turn with nature" because it happens at an inappropriate stage in the natural life cycle. Such deaths violate many of our assumptions about the world, particularly those related to our worldviews. Losses of this sort are often associated with powerful feelings of injustice, intense anger, and anguish because of the termination of a life that had unrealized potential. Because of the person's youth, survivors may experience more numerous and poignant secondary losses, such as seeing the person taken from life before achieving important goals (e.g., seeing his business succeed) or before fulfilling responsibilities that were important to him (e.g., raising his young children). Moreover, bereaved persons are also likely to mourn for other survivors who are dealing with the death of the same person. As one woman commented following the death of her husband, "I grieve for my husband, but I also grieve for my son. He was hoping to get a baseball scholarship to college. My husband coached his team for many years and practiced with him every weekend. Now there is no one to fill this role, and my son is thinking of dropping out of baseball. The loss to my son is incalculable. He has not only lost his father; he lost the confidence he had that he would make it to the top."

Additional Factors

Many additional characteristics of the death can exacerbate a mourner's distress (Rando, 2013). Some of these have to do with the perpetrator's behavior. If it is clear that the death resulted from the actions of a specific person, survivors typically become angry if he does not acknowledge what he did. Survivors also find it deeply troubling when the perpetrator expresses no remorse for what has happened. In many cases, perpetrators' lawyers may have advised them not to admit responsibility or blame for the incident that resulted in the loved one's death. Survivors may not be aware of this, and may believe that the defendant is "getting away with murder." As one mother expressed after her son's car was sideswiped by a truck driver high on amphetamines, "If he would have just looked me in the eye and said he was sorry for what he did, it would have brought me a lot of comfort."

Sometimes the survivor will encounter the perpetrator somewhere in the community— the grocery store, the movie theater, the park. One woman lost her 7-year-old daughter when the dentist administered too much anesthesia. "He killed my daughter, and is still practicing dentistry. But today at the park, I saw him pushing his own daughter on a swing, without a care in the world."

Other characteristics of the death that can complicate the mourning process include waiting for confirmation of the death; failing to recover the body; finding the injured or dying person still alive; and being notified about the death insensitively. Additional experiences that can exacerbate grief include having upsetting encounters with police, emergency medical staff, doctors, or nurses at the hospital, or personnel at the medical examiner's office or the funeral home. These experiences can become part of the survivor's narrative of the death, and are therefore legitimate targets for intervention in the therapy.

The process of identifying the loved one's body or viewing the body for the first time can result in long-term traumatization of the bereaved. When people receive notification that a loved one has died, several scenarios may ensue. In some cases, survivors are told that a member of the family must identify the body. In other cases, survivors are strongly discouraged or even prohibited from viewing the body, even if they have a strong desire to do so. This directive may come from officials at the police department or coroner's office, who usually prohibit contact with the body when there is an ongoing criminal investigation. There are also cases in which one or more family members may strongly advise a mourner not to view the body. As one father explained following the death of his daughter in a shooting accident, "Jennifer's skull was shattered by the impact of the bullet. Nonetheless, my wife expressed a strong desire to be with Jennifer. I did everything I could to dissuade her. I wanted her to remember our daughter the way she was." Alternatively, a family member may encourage another to view the body, even if that person does not wish to do so.

Available research suggests that there are strong individual differences in survivors' desire to view the body, and in the impact of viewing the body on later adjustment (Chapple & Ziebland, 2010). Particularly after the death of a child, parents often have an overwhelming desire to be with their child's body, and to retain their role of caring parents. As one researcher described it, "We were surprised that so many expressed such an intense need to see, touch, hold, talk, or sing to the body" (Bower, 2010, p. 10). Many parents appear to draw comfort from such activities as washing and dressing their child. Survivors also value being with their loved one's body because it provides an opportunity for them to say goodbye. Still others felt that they would not be able to accept the reality of the death unless they view the body.

In many cases, survivors are extremely distressed that officials or other family members do not permit them to have time alone with the deceased. Instead, they are required to endure the presence of a police officer or someone from the coroner's office.

The first time bereaved persons encounter their loved one's body is usually at the funeral home. Even in cases where there is little visible damage, it is common for survivors to feel disconcerted by their loved one's appearance, frequently commenting that "It didn't look like him at all." In cases where there is more damage to the body, many are unprepared for the shock they experience when they view the body. As one mother indicated, "The funeral director did a good job, but there was only so much he could do. I brought my daughter's favorite dress, but we couldn't use it because it did not hide the bruises on her neck and arms, or the autopsy scar on her chest."

In cases involving sudden, traumatic loss, survivors typically benefit from viewing the body, even in cases where the body is badly damaged (Bower, 2010; Chapple & Ziebland, 2010). Those who decided to view the body had better outcomes and were less likely to regret their decision than those who chose not to view the body, who were more likely to regret their decision.

Overall, evidence suggests that the determining factor about whether viewing the body is ultimately a good idea may have to do with whether the survivor is encouraged, or at least permitted, to do what she chooses. Those who choose to view the body are likely to believe that they made the right decision, especially as time passes. Regrets are more often experienced by individuals who decide not to view the body. A central dynamic of trauma is loss of control, so when survivors are able to resume control following a terrible event or experience, recovery can begin. Being thwarted in one's preferences about viewing the body or spending time with the deceased continues the experience of loss of control.

In our experience, no matter how upset a survivor may be about what happened when he viewed the body, he is unlikely to raise these issues with members of his support network. Consequently, creating space in therapy where these issues can become legitimate topics of discussion and intervention can be highly beneficial to the client.

MODE OF DEATH

How does the mode of death influence the impact of a traumatic death? Are mourners who lose loved ones to suicide, for example, likely to experience more intense and prolonged distress than those who lose loved ones in motor vehicle accidents? Most of the studies assessing mode of death have focused exclusively on parents who lost children (Dyregrov et al., 2003; Murphy et al., 1999; Murphy, Johnson, Wu, Fan, & Lohan, 2003), although a few have examined survivors who lost spouses, siblings, parents, or friends (Cleiren, 1993; see Sveen & Walby, 2008, for a review). Those studies that have compared the impact of different modes of death have found fewer differences than they expected.

A study by Murphy and her associates compared parents who lost a child through homicide, suicide, or accident. They assessed parents four times over a 5-year period. Parents of children who were murdered reported a significantly higher number of PTSD symptoms than parents whose children committed suicide or died in accidents. Otherwise, there were very few differences in parents' psychological reactions as a function of the mode of death. These investigators found that 5 years after the loss, parents' responses on objective measures of mental distress and trauma were two to three times higher than those from normative samples of adults, regardless of the children's mode of death (Murphy et al., 1999; Murphy, Johnson, Chung, & Beaton, 2003; Murphy, Johnson, Wu, et al., 2003).

Dyregrov and colleagues (2003) studied parents who lost children to suicide, accident, or SIDS. They interviewed parents 1½ years after the deaths. They found that the majority of these bereaved parents evidenced severe psychosocial distress on virtually all measures used. Parents bereaved as a result of suicide or accidents evidenced significantly more problems than those who lost infants to SIDS. In particular, parents whose children committed suicide or who died in accidents were more likely to experience intrusive thoughts. Dyregrov and colleagues noted that the results of the study do not support the idea that loss of a child by suicide is worse than loss by other modes of death. In addition, they emphasized that although distress scores were reliably lower for parents of infants dying of SIDS than for the other groups, they nonetheless manifested very high distress. Taken together, the results of these two studies indicate that the sudden, traumatic death of a child brings about enduring distress among surviving parents, regardless of the cause of death.

Despite these findings, we believe it is important to provide information about the psychological ramifications of distinct modes of death. This material will help practitioners to respond to clients with greater awareness of the issues they are facing. Below, we highlight issues that affect the mourning process in response to acute natural death, accidents, disasters, military combat, homicide, and suicide. Each mode of death incorporates one or more of the characteristics of deaths described earlier in this chapter.

Acute Natural Death

Deaths brought about by acute natural causes, such as heart attack, stroke, aneurysm, acute illness, or infection, confront survivors with an unanticipated loss. For example, a spouse may suddenly die of a heart attack, or a child may die because of meningitis. Although survivors of such losses usually experience fewer intrusive, disturbing memories than do survivors of other kinds of traumatic deaths, this is not always the case. For instance, if the loved one is hooked up to tubes and gasping for breath during his final moments of life, these images can return to the mourner as intrusive reminders.

In deaths that result from acute natural causes, clinicians and other providers must be sensitive to whether the survivors view the deaths as preventable, since such perceptions can complicate the mourning process. Some mourners may believe that a loved one is responsible for the death—for example, when a person failed to take necessary medication, exercise, or eat a healthy diet. Others may place responsibility on members of the medical staff who they believe did not do enough to save their significant other. In these situations, some survivors may struggle with powerful feelings of anger after the loss. Still others may blame themselves. For example, a mother may blame herself for her child's death if the child had a high fever but she did not take him to the emergency room. In such cases, feelings of guilt are likely to plague the survivor.

Accidents

Motor vehicle crashes are the most prevalent cause of traumatic death. Survivors may also face such deaths as a result of firearms, falls, drowning, fires, choking, animal attacks, hazards at the workplace, and medical malpractice, among numerous other types. Most, but not all, of these accidents occur suddenly and without warning. Accidents occur at disproportionately higher rates among children, adolescents, and young adults (Heron, 2012), enhancing the likelihood that accidental deaths will be perceived by survivors as untimely. Motor vehicle crashes are more than twice as likely to claim the lives of African American or Hispanic male teenagers as those of European American teens (Armour, 2006). Accidental deaths are often associated with violence, mutilation, and destruction. In many cases, those who lose a significant other in an accident struggle with gruesome images of what happened, as well as fears that the deceased may have suffered.

We normally think of an accident-related death as constituting a sudden loss. Yet, as Armour (2006) has indicated, over half of those who die in motor vehicle crashes die en route to the hospital or during the first few weeks of hospitalization. In such cases, what does or does not take place in the hospital often becomes a critically important part of the dying-and-death story with which the survivor must contend (Rando, 2013). A survivor often finds the hospital experience to be profoundly disturbing. The traumatic event may have bruised and battered the loved one. He may be hooked up to tubes, ventilators, and other life support machines. The family members may have difficulty obtaining medical information. They may have agonized about whether health care providers are doing everything possible for their loved one. In many cases, the hospital staff is not able to control the patient's pain or keep him comfortable. Witnessing their loved one's suffering in such a setting not only exposes mourners to intense emotional distress, but can also provide an additional source of disturbing images, smells, and sounds that can resurface later. Depending on what they are told, family members may alternate between hope and despair. In a case where heroic measures such as cardiac paddles are used, survivors may experience anguish if the deceased had to endure these procedures but dies anyway (Rando, 1993).

Another potential source of traumatization is that family members are often required to make a decision about taking a loved one off life support. Regardless of the extent of their loved one's injuries and their implications for future quality of life, most people find it agonizing to take someone they love off life support and watch him die. It is also common for survivors to experience doubts in the future about whether they made the right choice.

Decisions about donating the loved one's organs can also be unsettling and retraumatizing. "I kept thinking about them cutting out her organs," said one father who lost his daughter in a bicycle accident. "I know it was for a good cause, but I still found it horrifying" he said. At this point in time, most survivors have not yet accepted their loved one's death, so assaults on the loved one's body are difficult to endure.

In a case where an accident comes about in part through the deceased's own behavior—for example, if she has been drinking and driving—survivors may experience intense anger toward their significant other. Such feelings may be accompanied by guilt over this anger, as well as guilt that the survivors were unable to influence the deceased's behavior and hence prevent the fatality. Such feelings are common among parents of teenagers or young adults, who often feel that if they had been more effective as parents, the tragedy would not have occurred. As one father indicated, "Our son had problems with alcohol and drugs. We tried to get him into treatment, but he was very resistant. One night after drinking several beers, he took the family car without our knowledge and was killed when the car went off the road. If we had been successful in getting him into a treatment program, this never would have happened."

In cases where the surviving mourner was also injured in the accident that caused the death, it may be very difficult to commence the mourning processes. If injuries are permanent, they may serve as a perpetual reminder of the other's death. Of course, there are also cases in which the death of a loved one comes about because of the mourner's behavior. For example, a father might decide to purchase a gun and keep it in his night stand. His decision could prove fatal if his 10-year-old son discovers the gun and is accidentally killed when it misfires. As discussed in Chapter 3, mourners typically experience powerful feelings of guilt even in cases where they played no role in their loved ones' deaths. Such feelings are paramount when a death comes about because of a survivor's poor judgment. Research shows that feelings that one could have done something to avoid the death are associated with increased PTSD risk and prolonged feelings of grief and depression (Kristensen et al., 2012).

In some cases, mourners perceive accidents as preventable. As Armour (2006) has indicated, the police classify a large percentage of deaths from motor vehicle crashes as due to the negligence of other drivers, suggesting that such deaths were preventable. Crashes in which perpetrators were speeding, driving under the influence of alcohol or other substances, or driving while using cell phones or texting are just a few examples. In such instances, the perpetrators may be arrested and face criminal prosecution. However, as described in Chapter 4, people who cause motor vehicle accidents are rarely held fully accountable for what they have done. They may receive small fines, or their licenses may be revoked for a few months, but in our experience they are almost never sent to prison.

In other cases, survivors may perceive an accident as a random event, in which the loved one was "in the wrong place at the wrong time." One man was killed in a motor vehicle crash on his way to work. He proceeded into the intersection when the light turned green, and was struck and killed by a driver who was trying to run the light. On the day of the accident, his boss had asked him to come in to work 10 minutes early. "If that request had not been made, my husband would still be alive," his wife said. As noted above, the belief that the death was random is painful, because survivors feel that they have no control over their lives and are at the mercy of fate or other people.

Survivors' struggles may relate very specifically to particular aspects of a death. Those who lose a loved one in a motor vehicle crash may develop profound anxiety about driving. If their loved one died in a crash caused by a truck driver, they may experience intense fear when a truck comes up behind them on the highway. They may also become particularly fearful when other loved ones are traveling by car. As one young man expressed it, "After my dad was killed in a car crash, my mom wanted me to transfer from the college I am attending now, which is about a 4-hour drive from our home, to a college in our home town. She told me that if I don't transfer, she doesn't want me to come home on weekends any more." Similarly, if the deceased loved one drowned, survivors may fear the water and refuse to go swimming or to accompany others to a beach or pool.

Disasters

Disasters are usually classified as one of two types: natural disasters, such as hurricanes or earthquakes; or human-induced disasters, such as the terrorist attacks against the United States on September 11, 2001. In most cases, survivors view natural disasters as unavoidable, although they may feel that attempts to warn them about the disasters or to contain the ensuing destruction were insufficient. Survivors are likely to view human-induced disasters as due to human callousness or malevolence, and perhaps preventable as well (Kristensen & Pereira, 2011). Consequently, they may experience feelings of rage and bitterness toward those they perceive to be responsible (Christ, Kane, & Horsley, 2011). Attributions of malevolence often challenge survivors' beliefs about the inherent worth of others.

Regardless of how disasters come about, they pose a unique set of issues for the mourners. Following a disaster, there is usually an agonizing period of waiting before survivors learn that their loved one has died. At that point, most mourners experience an overarching need to gain possession of their significant others' body. They may encounter many obstacles, such as bureaucratic processes of the county, state, or nation, as well as coroners' inquests. It can take weeks, or even months, to recover the body. Depending on the nature and magnitude of the disaster, the body may never be found, or it may not be found in recognizable form. In cases where the body is not intact or is not recognizable, survivors often struggle with intense anguish about whether their loved one suffered in her final moments. In those cases where there is no opportunity to see and recognize the body, it is harder for survivors to accept the reality of the death. Understandably, the absence of the body is likely to fuel disbelief, making it extremely difficult for the mourning process to begin.

In the course of a disaster, bereaved survivors may experience threats to their own lives or may witness gruesome scenes involving the deaths of others. Survivors who are exposed to the disaster that claims their loved one's life show more PTSD and prolonged grief symptoms than do those who were not exposed (Johannesson, Lundin, Hultman, Frojd, & Michel, 2011).

Following a disaster, survivors are also likely to encounter many secondary losses in addition to the death of their loved ones. As a result of Hurricane Katrina, the tsunamis of 2005 and 2011, the 2010 earthquakes in Chile and Haiti, and the 2011 earthquake in Japan, for example, many people faced multiple enormous losses—their homes, neighborhoods, possessions, money, and/or jobs. These losses typically bring the mourners into contact with insurance companies, federal agencies, and/or relief and assistance agencies, which they may experience as nonresponsive and highly bureaucratic. The lack of an adequate or appropriate response can cause a "second injury" (Symonds, 1980) that may exacerbate survivors' distress and must be addressed as well. A recent book on treatment for survivors of disaster (Dass-Brailsford, 2010) provides helpful information about what survivors experience and how they can be assisted.

A major disaster is also likely to be covered in the mass media for months and sometimes years following the event, as well as commemorated or at least noted annually, evoking painful and disturbing thoughts and images. Following the 9/11 catastrophe, for example, images of the collapse of the Twin Towers were televised repeatedly. Moreover, the attacks have been commemorated on a yearly basis. Finally, in those cases where the disaster affects the entire community, survivors can be overwhelmed by the loss of many individuals who played an important role in their lives. This was true in 9/11, when surviving firefighters and their family members faced the deaths of dozens of their friends and co-workers. Many firefighters reported that attending multiple funerals and commemorative events was extraordinarily difficult (Christ et al., 2011). It was also the experience of the Newtown, Connecticut community, when numerous funerals of young children and their teachers followed the horrific school shooting. As described earlier, this type of situation can result in a state of *bereavement overload*, in which the sheer number of deaths makes it difficult to mourn any one death. Opportunities for social support are often limited in such settings, since most of a person's usual support providers are either deceased, or stretched to the breaking point as they try to deal with their own losses.

Military Combat

Surprisingly few studies have focused on the impact of losing a loved one as a result of military action. Much of what we know about how such losses affect survivors comes from studies conducted in Israel (see, e.g., Rubin, Malkinson, & Witztum, 1999). For the most part, these studies have focused on Israeli parents who lost a son in a war. An interesting feature of this work is that it has examined the long-term impact of war deaths. For example, Rubin (1990) studied parents who had lost a son in a war on average 9 years earlier and compared these respondents to parents who had lost a 1-year-old son to illness (see also Malkinson & Bar-Tur, 1999; Rubin, 1992). Parents who had lost a son in a war manifested higher levels of grief, and they remained attached to their sons despite the passage of time. This body of research suggests that the emotional ramifications of war deaths can last for years. In these studies, parents rarely discussed their feelings with others and typically bore their grief alone. Of course, it is not clear whether these findings will generalize to those who have experienced the death of a loved one in other military conflicts, such as the wars in Iraq and Afghanistan. The generalizability of these findings may depend in part on the nature of each war and the extent of public support for it.

A recent study by Morina, von Lersner, and Prigerson (2011) focused on how young adults were affected by the deaths of their fathers as a result of fighting in the Kosovo War. These investigators interviewed a large number of bereaved young adults and nonbereaved young adults. Interviews were conducted a decade after the war. Bereaved participants scored higher than the nonbereaved on several indicators of mental distress, including depression, anxiety, and PTSD.

How do war deaths differ from other kinds of losses, and what are some of the unique stressors survivors face? Harrington-Lamorie and McDevitt-Murphy (2011) conducted an excellent review of the information available on these questions. As these authors explained, the U.S. Department of Defense categorizes war deaths as resulting from hostile action, accidents, homicide, illness, suicide, terrorist attack, or undetermined. Over the past 10 years, the leading causes of death in the Iraq and Afghanistan wars have been hostile actions and accidents.

It is clear that factors known to enhance the negative psychological impact on survivors characterize the majority of war-related deaths. Combat deaths as well as accidents are likely to involve violence and mutilation. In addition, such deaths are almost always untimely. The average age of soldiers killed in combat is 24 years. Consequently, deceased soldiers who were married are likely to leave behind young families. Surviving military spouses, typically in their 20s, are unlikely to have experience dealing with death (George, Elliott, Jennings, Cleland, & Brown, 2009). Moreover, it may be difficult for them to identify other young people who have experienced the death of their spouses. This contrasts markedly with the situation facing older people who lose their spouses. Even if a spouse dies unexpectedly and under traumatic circumstances, the surviving spouse has the opportunity to spend time with members of her cohort who share some similar concerns. This isolation may be offset to some degree by the military community, which can provide important support to spouses and families whose loved ones die in combat-related incidents. One important resource for such families is the Tragedy Assistance Program for Survivors (*www.taps.org*).

Several complicating factors are typically present for a spouse or family following a wartime death (Harrington-Lamorie & McDevitt-Murphy, 2011). In most cases, a lengthy period of separation precedes such a death. The separation itself may include stressful elements, such as the necessity of serving as a single parent and living under the constant threat that the loved one may be killed. These chronic stressors become the backdrop against which the death occurs and must be mourned.

After the death, those who lose a loved one in combat go through many of the same experiences as those who lose loved ones in disasters or terrorist attacks, such as dealing with the notification, waiting for information about whether the body has been recovered, and if so, learning the condition of their loved one's remains.

After the funeral, survivors of wartime deaths immediately face a multitude of hurdles (George et al., 2009). The bereaved spouse must navigate a complex bureaucratic system in an attempt to obtain government benefits, as well as the return of personal property. These matters may take considerable time to be resolved, which can make it difficult for mourning to proceed. Other issues that require attention in the immediate aftermath of the death include decisions about housing, relocation, and employment (Harrington-Lamorie & McDevitt-Murphy, 2011). A particularly challenging issue for a surviving spouse involves the formation of a new identity. As Harrington-Lamorie and McDevitt-Murphy (2011) have indicated,

> Spouses often feel the loss of an identity as a "military spouse," loss of a way of life as a "military family," loss of housing (if on a base or post), loss of friends through the unit or command, and a loss of feeling connected to the greater military community. . . . Many were afforded little opportunity to develop their own careers, hobbies and support networks outside of the military due to frequent moves and the demands of the military occupation on the family. (pp. 267–268)

The survivor's attitude toward the war or mission constitutes another set of issues that can complicate the mourning process. Did the surviving spouse, parent, or child agree with the deceased's decision to enter the military and to participate in this war? If not, the survivor may harbor resentment toward the deceased for putting himself in such a dangerous situation. If the war was unpopular, this may also reduce the likelihood that a survivor will receive social support outside military circles. Attitudes toward how the military treated her loved one can also play an important role. Some survivors may feel resentful that the military did not do everything it should have done to protect the decesaed. Others may feel that the sacrifice made by their loved ones was not appropriately acknowledged or appreciated.

Feelings of resentment that the military could and did not protect their loved one are likely to be paramount in cases of military suicide. In 2012, the number of suicides among active duty troops was 349. This number exceeded the 229 soldiers who were killed in combat that year in Afghanistan (Londono, 2013). In addition to feeling betrayed by the military for failing to keep their loved ones safe, survivors may also feel betrayed by the deceased. Whereas some soldiers kill themselves while in combat, others take their lives while they are making the transition to civilian life. One widow stated, "My husband chose death over coming home to me and the kids. That is hard for me to forgive."

It is virtually impossible for survivors of military deaths to escape ubiquitous reminders of a continuing war because of media coverage. In addition to serving as a trigger for their distress, the content of a news story may be deeply disturbing. For instance, a parent may be sickened to hear that additional troops, equipment, and supplies are being shipped to fortify resources in the area where her son was killed.

In Chapter 3, we have mentioned the notion of *moral injury* (Litz et al., 2009). This experience of having violated one's own moral code is relevant to military service members. They may be mourning the loss of fellow combatants for whose death they feel some responsibility or other moral involvement.

As noted above, there is frequently a delay in notification following the loss of a loved one in military conflict. Powell, Butollo, and Hagl (2010) conducted a study to determine the psychological impact of having a loved one who is missing but has not yet been declared dead. These investigators studied two groups of wives who had survived the war in Bosnia and Herzegovina: those whose husbands' deaths were confirmed, and those whose husbands were still listed as missing because of the war. The wives with unconfirmed losses had higher levels of traumatic grief and severe depression than those whose husbands were confirmed dead. The authors indicate that many health care providers may not be aware of the extreme vulnerability of mourners with unconfirmed losses.

Homicide

Homicide differs from other modes of traumatic death with regard to the depths of rage, horror, and vengefulness it typically unleashes in survivors. As Armour (2006) has stated, homicide "violates every norm about what a civilized society stands for" (p. 67). It is typical for survivors to be frightened and confused by the intensity of their rage and their preoccupation with vengeance. As noted above, there is some evidence that those bereaved by homicide exhibit higher levels of PTSD and grief symptoms than do survivors of suicide or accidents (see Kristensen et al., 2012, for a review). Parents are also more likely to show declines in marital satisfaction, and to have the most difficulty accepting their child's death (Murphy, 2008; Murphy, Johnson, Wu, et al., 2003). Rynearson and McCreery (1993) found that homicide survivors were more likely to experience frequent and intense replaying of the events surrounding a murder, even if they were not present when the murder occurred.

Armour (2006) has emphasized that, as is the case with motor vehicle crashes, homicide is far more prevalent in some groups than in others. For example, African American males are six times more likely to be victims of homicide than European American males. If the survivors are also African Americans, their mourning could well be complicated further by the effects of racism in our society. Minority groups may find mainstream resources such as support groups more difficult to access. In addition, resources such as books and websites may be less relevant to their experiences and needs.

The murder of a loved one also results in even more negative views of the world among survivors than losing loved ones in an accident (Wickie & Marwit, 2000–2001). Those whose loved ones are murdered also experience powerful feelings of betrayal and alienation (Riches & Dawson, 1998). Because of the intensity of their emotions, it is common for homicide survivors to feel helpless and out of control. As one daughter described the situation her family faced, "[We] are all in this deep hole . . . we are just getting deeper and deeper and there is nowhere to go but down" (Armour, 2006, pp. 69–70).

Another prevalent problem following homicide is that mourners live with pervasive anxiety and fear. Survivors often become hypervigilant, determined to avoid violence for themselves and their remaining loved ones. They typically feel extremely vulnerable to potential assaults, and restrict their contact with people and situations with which they are not intimately familiar.

Homicide survivors often experience an endless number of intrusions and frustrations at the hands of the criminal justice system. As we have discussed in an earlier chapter, survivors are often initially hopeful that the system will hold a perpetrator accountable for his actions. They believe that the judicial system exists to protect the rights of the murder victim and surviving loved ones. Because murder is a crime against the state, it is the state that prosecutes alleged murderers. This means that the survivors will have virtually no control over the court proceedings. In many cases, the court will withhold from them the very information they are seeking so that they can understand what happened. For example, the court may regard as evidence information about the crime as well as the extent of their loved one's injuries, and therefore withhold it from the survivors until after the trial (Armour, 2006).

In an eloquent discussion of these issues, Redmond (1989) described the profound difficulties that she had in dealing with the criminal justice system. As this mother expressed it, "There is one closed door after another . . . you can't show any emotion in the courtroom, can't get a trial date set, can't get a first degree murder charge" (p. 40). Court proceedings can result in a drain on survivors' personal and economic resources as they make such decisions as how much time they should take off from work or whether they should hire a private investigator. If the state obtains a conviction and the murderer is incarcerated, many survivors feel compelled to monitor the situation. They are concerned that the sentence will be whittled away by appeals, early release, or other forms of legal maneuvering. These processes can affect survivors' worldview, particularly their beliefs in justice and in fairness.

Many survivors do not have enough emotional energy to deal with both the criminal proceedings and the mourning processes simultaneously (Rando, 1993). For this reason, they often intentionally inhibit full mourning until the trial has ended. It often takes several years for legal proceedings to be resolved. This means that complicated mourning becomes a way of life for these survivors until they can turn their attention to their delayed mourning. Unfortunately, problematic adaptations may have developed in the interim. In addition, other family members and close friends may be ahead in their own mourning (because of not having to suppress it) and may have difficulty understanding the survivor's emotions and symptoms. They may thus respond in unsupportive ways that can unintentionally shame or isolate the survivor.

Armour (2006) has pointed out that in a significant minority of cases, a murder is not solved and the assailant is never apprehended. This places stress on survivors who, in some instances, may live in fear that the murderer will return to harm them or their family members. When the assailant is not captured, they may constantly wonder, as they encounter friend and stranger alike, whether this is the person responsible for their significant other's death.

In many cases, homicide survivors will also be required to deal with the media. In their efforts to procure a story, reporters are often persistent and at times intrusive. Survivors' privacy is often stripped away, as details of their lives and that of the deceased become public. The news stories may include graphic details that are profoundly disturbing to survivors. TV and news stories are likely to appear not only at the time of the murder, but also at various points during the legal proceedings. Images can appear unexpectedly for a long time afterward. In a single instant, a news article, feature, or media clip can bring back all the anguish associated with the murder.

Like suicide survivors, homicide survivors are likely to have difficulty maintaining social support. These problems stem largely from the violence and horror associated with murder. It may be particularly difficult for survivors of homicide to initiate, or even to attend, social events. They often feel that their presence will make others uncomfortable. They may also feel that because of the murder, their friends and neighbors regard them negatively, viewing them as singled out for one of the worst imaginable outcomes. As one wife expressed it, "I feel like I have a big M on my forehead for murder" (Armour, 2006, p. 71). Of course, the behavior of potential support providers can also bring about difficulties. Most people experience trepidation at the prospect of interacting with someone whose loved one was murdered. In addition, supporters may be motivated to protect themselves from the belief that such an event might happen to them. In order to maintain their own feelings of security, they are often inclined to view the death as preventable. In so doing, they may attribute blame to the deceased and/or the survivors. Although this process may provide some peace of mind for potential support providers, it occurs at the expense of survivors. In many cases, they experience stigmatization and alienation, which can reduce their feelings of connection and intimacy with others.

Rando (1993) has suggested that working with homicide survivors places more demands on therapists than does working with those who have lost loved ones through other modes of death. She indicates that this is true in part because of the intense affect associated with this type of loss, and in part because therapists find such deaths so threatening: "The horror of the act and the awareness on some level that the victim could just as easily have been the caregiver's own loved one fuel discomfort, as do the intensity and duration of the reactions with which these mourners present" (p. 552). According to Rando, homicide survivors often report that members of the mental health field have treated them insensitively, reflecting how fear or other strong feelings can overpower even the best intentions to provide good care.

Suicide

Many practitioners believe that deaths caused by suicide pose greater problems for survivors than deaths that come about in other ways (see, e.g., Worden, 2009). Earlier in this chapter, we examined two studies that found relatively few differences between survivors of suicide and those of other modes of traumatic death, thus calling these beliefs into question (Dyregrov et al., 2003; Murphy, Johnson, Wu, et al., 2003). More recently, Sveen and Walby (2008) examined 41 studies that compared suicide survivors with those who were bereaved in other ways. No significant differences emerged in symptoms of mental health, such as depression, anxiety, or anger. They did find significant differences on some variables believed to differentiate between survivors of suicide and of other kinds of loss: rejection, shame, stigma, concealing the cause of death, and blaming others. Their results were inconsistent for other variables commonly believed to be more prevalent following suicide, such as guilt, relief, impaired functioning, and social support.

In an excellent discussion of these issues, Jordan and McIntosh (2010) have pointed out that all of the studies included in Sveen and Walby's (2008) analysis utilized quantitative measures and comparison groups. They felt that the validity of the conclusions would be enhanced if qualitative studies, as well as their own clinical experience, were considered. Jordan and McIntosh maintain that there is clear evidence for differences between survivors of suicide and those of other kinds of loss in regard to rejection, shame, stigma, need to conceal the body, and tendency to blame others. They found some support for differences associated with such variables as anger, guilt, search for an explanation or desire to understand why, relief, shock/disbelief, social support issues, and family system effects. (See Jordan & McIntosh, 2011, for a more detailed discussion; see also Jordan, 2001.) Jordan and McIntosh assert that these variables reflect prominent themes in the subjective experience of survivors, and argue that an understanding of these factors is critical for treatment providers. Below, we consider these themes in more detail.

In many cases, suicide survivors regard suicide as intentional rejection; in a sense, the deceased person has chosen death over life with the mourner. A bereaved survivor may also feel betrayed by her loved one's decision to end his life. The mourner may feel that she meant nothing to the deceased. In addition, the survivor often feels that the suicide invalidates everything positive that had transpired in the relationship. In such a case, the survivor's inability to realistically remember her loved one or the relationship may compromise her mourning. Feelings of shame, humiliation, inadequacy, shattered self-worth, and rage related to these feelings often accompany beliefs that the survivor was not important to the deceased.

Given the feelings of humiliation and guilt that so often accompany suicide, it is not surprising that survivors may attempt to disguise the cause of death. For example, a family may present a loved one's cause of death as a drug overdose, a motor vehicle crash, or an undiagnosed illness. In a review of the literature on suicide, Jordan (2001) concluded that such behavior is surprisingly common, occurring in over 40% of cases. Rando (1993) has pointed out that the survivors often defend this behavior as protecting surviving family members, particularly children. However, such a secret is likely to interfere markedly with sharing feelings of grief, both within the family and with others in the social network (Armour, 2006; Rando, 1993); hence it will probably have a negative impact on the mourning process. In addition, it is likely to reinforce the experience of shame.

As noted above, survivors of suicide are more likely to blame others than those who lose loved ones in other ways. In some cases, they may blame therapists, physicians, or other health care providers for what has happened. Family members may direct blame toward close friends or the life partner of the deceased for not preventing the suicide. It is also common for family members to blame one another in the aftermath of suicide. For example, a woman whose son killed himself may blame her husband because of the harsh discipline he employed.

The tendency of survivors to blame others is closely tied to feelings of guilt. It is common for them to ask themselves, "Why didn't I know? What did I miss? If only . . ." Many survivors are consumed with guilt because they had no idea that their significant other was capable of this act. They struggle to understand how their loved one could have ended her life in this way. They may look back and see clues that make sense in retrospect, but that were impossible to recognize prior to the death. Sometimes a survivor may believe that he caused a suicide directly; for example, a father may believe that he precipitated his daughter's suicide by taking away her privileges. In other cases, a suicide may occur following an altercation between a survivor and her loved one. Those who believe that they somehow brought about the suicide carry a heavy load. In other cases, survivors blame themselves for not anticipating the suicide, or not doing more to prevent it. For example, a parent may regret not making a stronger effort to get his son into psychiatric treatment.

Rando (2014) has noted that, in many cases, survivors are tormented by questions they wish they could ask their loved ones. As Rando has explained, "the inability to do this and receive answers can result in unfinished business that they need to address. Many of the survivor's unanswered questions concern the choice to commit suicide. Such questions might include 'How could you do this to yourself? How could you do this to those who love you? Didn't you know, or didn't you care, about what this would do to us? How could you be so selfish? Why didn't you give us a chance to help? Didn't you know I loved you? How could you sentence me/ us to all this pain and all these problems, while you're now at peace?'"

Rando (2014) has pointed out that, in some cases, a suicide note may answer some of these questions. She indicated that such a note can be beneficial if it does one or more of the following:

- Absolves the survivor of responsibility.

- Makes it explicit that the person was determined to end his life, that it was considered rather than impulsive, and that there was nothing the survivor could have done to prevent it.

- Recognizes that the death will be difficult for the survivor, tells the survivor why he felt that suicide was the only choice, and asks the survivor to understand even if she doesn't agree.

- Conveys his love for the survivor and expresses regret that things ended this way.

- Acknowledges that the survivor was a good parent, spouse, partner, sibling, child, friend, or other loved one.

- Asks for the survivor's forgiveness.

- Helps the survivor understand what happened.

Although some suicides occur for no apparent reason or with no apparent precursors, most do not. In some cases, the deceased may have threatened suicide in the past, or perhaps even made previous attempts. Under these conditions, survivors' guilt may be intensified. In other cases, the suicide may represent the culmination of a long history of problems in many domains of the deceased's life. The deceased may have struggled with depression, anxiety, or addictions, and may have tried unsuccessfully to deal with these problems. In such a case, mourners' emotional reactions may be complex and multifaceted: gratitude that the loved one is no longer suffering, profound sadness that nothing helped, relief at being free of the burdens and demands of an emotionally disturbed and self-destructive person, and guilt for feeling relieved (Jordan, 2001). As Cleiren (1993) has pointed out, it is important to recognize the enormous differences in the ways survivors view a suicide death: "For some bereaved, the suicide came undeniably as a solution to an unbearable situation, and created new opportunities and freedom of movement. For others, it meant personal failure or made no sense at all" (p. 250). (See Sands, Jordan, & Neimeyer, 2011, for more information about individual differences in reactions to the suicide of a loved one.)

There is some evidence that family problems are more common among those whose loved ones have completed suicide (see, e.g., Armour, 2006; Jordan, 2001; Jordan & McIntosh, 2011). It is important to recognize that in the case of a suicide, family dynamics are often highly problematic before the death occurs. Prior to the suicide, family members are often (although not always) locked into destructive patterns of behavior and communication. Problematic family dynamics may have contributed to the distress of the person who subsequently kills himself, or may even precipitate the suicide. Similarly, continual displays of disruptive and self-defeating behavior by that person may have had a negative impact on the mental health and functioning of other family members. Even in those cases where the family is functioning well prior to the suicide, the death is likely to have a detrimental effect on family interactions. There is typically an increase in hostility, recrimination, blame, and guilt induction (Jordan, 2001).

As we discuss in Chapter 10, it is common for survivors of traumatic death to have difficulty maintaining effective support. There is some evidence to suggest that survivors of suicide have more pronounced difficulties. These support problems stem in large part from the negative attitudes others hold toward them. In a review of this literature, Jordan (1991) reported that others typically view those who have lost loved ones to suicide as less likeable, more psychologically disturbed, more in need of professional help, more blameworthy, and more ashamed than those whose loved ones died in other ways.

CLINICAL INTEGRATION

Dr. Jack Brown had been meeting with Suzanne for about 10 weeks now. He was using the integrated treatment approach for traumatic bereavement with her. Although he was familiar with the approach after having used it with other clients, he decided to seek out ongoing peer consultation from a colleague for this particular therapy. He was anxious to speak with his colleague, Caitlin, today as he noticed a growing sense of dread in anticipation of his next session with Suzanne.

"So," said Caitlin when they sat down in her office for their semimonthly consultation, "what do you know about this dread you've been feeling?"

"Well, I often feel a heaviness before I meet with Suzanne—like an inner awareness that the session is going to be really hard work, as well as some anticipation or worry that all our work will be futile. Suzanne is still so overwhelmed with both grief and traumatic stress symptoms; I worry that anything I do is not only too little, but will actually make things worse."

"And if I remember correctly, you're now focusing on some exposure work. Is that right?"

Jack nodded.

"I wonder if the anticipation of things getting worse might be a reflection of being in touch with Suzanne's pain—the very pain she's been avoiding."

Jack took a breath. "Yeah. I know we need to go there, and I'm wondering if I'm up to it."

"You doubt your ability to be helpful. Feeling overwhelmed?"

"Really overwhelmed," Jack agreed.

"Maybe you're feeling a lot of what Suzanne herself is feeling?"

Jack agreed again.

"Let's say we assume for now that your thoughts and feelings are a window into Suzanne's experience. If so, what does your experience tell you about where your client is in all of this?" Caitlin's tone was compassionate yet confident, and seemed to indicate her faith in Jack.

"There's just so much—so many feelings, thoughts, symptoms. I guess I understand the avoidance. If she avoids, then she won't have to face all of the pain. If I avoid with her, then I won't have to discover it's too big to handle . . ." Jack paused for a long moment. " . . . or discover that I've made her go through that pain for nothing."

"You'll make her go through the pain." Caitlin repeated his words deliberately. "It sounds as if you're feeling responsible for her pain."

"Yeah, I guess I am. And I can see how this could be a reflection of Suzanne's feeling responsible for her daughter's pain and death. This is one of the realizations she's been avoiding, I think. Even though her guilt lives with her, under the surface, she hasn't spoken this out loud—not fully, anyway."

"And what do you know about that?" urged Caitlin.

"Well, I know that before her daughter's death, Suzanne prided herself on being a great mother. She is a religious person—Catholic—and felt as though she was put on this earth to be a mother, to raise kind, compassionate, strong children, and to take care of other children as well. She reports that she and Sarah had a warm, close relationship. So I think that, in addition to other needs, her sense of identity has been violently assaulted by what happened. 'How can someone who was put on this earth to mother fail to protect her own daughter?' And then she experiences tremendous guilt for failing her daughter, which is how she sees it."

"So Suzanne is dealing with the question 'If I'm responsible for my daughter's death, then who am I, and how do I live with myself?'" Caitlin was again reflecting on Jack's own words.

"Yeah."

"And you mentioned 'among other needs.' What are the others?"

"Well, self-trust. Her daughter's suicide was a shock to her; she didn't see it coming, and now she doesn't trust her judgment or intuition at all. And, of course, her esteem. She believes she's a bad person, and that she is no longer worthy of being supported by the God she believes in, which is a significant secondary loss for Suzanne in all of this."

After a pause, Caitlin said, "It sounds as though you're in touch with much of what Suzanne is experiencing. I want to encourage you to use that as a window into Suzanne's experience as we did here today. And I want to remind you that you've done a thorough assessment and have expressed your belief that your client has the resources to get through this. I believe you have the clinical skill to help her through." Caitlin smiled at Jack. With that, he felt himself begin to relax as the sense of being overwhelmed slightly diminished.

CONCLUDING REMARKS

In this chapter, we have described the phenomenology of traumatic bereavement as it relates to factors surrounding the death. Recognizing many of the risk factors involved with traumatic bereavement, and understanding how these factors may affect the processes of mourning and trauma adaptation, will assist us in our work of helping survivors. First, this breadth of knowledge fosters empathic attunement with our clients. Second, it allows us to assess the unique challenges and stressors that an individual client may be confronting. Third, it helps us listen for specific themes that mark a client's subjective experience of her traumatic loss.

The example of Suzanne's horrific experience incorporates several of the risk factors named in this chapter. Suzanne experienced a suicide; she experienced the untimely death of her child; and she discovered her daughter's body. Suzanne perceived the death as preventable and blamed herself for not having seen the warning signs. Unfortunately, it is not uncommon for bereaved survivors to experience multiple risk factors related to the death, as was the case for Suzanne.

CHAPTER 6

Person-Related Factors

Karen lost her teenage son, William, when a drunk driver who ran a red light struck his car broadside. In a similar situation, a drunk driver killed Juan, Sonia's teenage son, as he was riding his bicycle home from school. Now, 3 years later, both women still experience intrusive thoughts about how the accidents unfolded and whether their sons suffered. Both struggle with guilt that they were unable to protect their sons. Both continue to mourn for their sons on a daily basis. In other ways, however, their reactions are very different.

Karen feels unable to go to the cemetery. When she tried to do so on William's birthday, she experienced waves of nausea and had to return home. The fact that the perpetrator still has not been brought to justice fills Karen with rage. She has devoted a substantial amount of time to following the criminal case against the driver and becomes distraught when there is a setback, such as a continuance. Karen also has difficulty leaving the house. She dislikes it when others ask how she is doing. She has never driven by the scene of the accident, even though it is less than a mile from her home; in fact, she goes out of her way to avoid it. She also becomes distressed when she learns about someone else dying because of a drunk driving crash. Consequently, she minimizes her exposure to local newscasts and newspapers.

Sonia visits the cemetery on a regular basis, as doing so helps her to feel close to her son. Unlike Karen, Sonia's feelings of sadness, rather than those of anger, are predominant. Although she is highly self-conscious when doing so, she is usually able to engage with others in social situations. Sonia frequently finds herself ruminating about Juan's death. When she hears a news story about a drunk driving crash, she feels a deep sadness, knowing that others are struggling with the same painful issues that she is. She also feels compelled to do whatever she can to decrease the likelihood of alcohol-related motor vehicle crashes. Recently she has become involved with a group attempting to get Breathalyzers installed in the cars of repeat drunk driving offenders. However, she reports having little energy to put into it.

How can we account for the striking individual differences in response to traumatic death? Even when survivors have experienced losses that appear to be similar, as was the case with Karen and Sonia, their reactions and responses may be very different. As we have explained in Chapter 2, CSDT describes psychological trauma as arising from an interaction between aspects of the event and aspects of the person. In this chapter, we elaborate on some aspects of the person that can contribute to traumatic bereavement. We focus on those factors that seem most significant, according to both extant research and our clinical experience. In some cases, the research we present focused on survivors of traumatic death. In others, the investigators studied a heterogeneous group of respondents whose loved ones died in different ways. We have included studies in the latter group that we believe will generalize to survivors of traumatic death. The focus is on recognizing the variables that can help us to understand the different responses of survivors to similar events.

GENDER

Men appear to have greater difficulty than do women in coping with the death of a spouse. A large number of studies have found that widowed men are more likely to become depressed and to experience greater mortality than are widowed women (see Miller & Wortman, 2002, and Stroebe, Stroebe, & Schut, 2001, for reviews). One possible explanation for these gender differences is that men may benefit more from marriage than do women, and thus the death of their spouses may affect them more adversely. Consistent with this view, several studies have shown that men rely primarily on their wives for social support, whereas women typically have many close friends besides their husbands (see Wortman & Boerner, 2011, for a review). Cleiren (1993) has reported that widowers are at relatively high risk for poor outcomes following the death of a spouse because their social activities decrease over time. His study also showed that widowers had great difficulty in maintaining and building social relationships following their wives' deaths. It will be interesting to see whether these differences become less pronounced as more marital relationships are characterized by gender equality.

Umberson (1987, 1992) has identified another mechanism that may account for gender differences in the reaction to the loss of a spouse. She found that women typically take more responsibility for their partners' health care, diet, nutrition, and exercise than men do. For example, married women are typically the ones who schedule medical appointments and monitor whether their spouse is taking prescribed medications. When men lose their wives, they experience these types of secondary losses at a time when they may need more support with basic health care regimens. Taken together, this research demonstrates the importance of talking with widowers about their support networks, and about how they handle matters pertaining to their physical health.

Studies of child loss have consistently found that, although fathers evidence considerable distress following the death of a child, mothers report significantly more distress than do fathers. This appears to be the case following perinatal deaths, deaths in infancy or childhood, and the deaths of older children. As described in Chapter 5, Dyregrov and colleagues (2003) conducted a study of the predictors of grief among parents who had lost children through suicide, accidents, or SIDS. Across all three samples, mothers evidenced higher levels of posttraumatic reactions and complicated mourning than fathers. Mothers also reported more intrusive thoughts, bodily symptoms, depression, anxiety, and grief than did fathers (Dyregrov & Matthiesen, 1987). Gender differences between parents also emerged in the previously discussed studies conducted by Murphy and her associates (Murphy et al., 1999; Murphy, Johnson, Wu, et al., 2003), which focused on parents who had lost a child as a result of accidents, suicide, or homicide. Regardless of gender, parents were devastated by the loss. Two years after their child's death, mothers' mental distress scores were up to five times higher than those of "typical" women in the

United States. Fathers' scores were up to four times higher than "typical" men in the United States. However, mothers scored higher than fathers on many other indices of mental distress, including depression, anxiety, somatic complaints, and cognitive functioning. Five years after the deaths, three times as many mothers (27.7%) met criteria for PTSD and twice as many fathers (12.5%) met criteria for PTSD compared with a normative sample (Murphy, Johnson, Chung, & Beaton, 2003). Women continued to show greater overall distress than men did as the study continued, and gender was one of the best predictors of changes in distress over time. The mental distress of fathers showed a greater decline over time than that of mothers (Murphy et al., 1999). Cleiren (1993) obtained similar results in his study of how people reacted to the death of a spouse, child, parent, or sibling as a result of motor vehicle crashes, suicide, or illness. He found that mothers were at far more risk for developing severe problems than were fathers, and that mothers scored higher on depression and health problems.

Available research has also found gender differences in the coping strategies that are most helpful in dealing with loss. In a treatment study conducted by Schut, Stroebe, van den Bout, and de Keijser (1997), for example, widows showed a greater decline in distress than widowers did after counseling that focused on day-to-day problems. In contrast, widowers showed a greater decline after counseling that facilitated emotional expression. According to Archer (1999), such findings reflect a sociocultural pattern of gender differences involving the inhibition of emotional expression by boys and men. Similar findings emerged from studies focusing on the death of a child. Mothers typically cope with such losses by seeking support or by communicating with other family members. Fathers attempt to conceal their feelings, which they claim is to support their wives. However, wives often complain that their husbands are not willing to share their feelings. Archer has stated that these findings "can be seen as part of a widespread pattern of male inexpressiveness" (1999, p. 245).

Murphy and colleagues (1999) reported an interesting shift in the symptom patterns for fathers and mothers starting in the second year of their study. At that point, mothers' symptoms declined. Fathers, who started out with lower distress than their wives did, reported slight increases in 5 of the 10 symptoms that were assessed. This suggests that men may "hold in" their grief initially in an effort to be strong for their families (Martin & Doka, 2000). Cleiren (1993) also reported that for a number of the fathers in his research, bereavement symptoms increased over time. Cleiren has similarly suggested that this pattern occurs because fathers initially take the role of principal comforters and supporters of their wives. He maintains that in many cases, this constitutes an additional burden for fathers.

A program of research by Doka and Martin (2010; Martin & Doka, 2011) has considerable relevance for understanding gender differences in reaction to loss. These investigators have found that there are two primary patterns of grieving. *Intuitive* grieving involves intense expression of emotions, often at the cost of role functioning. Intuitive grievers often experience their grief as "waves of affect." Because it is important to them to express their grief, they make an effort to find outlets to do so. *Instrumental* grievers direct energy away from the expression of feelings. In most cases, their affect is more muted than that of intuitive grievers. They tend to express their emotions in concrete ways, such as setting up a scholarship fund to honor the memory of a deceased child.

According to Martin and Doka, intuitive and instrumental patterns of grief should be regarded as the two ends of a continuum. They emphasize that there are no pure intuitive or instrumental patterns of grief. In fact, many people have a blended style of grieving, sometimes expressing their feelings and sometimes channeling them into constructive activities.

These investigators have noted that the intuitive style is widely viewed as "feminine," while the instrumental pattern is regarded as a masculine grieving style. In our culture, it is common to pathologize the masculine style and to portray men as ineffectual mourners. As Martin and Doka (2011) have emphasized, such a characterization is inappropriate. They note that while containing one's emotions is more prevalent among men, it also occurs among women (see Doka & Martin, 2010, for a more detailed discussion). Interestingly, they note that women who are instrumental grievers are more likely than men with the same style to be criticized for not expressing their feelings following a loved one's death. Because women are expected to express their feelings, they may be judged harshly when they do not.

RELIGION AND SPIRITUAL BELIEFS

Over the past decade, there has been increasing interest in studying the role that religion may play in coping with the death of a loved one. As Park and Halifax (2011) have emphasized, "religion and spirituality continue to thrive throughout the world and there is little evidence of its abatement" (p. 356). According to public opinion polls, nearly 90% of people in the United States describe themselves as religious or spiritual. Over 90% say that they believe in God; approximately 70% state that they are members of a church or synagogue; and 90% report that they pray regularly (see Becker et al., 2007; Kelley & Chan, 2012).

Evidence suggests that religious beliefs and practices are widely used by bereaved individuals, and that the majority of the bereaved regard them as helpful. For example, in their study of coping with the violent death of a child, Murphy, Johnson, and Lohan (2003b) found that 70% of the sample identified prayer as an important coping resource. The assumption that religious beliefs are beneficial is also widely held among treatment providers (Wortmann & Park, 2008).

Most studies report a positive relationship between religious beliefs or practices and some indicators of adjustment to the loss (for reviews, see Becker et al., 2007; Hays & Hendrix, 2008; Wortmann & Park, 2008). However, there is a consensus that the results of these studies should be interpreted with caution. This research has been plagued by methodological problems, such as reliance on weak experimental designs and lack of consensus regarding how religion should be conceptualized and measured. Wortmann and Park (2008) have indicated that the measures of religion used in most studies are too broad and "do not adequately capture the complex nature of religion in people's lives" (p. 705). When the specific facets of religious beliefs are examined, we find several intriguing lines of research that have clear relevance for clinical practice.

As Park and Halifax (2011) have emphasized, religious and spiritual traditions "offer a panoply of coping resources for dealing with death" (p. 359). One such resource is prayer. Available evidence suggests that an increase in one's frequency of prayer is helpful in coping with the death of a loved one (Wortmann & Park, 2008). A second is religious social support, which includes support from clergy and members of a congregation. Religious social support can impart a sense of belonging to a broader community of individuals with similar religious views. In addition, religious social support can help the bereaved find solace and comfort, which can assist them in coming to terms with their loss (Wortmann & Park, 2009). A number of studies have shown that religious social support during bereavement has a positive impact on psychological well-being (see Hays & Hendrix, 2008, for a review). For example, Thompson and Vardaman (1997) found that religious social support was beneficial to families who had lost loved ones to homicide.

A third way in which religious beliefs might influence adjustment to the death of a loved one is by affecting how survivors cope with the loss. In a study focusing on respondents whose partners had died of AIDS, those with religious beliefs were more likely to use positive appraisal and effective problem-solving techniques (Richards, Acree, & Folkman, 1999; Richards & Folkman, 1997). There is also evidence to suggest that religious beliefs can facilitate finding meaning in a loss (Park & Halifax, 2011; Wortmann & Park, 2009). Drawing from many studies in this area, Wortmann and Park (2009) concluded that meaning making is the major pathway through which religious beliefs influence the mourning process. In one study of parents who lost an infant to SIDS, the more important religious beliefs were in the parents' lives, the more they were able to find meaning in their children's deaths (McIntosh, Silver, & Wortman, 1993). Murphy, Johnson, and Lohan (2003b) found that the use of religious coping strategies such as seeking God's help was associated with finding meaning in the loss of a child from suicide, homicide, or an accident 5 years after the death occurred. Finding meaning, in turn, was associated with less mental distress and higher marital satisfaction. As described in Chapters 3 and 10, however, many survivors of traumatic loss are unable to sustain their faith or find meaning in the loss.

Coping strategies such as maintaining a rewarding connection through prayer, utilizing proffered support of the faith community, and drawing on religious beliefs to find meaning in the loss are referred to as *positive religious coping* (Cowchock, Lasker, Toedter, Skumanich, & Koenig, 2010). Several investigators have maintained that it is equally important to assess *negative religious coping*, which is sometimes called *religious struggle*. Feelings of anger toward God, feelings of abandonment or betrayal, or feelings that one is being punished for sins are all believed to reflect negative coping or religious struggle. Some researchers have found that those who expect to be comforted by their religious beliefs, but ultimately are not, are at heightened risk for negative coping or religious struggle.

Labeling beliefs such as anger toward God as *negative coping* is not helpful to mourners. It is clear that those who have experienced sudden, traumatic losses are more likely to struggle with their religious beliefs than those whose loved ones died of natural causes (Chapple, Swift, & Ziebland, 2011). As we have discussed in Chapter 3, it is extremely common for survivors of such losses to experience a crisis of faith, and to believe that now that their loved one has died, life holds no meaning. Religious struggle has been identified as a powerful predictor of poor outcome following the death of a loved one (Cowchock et al., 2010). Thus individuals engaged in religious struggle are likely to benefit from therapeutic support in dealing with these issues. This work can be facilitated by doing an assessment of each client's spiritual beliefs. For example, clients might be asked to articulate their views on the afterlife, or to discuss why they think bad things happen to good people.

According to Tedeschi and Calhoun (2006, 2008), there are some cases in which people emerge from their religious struggle with spiritual lives that are more meaningful and satisfying than before the loss. Tedeschi and Calhoun use the term *posttraumatic growth* to refer to positive changes that may occur through a struggle with life events like the death of a loved one. The posttraumatic growth construct may offer clinicians some useful hypotheses to explore, despite problems with its measurement (Wortman, 2004).

Tedeschi and Calhoun (2006, 2008) have emphasized that the loss event itself is not what promotes growth. Rather, the survivor's struggle with the painful ramifications of the loss is the catalyst for growth. They use the metaphor of an earthquake to describe this process, noting that a traumatic event, like an earthquake, can severely shake, threaten, or reduce to rubble many of the schematic structures that have guided a person's life. They state that life events are most likely to promote growth if they challenge an individual's assumptions about the world.

Tedeschi and Calhoun (2006, 2008) maintain that five different types of experiences indicate personal growth (see Tedeschi & Calhoun, 2008, for a more detailed discussion). The first is the emergence of new possibilities. For example, some women who lost their husbands stated that they were able to learn new skills, such as how to handle finances; they felt proud that they were able to do so. Second, a death sometimes brought about a positive change in relationships. For example, many parents who had lost children reported greater compassion and connection to other human beings, especially those who had experienced a similar loss. Survivors of traumatic loss may also report that they no longer take their loved ones for granted. As one bereaved parent expressed it, "I always tell the people I love that I love them." Third, many survivors reported an increased sense of personal strength. As one bereaved person explained, "I've been through the absolute worst that I know. And no matter what happens, I'll be able to deal with it" (quoted in Tedeschi & Calhoun, 2008, pp. 33–34). A fourth type of change is a greater appreciation for life. This is often accomplished by a shift in priorities, as when a parent decides to come home from work earlier so that she can be more involved in her children's activities. Finally, Tedeschi and Calhoun have emphasized that people often report changes in their religious and spiritual orientation. For example, an encounter with the death of a loved one may lead a person to a more meaningful or satisfying religious or spiritual life. As one survivor expressed it, "the understanding that God is going to get you through anything that happens to you . . . gives you a different outlook on life . . . that takes away a lot of fear and trepidation that most of us walk through life with" (Tedeschi & Calhoun, 2008, pp. 33–34).

Currier, Mallot, Martinez, Sandy, and Neimeyer (2012) have maintained that the violent deaths of loved ones will challenge survivors' assumptive worlds more than deaths that come about through natural causes. They have suggested that as a result, violent deaths are more likely to precipitate positive life changes. These investigators found that survivors who lost loved ones to violent deaths reported more psychological distress, but also scored higher on indices of posttraumatic growth, than either those who experienced nonviolent deaths or those who did not experience the death of a loved one.

It appears that the concept of posttraumatic growth has been embraced by researchers and clinicians working in the field of bereavement, as well as in other fields involving human adversity. An important question is whether the available data can and should be taken as valid. One criticism that has been raised about this work concerns the validity of respondents' statements about the growth they have shown. If a study participant states that the death of his child has made him stronger, should this be taken at face value? A respondent may wish to convince others, and perhaps himself as well, that something positive has come out of all of the anguish his family has experienced. In fact, research suggests that people in a survivor's life—family, friends, and professionals—may "pull" for expressions of positive change, in part by reacting negatively to expressions of distress (see, e.g., Silver, Wortman, & Crofton, 1990).

Results from a study focusing on the long-term impact of losing a spouse or child in a motor vehicle crash (Lehman et al., 1987), described in Chapter 1, casts some doubt about whether respondents' self-reports about personal growth are valid. In this study, people were asked whether anything positive had come out of their spouse's or child's death; 74% of respondents reported at least one positive change, with the majority reporting only one. The most common ones were increased self-confidence and focusing more on enjoying the present. In their review of the literature regarding posttraumatic growth, Tedeschi and Calhoun (2006, 2008) cited this study as indicative that people indeed experience posttraumatic growth following the traumatic death of a loved one.

When we look at the study data as a whole, however, two issues emerge. First, at least in this study, the one or two positive comments made by the respondents were dwarfed by the negative changes that they reported. If a person says that she is focusing more on enjoying the present—but sees the world as a more dangerous place, is struggling with symptoms of depression and PTSD, is going through a divorce, cannot concentrate at work, and is experiencing impaired quality of life—is that growth?

Second, the results reflect clear inconsistencies between respondents' statements about personal growth and other measures included in the study. Tedeschi and Calhoun (2006, 2008) have emphasized that warmer, more intimate relationships with others is one of the most important elements in posttraumatic growth. Only 20% of Lehman and colleagues' (1987) respondents indicated that they emphasized family more as a result of the accident. In comparison to controls, those who lost a spouse reported feeling more tense, upset, unhappy, and emotionally worn out when reflecting on their current experiences as a parent. These same findings emerged when respondents who lost a child were asked to reflect on their experiences as a parent to surviving children. Moreover, those who lost a child tended to feel more bothered, tense, and neglected than controls when thinking about their daily life with their spouse. As noted earlier, they were also more likely to seek and obtain a divorce.

In the Lehman and colleagues (1987) study, the traumatic death of a spouse or child also had an adverse impact on relationships with friends and relatives. Those who lost a spouse reported spending less time with their friends, having more arguments with them, and feeling more hurt and offended by them than controls. Those who lost a child indicated that they were less likely to talk with their relatives about their feelings or problems. They reported that in many cases, they felt angry or disappointed in their relatives and expressed agreement with the statement that they were "more likely to want to do the opposite of what their relatives wanted in order to make them angry." In this study, therefore, warmth and intimacy did not increase and, in fact, the impact on respondents' relationships with family and friends was decidedly negative (see Wortman, 2004, for a more detailed discussion).

In many cases, people try to comfort the bereaved by mentioning positive things that have come about as a result of the death. As Mehren (1997) has indicated, bereaved parents are hurt and offended by such remarks, as they imply that whatever good things emerge from the situation, such as increased compassion, are worth losing the child. As Mehren has indicated,

> It annoys many of us when people tell us we'll be better people because of all the sorrows we're going through. While we must grasp for any small blessings we can salvage, we'd rather be our rotten old selves and have our babies back. Besides, it's not like we were ax murderers to begin with! (p. 93)

As a result of challenges to their ideas, Tedeschi and Calhoun (2008) have stated that it is not a foregone conclusion that those who struggle with the ramifications of their loss will ultimately experience personal growth. Taken together, the research cited above emphasizes the importance of remaining open to alternative possibilities when our clients talk about personal growth. Our society clearly champions people who are strong in the face of adversity. As health care providers, will we be disappointed if a particular client does not manifest growth? Will survivors of traumatic loss experience feelings of inadequacy and shame if they are not able to find something good in what has happened?

It is critically important that clinicians not bring an expectation of growth to their clients, thus creating an environment in which they can fail. This body of work suggests that clinicians should create a space where clients can fully express and discuss issues surrounding these and other religious and spiritual beliefs. In Chapter 10, we offer specific suggestions regarding how to assist clients in this endeavor.

PERSONALITY AND COPING STRATEGIES

Personality refers to dispositional tendencies toward such states as optimism, self-esteem, anxiety, and emotionality. There is clear evidence that these and other aspects of personality predict adjustment to the death of a significant other (see Robinson & Marwit, 2006, for a review). For example, Riley, LaMontagne, Hepworth, and Murphy (2007) found that mothers who were more optimistic by nature reported less intense grief reactions. Similarly, in a study of mourners whose loved ones died of cancer or AIDS, Nolen-Hoeksema (2001) found that those who scored high on *dispositional optimism* (i.e., a tendency to be optimistic in most circumstances) showed a greater decline in grief symptoms following the loss of their significant other and were more likely to find meaning in the loss. It is clear that personality traits can exert their influence by affecting the coping strategies a survivor employs. For example, those who are generally optimistic may be more able to elicit support from their family and friends.

Evidence also suggests that self-esteem is associated with adjustment following loss. For example, Murphy and colleagues (1999) and Murphy, Chung, and Johnson (2002) found that for both mothers and fathers, self-esteem measures taken 4 months after their child's violent death were strong predictors of reduced mental distress throughout the five years of the study. Perhaps those with higher self-esteem were better able to restore their trust in themselves and others and to maintain their connection with others, allowing them greater access to social support. Similarly, Boelen, van den Hout, and van den Bout (2006) reported that negative beliefs about the self were strongly related to levels of complicated grief. Murphy and colleagues (1999) have suggested that clinicians should attempt to assist bereaved clients in gaining and/or maintaining feelings of self-esteem. Some therapists may not recognize the importance of this for traumatically bereaved clients. Another personality variable that contributes to a poor outcome following the loss of a loved one is *neuroticism* (Wijngaards-de Meij et al., 2005). People who score high on neuroticism are more likely to develop negative cognitions, which increase the likelihood that they will get stuck in the mourning process.

Sudden, traumatic death usually has an adverse effect on *affect management* (a self capacity that involves staying grounded in the face of strong feelings, described further in Chapter 10). Prigerson, Shear, Frank, and Beery (1997) found that difficulties in regulating one's emotions enhanced vulnerability to complicated grief. An individual who has never developed this self capacity (usually because of childhood family dysfunction or attachment challenges) may struggle more following a traumatic death than one who has.

Traumatic bereavement can also impair ego resources described within CSDT, such as initiative, judgment, ability to manage boundaries, ability to foresee consequences, and decision making. Again, the individuals at greatest risk for longer-term problems in these realms are those who may not have had the opportunity to develop these resources in childhood.

KINSHIP RELATIONSHIP TO THE DECEASED

Several studies have shown that the death of a child leads to more intense and prolonged grief and depression than the death of a spouse, sibling, or parent does (Cleiren, 1991, 1993; Cleiren, Diekstra, Kerkhof, & van der Wal, 1994; Leahy, 1992; Nolen-Hoeksema & Larson, 1999). In an important study, Cleiren (1993) examined mourners who had lost either a child, spouse, sibling, or parent. These losses resulted from suicide, traffic accidents, or long-term illness. He found that the kinship relationship to the deceased was by far the most important factor studied, determining mourners' adaptation to a substantial degree. His results showed that the group at greatest risk for a poor outcome was mothers, followed by husbands, fathers, and sisters of the deceased. As Cleiren (1993) expressed it, "Regardless of the age of their child or their own age, the loss [of a child] seems to create a permanent vacuum in their [mothers'] lives" (p. 253).

Li, Laursen, Precht, Olsen, and Mortensen (2005) studied a large cohort of people in Denmark. They conducted follow-up interviews with respondents who had lost a child, and a control group who had not suffered such a loss. Bereaved parents had a significantly higher risk of admission to a psychiatric hospital. This was particularly the case for mothers, who continued to show an elevated risk of psychiatric hospitalization for 5 years or more after the death. Li, Precht, Mortensen, and Olsen (2003) have also found an increased risk of mortality among parents after the loss of a child from unnatural causes.

A study by Rogers, Floyd, Seltzer, Greenberg, and Hong (2008) provides corroborating evidence regarding the long-term impact of child loss. They obtained information from a large number of parents who had lost a child and from a control group of individuals with similar backgrounds. Approximately 18 years following the child's death, bereaved parents reported more depressive symptoms, poorer well-being, more marital conflict, and more health problems than members of the control group did. Cause of death did not significantly influence these results, suggesting that the death of a child is devastating under almost any circumstances. In this study, both mothers and fathers showed high levels of enduring distress.

To our knowledge, Cleiren (1993) is one of the few investigators to study the impact of losing a brother or sister. He found that women who lost a sibling were at risk for a poor outcome. He reported that in contrast, men showed a much more favorable adaptation to the death of a brother or sister. According to Cleiren, these gender differences may have occurred because women are more likely to feel a greater sense of connection to and responsibility for their siblings than are men.

Marshall and Davies (2011) maintain that in many cases, the loss of an adult sibling is a *disenfranchised* loss; this means that others do not recognize the loss, its severity, or its meaning to the bereaved person. They cite data indicating that the average adult "has contact with a sibling once or twice a month for 60 or 70 years after leaving home" (p. 111). Nonetheless, most people who lose a sibling find that friends, co-workers, and even family members fail to acknowledge the loss or offer support. Moreover, in addition to dealing with their own grief, many adults who lose a sibling must support their parents, who are dealing with the loss of a child (see Marshall & Davies, 2011, for a more detailed discussion).

In recent years, there has been increasing interest in understanding how the traumatic death of a child affects surviving siblings. Buckle and Fleming (2011) maintained that surviving siblings face "wide-ranging and enduring consequences following the death of a brother or sister" (p. 93). Like their parents, they may experience the demise of the feelings of security that their family provided. Siblings often feel that their parents are focusing more attention on the deceased child than on them. Moreover, parents' comments about their child who died (e.g., "She was always such a good girl" or "He was so gifted") may engender feelings of anger and resentment (Handsley, 2001). Such families often find themselves in a vicious cycle: Parents' grief renders them less effective in dealing with surviving children, and the absence of attentive and consistent parenting contributes to the symptoms displayed by surviving siblings. This in turn adds to the parents' distress, making it even more difficult for them to relate effectively to their surviving children.

Another death that is often disenfranchised is the loss of a child during pregnancy. It is common for parents, particularly mothers, to experience feelings of guilt and emptiness as well as grief (Adolfsson, Larsson, Wijma, & Berterö, 2004; Jaffe & Diamond, 2011). Outsiders often fail to understand what was lost or to appreciate the impact of the loss. Consequently, couples often feel alone in their grief. This is also true for couples experiencing stillbirth or neonatal death. Bereaved parents often receive comments from others that minimize their loss—for example, "It was only a baby you didn't know."

In fact, Buchi and colleagues (2007) found that 2–6 years after the death of a premature baby (24–26 weeks' gestation), parents, especially mothers, were experiencing grief symptoms and significant emotional distress. According to these authors, clinicians should be aware that the death of a preterm infant can trigger a painful long-term process of mourning.

NATURE OF THE RELATIONSHIP WITH THE DECEASED

Historically, clinical writings on loss have maintained that prolonged or chronic grief results from conflict with or feelings of ambivalence toward the deceased (see, e.g., Bowlby, 1980; Parkes & Weiss, 1983). This hypothesis derives from psychoanalytic theories of grief (e.g., Abraham, 1924/1927). Supposedly, survivors who have ambivalent or conflictual relationships with their deceased loved ones have to cope with powerful angry or contradictory feelings toward them. In theory, this makes it more difficult for the survivors to process and accommodate the loss. Although this view may be widely accepted among practicing clinicians, well-controlled studies fail to support it. Wheaton (1990), a sociologist, advanced a hypothesis about the relationship between marital quality and reaction to spousal loss that is in direct opposition to the psychodynamic approach. He argued that those who are involved in conflictual marriages should show an improvement in their mental health following the death, in comparison to those who are not involved in such marriages, because they are exiting a stressful role. He conducted a study that provided strong support for this view.

Carr and colleagues (Carr, 2008; Carr et al., 2000) assessed respondents prior to losing their spouses and again 6 and 18 months later. They found that adjustment to widowhood was most difficult for those whose relationships had the highest levels of warmth and closeness. Those who were involved in conflictual relationships prior to their spouse's death showed low levels of yearning for their spouse throughout the study. Van Doorn, Kasl, Beery, Jacobs, and Prigerson (1998) and Prigerson, Maciejewski, and Rosenheck (2000) also found that people in close, supportive marriages were at elevated risk for complicated grief following the death of their spouse. Although these studies did not focus exclusively on respondents who experienced sudden, traumatic loss, the findings suggest that therapists should recognize that bereaved individuals who had warm and loving relationships might be at greater risk for traumatic bereavement.

Clinicians have also maintained that excessive dependency on one's spouse is a risk factor for intense and prolonged grief (see, e.g., Lopata, 1979; Parkes & Weiss, 1983; Rando, 1993). *Excessive dependency* is characterized by overreliance on another person in order to feel secure and manage daily affairs (Rando, 1993). Rando (1993) has stated that such individuals feel completely devastated if the loved one dies. Empirical evidence indicates that individuals are indeed at risk for poor outcome if they are highly dependent on their spouse (Bonanno et al., 2002). In one study, widowhood was associated with elevated anxiety among those who were highly dependent on their spouses (Carr et al., 2000). Johnson and colleagues (2007) obtained similar findings. Those who were highly dependent on their spouses were more likely to develop symptoms of complicated grief (see also Johnson, Zhang, & Prigerson, 2008). Women who depended on their husbands for assistance with daily tasks were particularly likely to have difficulty coping with their husband's death.

In an interesting line of research, Carr (2008) examined the connection between quality of a marital relationship and interest in remarriage following the death of a spouse. She found that interest in dating was determined in part by gender and in part by the nature of the mourner's relationship with the deceased spouse. Greater marital conflict was associated with less interest in dating. Widowers were much more likely to express interest in a new relationship than were widows. Men who had been the most emotionally reliant on their spouse expressed the greatest interest in remarriage. The reverse was true for women: The more emotionally reliant they had been on their husbands, the less interested they were in pursuing subsequent relationships. These findings have implications for understanding why some clients may be more interested in dating than others.

ATTACHMENT STYLE

In recent years, scholars have begun to examine the impact of attachment style on reactions to the death of a spouse. Drawing from the work of John Bowlby (1980), Mikulincer and Shaver (2008) indicated that attachment security is crucial for maintaining emotional stability and forming mutually rewarding and long-lasting close relationships. Bowlby (1973) hypothesized that if caregivers are consistently available and are responsive to a child's needs, the child is likely to develop a secure attachment style.

Bartholemew and Horowitz (1991) developed a model of attachment styles that has been highly influential. This model is based on the idea that attachment styles reflect people's beliefs about their partners and themselves. Specifically, attachment styles are determined by whether people judge their partners to be generally accessible and responsive to requests for support, and also whether they judge themselves to be the kind of person that others wish to support. People who judge their partners and themselves positively are characterized as *secure*. Secure individuals find it easy to become emotionally close to others, and don't worry about whether others will like or accept them. People who rate themselves positively but their partners negatively are characterized as *dismissive–avoidant*. These individuals deny needing close relationships and avoid attachment to others. People who rate themselves negatively but rate their partners positively are characterized as *anxious–preoccupied*. People with this style seek high levels of intimacy but tend to become too dependent on their partners. People who rate themselves negatively and their partners negatively are characterized as *fearful–avoidant*. These individuals are uncomfortable getting close to others, and worry that they will be hurt if they allow themselves to get too close to others.

Mikulincer and Shaver (2008) have suggested that secure attachment increases the likelihood of adjustment to a loss. According to these authors, securely attached people are able to experience and express feelings of grief and distress without becoming overwhelmed. A secure attachment style also serves as an important resource for tolerating separation, for making effective use of social support (Field & Wogrin, 2011), for regulating physiological and behavioral states, and for exploring the world (Shear & Shair, 2005). An individual who does not have a secure attachment style typically experiences the loss of a partner as a devastating event that triggers intense and pervasive stress. The situation is even more stressful when the deceased was the primary attachment figure—the one to whom the mourner would have turned for support in times of duress (Shear & Shair, 2005). According to Mikulincer and Shaver, individuals without a secure attachment style have great difficulty with the mourning process. They experience intense anxiety, depression, and anger. Those with anxious–ambivalent styles may be especially likely to show greater clinging and loneliness (Parkes, 2009). Their overwhelming negative affect presents an obstacle to mourning.

Although few studies have tested these ideas, available research supports Mikulincer and Shaver's (2008) hypothesis that there is a relationship between a person's attachment style and her reaction to the loss of a loved one. For example, Waskowic and Chartier (2003) found that following the death of their spouse, securely attached people were less angry, were less socially isolated, felt less guilty, had less death anxiety, and ruminated less than insecurely attached people.

Lobb and colleagues (2010) have maintained that poor outcome following the death of a loved one stems from insults to a child's sense of security that can result from weak parental bonding. Childhood separation anxiety, as well as high levels of strict parental control, have been shown to impede adjustment to subsequent loss (Johnson, Zhang, Greer, & Prigerson, 2007; Vanderwerker, Jacobs, Parkes, & Prigerson, 2006). Silverman, Johnson, and Prigerson (2001) showed that childhood abuse or serious neglect—experiences likely to interfere with the development of secure attachments and self capacities—put people at risk for poor outcomes following the death of a loved one. Other studies have also provided evidence that those who have insecure or anxious attachments to their partners show the most intense and prolonged grief (for more detailed discussions, see Shaver & Tancredy, 2001; M. S. Stroebe et al., 2005; Zhang, El-Jawahri, & Prigerson, 2006).

Bowlby (1973, 1980) noted that in some cases, parents discourage displays of what they perceive as negative emotions (e.g., crying), and encourage premature or unreasonable independence. According to Bowlby, such children are likely to develop an avoidant attachment style. People with this style try to suppress and deny attachment needs. Following the death of their partner, such individuals are typically unwilling or unable to express thoughts, feelings, or memories related to the deceased loved one. They also tend to downplay the importance of their loss. This impedes the commencement of the mourning process. In fact, Zech and Arnold (2011) have argued that avoidant individuals are less likely to enter therapy, given their tendency to minimize their distress.

Mancini, Robinaugh, Shear, and Bonanno (2009) have discussed the potential role of both generalized attachment style and the specific nature of the attachment to the deceased in shaping bereavement responses. In examining data from bereaved spouses, they found that attachment avoidance, attachment anxiety, and marital quality predicted complicated grief symptoms at both 4 and 18 months after the death. Interestingly, those individuals with a dismissive–avoidant style and high self-reported marital quality reported significant reductions in complicated grief symptoms over time. This finding is consistent with Fraley and Bonanno's (2004) work, which found among 59 bereaved adults that persons with a dismissive–avoidant style showed a similar symptom picture to those with a secure attachment style. This group contrasted with the fearful–avoidant group, whose members had a difficult time adapting to their losses. Thus it seems important to consider the mourner's generalized attachment style, as well as the attachment needs that characterized the mourner's relationship with the deceased.

Zech and Arnold (2011) have provided a thoughtful discussion of the therapeutic implications of these various attachment styles. They maintain that anxiously attached clients are likely to be emotionally hyperaroused much of the time, whereas avoidantly attached clients may be hypoaroused (i.e., numb and shut down). Zech and Arnold argue that if therapists try to engage either type in exploring deep feelings surrounding the loss, this "can potentially result in both types of clients being outside their 'window of tolerance'" (p. 29). They suggest that the ramifications of this process are unfortunate. Anxiously attached clients can easily be destabilized in therapy. They are likely to ruminate about their loved ones, which will result in an increase in their distress. Avoidantly attached clients may feel that as a result of the treatment, they are being flooded with unwelcome, distressing emotions. They may take any opportunity to distract themselves from their distress, or may drop out of treatment. Zech and Arnold offer guidance regarding how clinicians can address these challenges.

Individuals who have experienced abuse or neglect in childhood may develop *complex developmental trauma* (Courtois & Ford, 2009), also referred to as *complex PTSD*. Its hallmark symptoms are somatization, revictimization, affect dysregulation, relationship difficulties, disruptions of identity, and dissociation (Pelcovitz et al., 1997). Disorganized attachment, also referred to as a fearful–avoidant/dissociative style (Lyons-Ruth, Dutra, Schuder, & Bianchi, 2006), is characteristic of persons with complex developmental trauma. Although it seems that individuals who evidence complex developmental trauma adaptations may be more likely to experience traumatic bereavement following a sudden death, research has not yet adequately examined this hypothesis.

Taken together, these findings underscore the importance of assessing such childhood adversities as strict parental control and harsh parenting, childhood neglect and abuse, and other challenging childhood experiences. Our treatment approach utilizes the framework of CSDT, which, based on attachment theory, offers a map for the assessment of aspects of the self affected by inadequate attachment experiences earlier in life. It also provides guidance for resource-building activities before proceeding to trauma processing, which may be particularly important for those with insecure attachment styles.

ADDITIONAL PERSON-RELATED VARIABLES

The limited available research supports the view that a history of prior traumatic events or a family history of psychopathology enhances vulnerability to complicated grief (see Auster, Moutier, & Lanouette, 2008, for a review). There is also research to suggest that the presence of other major stressors can interferes with the resolution of grief. These might include serious health problems, caregiving responsibilities for an elderly parent or other loved one, behavioral problems of a child, or financial difficulties (see, e.g., Ott, 2003; van der Houwen et al.,

2010; Zisook & Shuchter, 1993). Clients who are dealing with such stressors may have difficulty becoming engaged in the treatment.

Clients who are dealing with other major stressors during the mourning process may find it more difficult to participate in a treatment that demands time and energy. Such stressors might include serious health problems, caregiving responsibilities for an elderly parent or other loved one, behavioral problems of a child, or financial problems.

Among parents who have lost a child, Li and colleagues (2005) found that parents who lost their only child had the greatest risk of admission to a psychiatric hospital. Consistent with these findings, Dyregrov and colleagues (2003) found that not having surviving children was a significant predictor of distress in all three of the samples they studied (loss of children via suicide, accident, or SIDS). Drawing from interview data, these investigators reported that among parents who had surviving children, parents of their children's friends helped to provide social support, inviting them into a social network following the death. In a study of parents who lost a child to natural causes, accidents, suicide, or homicide, Wijngaards-de Meij and colleagues (2005) found that the more children there were in a family after a death occurred, the fewer grief symptoms the parents reported. In addition, families in which the mothers became pregnant following the deaths showed a greater decrease in depression than families in which the mothers did not become pregnant. Rogers and colleagues (2008) obtained similar findings. They found that parents who had other children at the time of the loss were less likely to experience marital disruption. These authors suggested that the presence of other children "can be a way of finding meaning through important life tasks" (p. 210).

From these studies of child loss, two additional demographic variables have emerged as significant: work and educational attainment. Wijngaards-de Meij and colleagues (2005) found that the more bereaved parents worked outside the home, the fewer grief symptoms they reported. Respondents with more years of education also reported less grief than those with less education. Dyregrov and colleagues (2003) obtained similar results: Not working outside the home and fewer years of education were predictors of distress among those who lost a child via accidents, suicide, and SIDS.

CLINICAL INTEGRATION

Evan's thoughts were swirling as he waited for Sonia to arrive for her session. Fifteen minutes earlier, Karen had walked out of his office after her therapy session; her clinical file still lay open on his desk. "Karen is doing well in therapy," he thought to himself, "but she is in such a different place from Sonia."

Evan found it difficult not to compare the two women. He saw them in back-to-back appointments every Wednesday afternoon. Both women had lost sons in car accidents. Both had been mourning for about 3 years. Both experienced trauma symptoms. And Karen was so angry—in a way that Sonia wasn't. Karen seemed to adapt to the loss of her son by avoiding reminders of his death as much as she could. The exception to this was her intense focus on the ongoing criminal trial of the man accused of killing her son. If avoidance seemed so necessary to Karen, how was she able to throw herself into the trial—itself a reminder of William's death? And just as Evan conjured up this thought, a light bulb went on:

"I get it! Karen is pretty comfortable with anger; it's the hurt and despair she's warding off. I was framing Karen's avoidance in terms of the actual death rather than in terms of her feelings. It makes sense that she would avoid some feelings and not others. It's as though her anger and the trial itself protect her from these other feelings, allowing her to be engaged with William's death without feeling so much pain. The anger is easier. The problem, of course, is she's feeling that pain anyway, and . . ."

Such were Evan's thoughts when Sonia tapped on his door. "Are you ready for me?"

Startled, Evan replied, "Yes, of course, come on in." Evan quickly adjusted, flipping Karen's file closed and turning his attention to Sonia, though Karen was still in the background. He had a new hypothesis. Whereas Karen was avoiding feelings of profound grief and despair, maybe Sonia was avoiding anger.

After checking in about the independent activities Evan had asked Sonia to complete a week ago, he turned their attention to a new topic. "Sonia, I remember that when I asked you about your upbringing in our first session, you described your father as an angry person—as emotionally volatile and scary to you and your sisters. I wonder if you can tell me a bit about how you responded to your dad's anger."

"Well, I remember a few things. I remember really hoping something would happen that would distract him, like hoping he would turn on the TV. I also remember being glad his anger wasn't directed toward me, and usually it wasn't. I tried to stay quiet and out of the way. If I was involved, it was to try to calm or appease my dad before he got angry and out of control. When he wasn't so angry, I loved being with him. He was just so unpredictable, and so I often felt like I was walking on eggshells. And I didn't have a lot of my own feelings; I was too busy monitoring his."

"It sounds like anger was a pretty scary feeling for you?"

"Yeah, it was."

"And maybe it still is?" asked Evan.

"Yeah, I guess it is."

"And it sounds as though feelings—your own feelings, that is—are pretty unfamiliar to you? You said you didn't have a lot of your own feelings?"

"I think that's true. I respond to others' feelings, but I tend to have a difficult time feeling much of anything other than depression myself, especially these days. Do you think my father has something to do with my grief for Juan?" asked Sonia.

"I do," responded Evan. "I think that you may have learned some things about relationships and feelings from your father. And my guess is that anger is difficult for you to experience and express." Evan paused before continuing. "I wonder if you have allowed yourself to experience the full force of your anger about Juan being gone."

This question opened up a new area of exploration for Evan and Sonia. Evan worked with Sonia to address possible obstacles to her capacity to experience her full range of feelings, anger included. After this session with Sonia, his therapy with Karen also opened into a new direction. He again thought about their similarities and differences, and specifically about their respective attachment styles. Whereas Evan believed both women were more or less securely attached, he conceptualized Sonia's style as tending toward anxious-preoccupied and Karen's as tending toward fearful-avoidant, although Karen certainly experienced a bond with her son. When that bond was severed to the extent that it was by his death, Karen turned away from a range of painful emotions and toward anger, which helped her to feel more powerful. Both women were finding ways to adapt that worked for them. Evan's job was to understand how these adaptations served them, as well as how they posed obstacles to moving through their traumatic bereavement in a more complete way.

CONCLUDING REMARKS

We have provided a comprehensive discussion of person-related risk factors in this chapter, in an effort to offer our fellow clinicians information about their clients that will make their interventions more effective. The issues discussed in this chapter—for example, personality and attachment style—help provide a framework for the thematic content we might listen for in our ongoing work with clients. If we can hold an awareness of those factors that have been shown both to facilitate and to challenge the mourning process and that of trauma accommodation, then we are in a better position to assess our clients' unique needs and to intervene accordingly. Assessing what is true and relevant for a particular individual demonstrates respect and allows for the creation and strengthening of a therapeutic alliance.

The example of Evan's work with two different clients who had lost sons in similar circumstances illustrates this process. Evan was able to assess and explore each woman's general style of relating, conceptualize how this influenced their challenges in mourning the loss of their sons, and use this information to "fill in" the content of the particular interventions and processes that we discuss in Part III. Like Evan, we will all benefit from having a framework from which to assess those variables and risk factors that may affect a particular client's experience, thereby deepening empathy and facilitating recovery.

CHAPTER 7

Treatment Research

Two days before the Thanksgiving holiday, Harriet witnessed her partner die of a massive heart attack. She and Gwen were home alone, and Gwen was carrying extra chairs into their dining room from a spare bedroom upstairs. Harriet heard a crash and ran into the dining room to see Gwen clutching her chest. She was lying on the floor, gasping for breath, as Harriet picked up the phone to call 911. The next thing Harriet remembered was being down on the floor with Gwen, calling out her name over and over after she became nonresponsive. When the paramedics arrived, they began chest compressions, used the defibrillator, and quickly transported her to the hospital—but Gwen was already gone.

For the next year, Harriet felt as though she were in a daze. She seemed to be thinking about Gwen all the time, yet avoided talking about her to others, including their adult children. Harriet was haunted by images of what happened that day and memories of her own feelings of helplessness. In an effort to keep these images at bay, she tried to stay busy. She hated turning in at night because of the intense emptiness that she felt lying in bed alone. She also steered clear of their dining room because it evoked painful memories of the terrible scene of Gwen's final moments. She decided to sell the house shortly after the first anniversary of Gwen's death. Harriet came to recognize that staying in the home where they raised their children together would be impossible for her. She had come to realize that she could not continue living there without Gwen.

In developing this treatment approach, our goal has been to integrate work on the treatment of grief with work on the treatment of trauma. In so doing, we have identified a number of treatment elements that we believe are important for treating the traumatically bereaved, such as building self capacities and prolonged exposure. Is there an empirical basis for these and other components that form the foundation of our treatment approach? In this chapter, we review the scientific evidence regarding efficacious treatments for survivors of sudden, traumatic loss. We begin by considering research and treatments pertaining to grief. We then examine several treatments that have been developed for PTSD. Although many practitioners regard grief counseling as effective, there is far more research evidence in support of trauma treatments. We discuss the implications of research in both areas for treating traumatic bereavement.

TREATMENT FOR GRIEF AND MOURNING

To learn more about grief research and treatments that might inform our approach, we draw from three topics. First, we trace the development of the most important and influential ideas about grief and its resolution. In so doing, we illustrate how beliefs about grief therapy have changed over the years. Theoretical orientations that were once central to our understanding of grief, such as Freud's (1917/1957) notion of grief work and the various stage models of grief resolution, are far less influential today. To a considerable extent, these early views have been superseded by theoretical orientations that, in our judgment, have more to offer practitioners working in this field. These include the models of the mourning process developed by Worden (2009) and Rando (1993, 2014); the stress and coping model (Lazarus & Folkman, 1984); the continuing-bonds approach (Klass et al., 1996); the role of positive emotions in the grief process; the dual-process model of bereavement (Stroebe & Schut, 1999; M. S. Stroebe et al., 2005); and the role of meaning in the mourning process (Neimeyer, 2001; Neimeyer & Sands, 2011).

Second, we take a look at research designed to assess grief counseling as it is practiced in the United States today. These studies have compared clients receiving grief counseling with those in a control condition, such as being placed on a wait list. Taken as a whole, this research provides little support for the effectiveness of grief therapy.

Finally, we discuss scholarly research on complicated grief. As Shear, Simon, and colleagues (2011) have described it, complicated grief is a painful condition in which the normal grieving process becomes derailed. The bereaved person experiences prolonged acute grief symptoms, has difficulty meeting role obligations, and struggles unsuccessfully to build a rewarding life without the deceased person. The goal of this body of work is to identify those individuals who are most in need of grief treatment and most likely to benefit from it. To the extent that those with traumatic bereavement experience complicated grief, this work illustrates the devastating physical and mental health consequences that face traumatically bereaved clients.

Classic Grief Theories: Overview and Description

Freud's Grief Work Perspective

One of the most influential approaches to loss has been the classic psychoanalytic model of bereavement, which is based on Freud's (1917/1957) seminal paper "Mourning and Melancholia." According to Freud, the primary task of mourning is the gradual surrender of one's psychological attachment to the deceased. Freud believed that relinquishing the love object involves a painful internal struggle. The individual experiences intense yearning for the lost loved one, yet is faced with the reality of that person's absence. As mourners review thoughts and memories, ties to the loved one are gradually withdrawn. Freud referred to this process, which requires considerable time and energy, as "grief work" or "the work of mourning." At the conclusion of the mourning period, the bereaved individual is said to have "worked through" the loss and to have freed herself from an intense attachment to an unavailable person. Freud maintained that when the process has been completed, the bereaved person regains sufficient emotional energy to invest in new relationships and pursuits.

The understandings that emerged from Freud's ideas have had a profound effect on grief treatment and have only recently been called into question (Bonanno & Kaltman, 1999; Stroebe, 1992–1993; Wortman & Boerner, 2011). For years, it was common for therapists to organize their entire treatment approach around the notion of loosening or breaking down bonds between the mourner and the deceased. Continued attachment to the deceased was referred to as unresolved grief (Klass et al., 1996). Rando (1993) has pointed out that a therapist who focuses on the importance of breaking the bond may see behaviors reflecting a continuing connection with the deceased, such as asking his advice on current life decisions, as maladaptive. Along similar lines, Valentine (2006) has emphasized that although "sensing the presence of the deceased" is very common (see our discussion in Chapter 12), treatment providers have often regarded it as a sign of continued attachment to the deceased and thus as indicative of pathology.

In a review of the literature on breaking down attachments to the loved one, Malkinson (2010) states that studies have not found support for the theory of relinquishing bonds. She argues that in many cases, studies have shown that inner relationships with the deceased often continue throughout one's life, and that such ties are often beneficial. In fact, as we describe below, available evidence suggests that treatments centered around breaking down bonds between the bereaved person and the deceased may actually be harmful (Klass et al., 1996).

Emphasis on Negative Emotions

In examining the mourning process as described by Freud, we are struck by the singular focus on negative emotions. Freud's model emphasized the importance of working through the emotional pain associated with the loss. Amid the despair and anguish that often accompany grief, positive emotions may seem unwarranted or even inappropriate (Fredrickson, Tugade, Waugh, & Larkin, 2003). When they are mentioned at all, positive emotions are typically viewed as indicating denial and as impediments to the mourning process (Deutsch, 1937; Sanders, 1993; see Keltner & Bonanno, 1997, for a review). With notable exceptions (e.g., Folkman, 1997b, 2008; Folkman & Moskowitz, 2000; Fredrickson, 2001; Lazarus, Kanner, & Folkman, 1980), theories focusing on the grieving process have failed to consider the role that positive emotions may play. Subsequent work, discussed below, has demonstrated unequivocally that positive emotions can facilitate the healing process.

Stage Models of Grief

One of the most widely held assumptions about the mourning process is that people proceed through a series of stages as they attempt to come to terms with loss. One of the most influential stage models was proposed by John Bowlby (1980). In his seminal work on grief, Bowlby integrated ideas from psychodynamic thought, the developmental literature on young children's reactions to separation, and work on the mourning behavior of primates. Bowlby maintained that during the course of normal development, individuals form instinctive affectional bonds or *attachments*. These are initially created between child and parent and later between adults. Bowlby was also the first to maintain that there is a relationship between a person's attachment history and how he will react to the loss of a loved one.

According to Bowlby (1980), these attachments are formed because of a need for safety and security. He suggested that threats to affectional bonds activate powerful attachment behaviors, such as intense anxiety, crying, and angry protest. Unlike Freud, Bowlby believed that the biological function of these behaviors is not withdrawal from the loved one, but rather reunion. However, in the case of a permanent loss, the biological function of ensuring proximity with attachment figures becomes dysfunctional. Consequently, the bereaved person struggles between the opposing forces of activated attachment behavior and the reality of the loved one's absence.

Bowlby maintained that in order to deal with these opposing forces, the mourner goes through four stages of grieving: initial numbness, disbelief, or shock; yearning or searching for the deceased, accompanied by anger and protest; despair and disorganization as the bereaved gives up the search, accompanied by feelings of depression and hopelessness; and reorganization or recovery as he accepts the loss, with a gradual return to former interests. By emphasizing the survival value of attachment behavior, Bowlby was the first to give a plausible explanation for responses such as anger or searching for the deceased during the mourning process. Drawing from this work, several theorists have proposed that people go through stages or phases in coming to terms with loss (see, e.g., Bowlby & Parkes, 1970; Engel, 1961; Parkes, 1972; Ramsay & Happee, 1977; Sanders, 1989).

Perhaps the best known stage model, preceding Bowlby's model by a decade, is the one Kübler-Ross (1969) proposed in her highly influential book *On Death and Dying*. This model was developed to explain how dying persons react to their own impending deaths. It posits that people go through denial, anger, bargaining, depression, and ultimately acceptance. This model generated considerable interest among professionals providing late-stage and end-of-life care.

Within a few years, practitioners working in the field of bereavement began to apply Kübler-Ross's stages of dying to individuals who were mourning the loss of a loved one. This approach captured the imagination of many grief practitioners. The book *On Grief and Grieving: Finding the Meaning of Grief through the Five Stages of Loss* (Kübler-Ross & Kessler, 2005), published shortly after Kübler-Ross's own death, facilitated the application of Kübler-Ross's ideas to the grief process.

Since that time, professionals with an interest in grief and loss have embraced Kübler-Ross's stages of grief. Her stages have been integrated into the curriculum of thousands of academic and professional institutions across the country. The five stages proposed by Kübler-Ross have become a mainstay not only in counseling, but in social work, hospitals, medical schools, nursing programs, and seminaries. We see these stages in popular media (e.g., the TV shows *Grey's Anatomy* and *The Simpsons*) as well as in self-help literature for the bereaved, appearing in magazines and books, and on influential websites.

Is there scientific evidence in support of stage models? With few exceptions (Maciejewski, Zhang, Block, & Prigerson, 2007), there are virtually no studies corroborating these models of the mourning process. Instead, well-designed studies have produced findings that do not support stage models (Barrett & Schneweis, 1981; Holland & Neimeyer, 2010). Robert Neimeyer (2001) has indicated that research has failed to identify a universal or normative pattern of mourning. As we have described in Chapters 5 and 6, there is considerable variability in the kinds of emotions people experience after a loss, and the order in which they are experienced. Nor do stage models help us understand why some people are devastated by a loss, while others emerge unscathed or even strengthened. Another criticism of stage models is that they place mourners in a passive role (Neimeyer, 1998). As we have described in Chapter 2, mourning is a process that requires the active involvement of the survivor. In addition, stage models focus almost exclusively on the survivor's emotional responses to the loss. There is consensus that cognitions and behaviors are equally important targets of interventions. Finally, stage models do not acknowledge the role of situational factors—aspects of the death and its surrounding circumstances—which influence the effects on survivors.

Stage models can have a negative effect on bereaved individuals, on those in their social networks, and on professionals who treat them. Each of these groups may use a stage model as a yardstick to assess how well a bereaved person is coping. Bereaved people may worry if they don't experience a particular stage, erroneously inferring that they cannot move forward until they do. As one woman explained, "I haven't felt much anger since my husband died. I asked my family to do things that would make me mad, so that I can go through the anger stage." Or health care providers may lead mourners to feel that they are not coping correctly if they do not experience a certain stage. A woman who lost her daughter in a drunk driving crash told her therapist that she did not feel angry. The therapist replied, "Why aren't you angry? You should be angry."

Stage models can also lead others to dismiss mourners' legitimate emotional reactions as "just a stage." One woman attended a family gathering shortly after her husband's death. Her sister asked repeatedly about how much insurance money she would receive. She finally rebuked her sister sharply, stating that she did not want to discuss the matter. Later she overheard her sister say to another family member, "Don't worry about Jill. She's just going through the anger stage." In fact, one of the most problematic aspects of stage models is that they have great potential to confuse, inhibit, misdirect, or pathologize mourners.

Ironically, some of the harshest criticisms of the stage model were made by Kübler-Ross herself. To her credit, she noted in her final book (Kübler-Ross & Kessler, 2005) that the stages should be applied flexibly because all people don't mourn in the same way. Unfortunately, many of her followers have paid little attention to these qualifications, and have tended to view her stages as a fixed sequence of responses. Shortly before her death in 2004, she stated that despite her best intentions, the stages she proposed have contributed to misunderstandings about the mourning process.

Why do treatment providers and laypersons alike cling to these models despite the absence of empirical support? Neimeyer (2001) has pointed out that stage models offer an apparent roadmap through turbulent terrains. It may be less frightening for people to go through the mourning process, or help others through it, if they know what is supposed to happen next. Such roadmap, however imperfect, may provide considerably more comfort than flying blind.

Classic Grief Theories: Impact on Clinical Practice

As Breen (2010–2011) indicates, "there is very little research describing grief counselors' understandings of grief and how they incorporate these understandings into their practices" (p. 286). However, there are reasons to believe that the classic grief models are continuing to hold sway over some practitioners. As Jordan and Neimeyer (2003) emphasize, "It is a truism that grief is unique to each individual, yet this wisdom is rarely reflected in the design and delivery of services to the bereaved" (p. 782). Breen and O'Connor (2007) state that "although the assumptions within the dominant grief discourse have been subject to robust empirical and theoretical challenges in recent years, they remain uncritically accepted by many service providers" (p. 205). On the basis of their review of studies of current practices of health care providers, they conclude that the prevailing construction of grief "remains a stage-based reaction, where recovery occurs within a relatively short time frame . . . and continued attachment to the deceased is pathologized" (p. 202). Similarly, Rando (1993) has maintained that while practitioners pay lip service to the idea that grief is an individual process, many are still likely to believe that having a continued relationship with the deceased indicates complicated or pathological mourning, and that they need to "help" the bereaved to detach from the deceased and move on. Bennett and Bennett (2000–2001) note that the concept of a progression from desolation through detachment to "recovery" persists in much of the literature written by and for grief counselors.

Our observation is that clinicians practicing today are becoming increasingly skeptical about the value of any stage approach. However, there is evidence to suggest that other health care providers, such as physicians, nurses, and social workers, are likely to endorse views that are consistent with a stage approach. In a systematic study of 23 highly rated and best-selling psychiatric nursing texts, Holman, Perisho, Edwards, and Mlakar (2010) reported that 87% of the texts stated that there are set stages or a predictable course of coping. Moreover, 65% of the texts mentioned a timeline specific enough to indicate a given number of weeks or months for the mourning process to be completed. There was no significant correlation between the age of a textbook and the presence of such statements, suggesting that these problems in how grief is conceptualized in these terms are not being resolved over time. Holman and colleagues find these results surprising, in light of the fact that the nursing profession has adopted an evidence-based approach to practice. They express concern that these beliefs may undermine nurses' ability to provide appropriate, supportive care that meets the unique needs of each patient.

The Mourning Process: More Recent Theoretical Developments

Largely in reaction to the classic grief models described above, subsequent bereavement experts have proposed views of the mourning process that are less dogmatic, more flexible, and more consistent with research evidence. Six distinct approaches to the mourning process have informed our treatment approach. First, both Worden (2009) and Rando (1993) have rejected the idea that grief should be regarded as a fixed series of stages. Both maintain that much can be gained by regarding mourning as a set of overlapping tasks (Worden, 2009) or processes (Rando, 1993, 2014). The second approach, the stress and coping model (Lazarus & Folkman, 1984), addresses why some people show intense and prolonged distress following the death of a loved one while others do not. The model also helps to clarify how risk factors, such as the circumstances surrounding the loss, can help account for the variability in individual responses to the death of a loved one. Third, the continuing bonds approach has focused on the connection between the mourner and the deceased. This model has posed a challenge to the idea that the bond between the mourner and the deceased must be severed. Studies indicate that in many cases, a continuing connection with the deceased can be beneficial (Klass et al., 1996). Fourth, we discuss research on positive emotions (Folkman, 1997a, 2001)—a topic rarely considered by those interested in grief and loss. Such emotions are surprisingly prevalent during the mourning process. Moreover, it is clear that positive emotions can facilitate the process in many ways. Fifth, Stroebe and her associates (Stroebe & Schut, 1999; M. S. Stroebe et al., 2005) have developed a theoretical approach to grief known as the dual-process model. They have emphasized that loss-oriented responses, such as experiencing intrusive images of the loved one's death, represent only part of the story of processing the loss. This model indicates that restorative activities, such as engaging in new pursuits or meeting new people, can play a vital role in the mourning process. Finally, as a way of emphasizing the uniqueness of each individual's grief, Neimeyer and his associates (Holland et al., 2006; Holland & Neimeyer, 2010; Neimeyer, 2001; Neimeyer & Sands, 2011; Shear, Boelen, & Neimeyer, 2011) maintain that the process of mourning is in many cases a search for meaning. This perspective is valuable because it helps therapists engage with clients whose ways of finding meaning in life have been disrupted, if not destroyed, by the loved one's death and its related losses. Each of these approaches to understanding and treating bereaved people is discussed below.

Moving beyond Stages: Worden's Tasks and Rando's "R" Processes

One shortcoming of the stage models is that they lack flexibility because each prescribes a specific sequence of responses to loss. Stage models also provide little guidance about how to help clients move forward with their mourning process. Two models have been designed to overcome these problems: Worden's task model (Worden, 2009; Worden & Winokuer, 2011) and Rando's (1993, 2014) "R" processes. Both of these approaches have been developed specifically to aid practitioners in intervening in the mourning process. Both are widely used in clinical settings, and practitioners generally regard them as helpful (see, e.g., Stroebe, Stroebe, Schut, & van den Bout, 1998).

Worden (2009) regards the grieving process as a series of specific tasks that should be addressed during treatment: to accept the reality of the loss; to process the pain of grief; to adjust to a world without the deceased; and to find an enduring connection with the deceased in the midst of embarking on a new life. According to Worden, a task approach is flexible because tasks can be addressed in different orders, depending on each client's needs. In addition, he emphasizes that tasks can be revisited and reworked over time. He also states that unlike stages, which must be passed through, the tasks convey to the mourner that there are things she can do to adapt to the loss. This may help the mourner to maintain hope that she will be able to cope with the loss and move forward with her life. As Worden puts it, "This can be a powerful antidote to the feelings of helplessness that most mourners experience" (p. 38).

Rando (1993, 2014) conceptualizes mourning in terms of processes rather than tasks. As we have described in Chapter 2, she identifies six specific processes: *Recognize the loss; React to the separation; Recollect and reexperience the deceased and the relationship; Relinquish the old attachments to the deceased and the old assumptive world; Readjust to move adaptively into the new world without forgetting the old;* and *Reinvest*. Although there is some overlap between these two approaches, Rando's "Rs" offer practitioners a more detailed and fine-grained analysis of the mourning process. Like Worden (2009), Rando maintains that the sequence of the "Rs" is not fixed. According to Rando, mourners may move back and forth among processes; such movement illustrates the nonlinear and fluctuating course of mourning.

Rando (1993) believes that keeping the focus on processes rather than tasks helps a therapist to focus on what a mourner is doing at present, thus providing more immediate feedback on where the mourner is in the process and how to intervene. These "R" processes form an important component of our treatment approach, and are discussed further in Chapter 12.

Understanding Variability in Response to Loss: The Stress and Coping Approach

Over the past two decades, a theoretical orientation referred to as the *stress and coping approach* (Lazarus & Folkman, 1984) has become highly influential in the field of bereavement. The basic assumption underlying this model is that exposure to stressful life events, such as the death of a loved one, can precipitate the onset of physical or mental health problems. Investigators using this approach were particularly interested in understanding why some people show great vulnerability to stressful life experiences while others do not (Wortman & Boerner, 2011).

The stress and coping approach highlights the role of cognitive appraisal in understanding how people react to loss. A person's *appraisal*, or subjective assessment, of what has happened is hypothesized to play a major role in determining her reaction to the stressor. The stress and coping model also calls attention to the critical role played by the survivor's coping resources. Individuals appraise events as stressful when they believe their coping resources are insufficient to deal with what has happened. Building clients' coping resources is a major focus of this treatment approach. Augmenting their resources enables clients to do the hard work of processing and mourning the loss.

To account further for why a given loss has more impact on one person than on another, stress and coping researchers have focused on the identification of potential *risk factors*, or factors that enhance vulnerability to the stressful event. Over the past decade, countless studies have demonstrated that risk or vulnerability factors dramatically affect reactions to the death of a loved one. As we have discussed in Chapter 5, some risk factors focus on circumstances surrounding the loss, such as whether the death was violent. Others are person-related factors like attachment history and gender, as described in Chapter 6. Knowledge of risk factors helps practitioners to tailor the treatment to the unique vulnerabilities of each client.

Breaking Down Attachments

According to the traditional view of the mourning process, it is necessary to disengage from the deceased in order to get on with life (Freud, 1917/1957; Volkan, 1971). As described above, these writers believed that for grief work to be completed, the bereaved person must withdraw energy from the deceased and thus free himself from that attachment. Until recently, relinquishing the tie to the deceased has been a major goal of grief therapy (see, e.g., Humphrey & Zimpfer, 1996; Sanders, 1989).

During the past decade, this view has been called into question (for reviews, see Stroebe & Schut, 2005; Wortman & Boerner, 2011). Indeed, it appears that an increasing number of researchers and practitioners now believe that it is normal to maintain a continuing connection to the deceased, and that such a connection may actually promote good adjustment following the loss (Attig, 1996; Klass et al., 1996; Neimeyer, 1998; Shmotkin, 1999). In their groundbreaking book *Continuing Bonds*, Klass and colleagues (1996) have also emphasized the potential value of maintaining a healthy connection with the deceased loved one. These investigators note that their training led them to expect grief resolution to be accompanied by breaking down attachments to the deceased. However, this was not what they found in their research or in their clinical work. For example, in their work with bereaved parents, they found that the process through which parents resolved their grief involved sustaining an intense connection with the child who died. They report that in almost all cases, parents were able to move forward only by maintaining the child as a significant presence in their lives.

In their study of how the death of a child as a result of accident, suicide, or homicide affected parents, Murphy and colleagues (1999) obtained similar findings. When asked what challenge they were facing at the present time, 76% of the respondents at 4 months, and 52% at 12 months, stressed the importance of maintaining ties with their deceased child.

In recent years, practitioners working within a continuing-bonds framework have come to recognize that encouraging such bonds is not always beneficial to a client. As we discuss in more detail in Chapter 12, it is important to identify what can be continued and what needs to be relinquished, given the reality of the death (Field, 2008; Rando, 1993, 2014). In an excellent discussion of this matter, Field and Wogrin (2011) emphasize the importance of transforming the bond from a physical one to one that is mental or symbolic. They suggest that a symbolic bond can serve as a "safe haven" for a bereaved client, which can facilitate the ability to move forward.

The Role of Positive Emotions

Until recently, grief therapy has been based on the implicit assumption that negative feelings must be "worked through." As noted above, it was also widely assumed that mourners rarely experience positive emotions. When they do emerge, such feelings are thought to reflect a failure to accept the loss and its ramifications.

In the 1980s, Wortman and her associates became interested in whether positive emotions were experienced by people who had encountered major losses, and if so, whether they might sustain hope and facilitate adjustment. Therefore, they decided to measure positive as well as negative emotions in a study focusing on loss of a child as a result of SIDS (see Wortman & Boerner, 2011, for a more detailed discussion).

This study provided clear evidence that positive emotions are prevalent following major loss. At 3 weeks following the death of their infant to SIDS, parents reported experiencing positive emotions such as happiness as frequently as they experienced negative feelings. By the second interview, conducted 3 months after the infant's death, positive affect was more prevalent than negative affect; this continued to be the case at the third interview, conducted at 18 months after the loss. Respondents were asked to describe the intensity as well as the frequency of their feelings. These measures were included so that the investigators could determine whether negative feelings, while no more prevalent than positive ones, were more intense. However, this did not turn out to be the case. At all three interviews, feelings of happiness were found to be just as intense as feelings of sadness. In fact, at the second and third interviews, respondents reported that their feelings of happiness were significantly more intense than their feelings of sadness.

Subsequent studies have corroborated that positive emotions are surprisingly prevalent during bereavement (Folkman, 1997a, 2001; Folkman & Moskowitz, 2000; Stein, Folkman, Trabasso, & Richards, 1997). Research has also demonstrated that the ability to display positive emotions is associated with the resolution of grief. Bonanno and Keltner (1997) conducted a study with people who lost a spouse. At 6 months after the loss, they asked respondents to talk about their relationships with their deceased spouse. Participants were videotaped during the interviews, and the videotapes were then coded for the presence of genuine laughs or smiles, which involve movements in the muscles around the eyes. The majority of participants exhibited positive emotion. Moreover, the presence of positive affect was associated with reduced grief at 14 and 25 months after the losses. Those who exhibited laughs or smiles also evoked more favorable responses in observers (Keltner & Bonanno, 1997). In addition to rating them more positively overall, observers rated those who engaged in laughs and smiles as healthier, better adjusted, less frustrating, and more amusing. These findings suggest that one way positive emotions may facilitate coping with loss is by eliciting positive responses from those in the social environment. On the basis of these results, Bonanno (2001) maintains that recovery is most likely when negative grief-related emotions are regulated or minimized and when positive emotions are instigated or enhanced.

Folkman (1997b, 2001, 2008) has also conducted important work on the role of positive emotions in coping with bereavement. Folkman proposes that when people are distressed as a result of a loss event, they can generate positive emotions by infusing ordinary events with positive meaning. This observation came about in an interesting way. In a study of caregiving partners of men with AIDS, Folkman (1997b) had initially focused exclusively on stressful aspects of the caregiving situation. Respondents were questioned about these aspects every 2 months. Shortly after the study began, several participants "reported that we were missing an important part of their experience by asking only about stressful events; they said we needed to ask about positive events as well if we were to understand how they coped with the stress of caregiving" (p. 1215). Consequently, Folkman added a question in which respondents were asked to describe "something you did, or something that happened to you, that made you feel good and that was meaningful to you and helped you get through the day" (p. 1215). Such events were reported by 99.5% of the respondents. Events focused on many different aspects of daily life, such as enjoying a good meal, receiving appreciation for something done for one's partner, or going to the movies with friends. Folkman has hypothesized that events of this sort generate positive emotion by helping people feel connected and cared about, by providing a sense of achievement and self-esteem, and by providing a respite or distraction from the stress of caregiving. She has suggested that engaging in activities that generate positive emotions, and positive emotions themselves, can help sustain coping efforts in dealing with a stressful situation. More recent empirical evidence is consistent with this prediction (Bonanno, Moskowitz, Pappa, & Folkman, 2005; Moskowitz, Folkman, & Acree, 2003).

The Dual-Process Model

As described above, the concept of grief work, or working through the loss, is central to grief treatment as it is practiced today. Grief work typically refers to such processes as confronting the reality of the death and its many ramifications.

Stroebe and Schut (2010) have argued that despite its dominance in the field of grief counseling, the grief work hypothesis has a number of serious limitations. First, drawing on bereavement practices in non-Western cultures, they maintain that confronting one's grief is not always necessary for adaptation to occur. Second, consistent with other bereavement researchers and practitioners, they indicate that the grief work approach "seems somewhat passive (as though the person is being put through, rather than dealing with . . . the effortful struggle that is so much part of grieving)" (p. 275). Finally, they state that those working within a grief work perspective fail to acknowledge the need for "dosage" of grief, given how arduous and exhausting the mourning process can be.

In order to address these shortcomings, Stroebe and Schut (1999, 2010) have developed the *dual-process model* of grief. They suggest that responses to the death of a loved one can be classified into two broad categories: *loss-oriented* and *restoration-oriented*. Loss-oriented coping refers to processing some aspect of the lost relationship. Examples of loss-oriented responses include experiencing the pain associated with the loss, reminiscing about life as it had been, or ruminating about the circumstances surrounding the death. Most past models of mourning have focused exclusively on loss-oriented coping.

Stroebe and Schut's (1999, 2010) focus on the benefits of restoration-oriented coping is highly compatible with the material on positive emotions discussed above. Such coping might involve doing new things, mastering new skills, taking on new roles or identities, or entering new relationships. Like positive emotions, restoration-oriented coping provides a respite from the intense pain associated with loss-oriented coping. Stroebe and Schut (2001a, 2010) have proposed that a bereaved person typically alternates between loss- and restoration-oriented coping. They indicated that oscillation between these types of responses is necessary for accommodating the loss. Restorative activities not only give the mourner a break from the difficult work of facing the loss, but also help replenish psychological resources such as energy and hope

(Folkman, 2001). Over time, there is usually a shift away from loss-oriented coping and toward restoration-oriented coping, such as developing new relationships.

The dual-process model has generated a great deal of interest among researchers and practitioners. Some clinicians who have developed interventions for the bereaved have used this model as an organizing framework (Richardson, 2010; Shear, Frank, Houck, & Reynolds, 2005; Shear, Gorscak, & Simon, 2006). One of the most significant aspects of this model is that it advocates exposing clients to the painful aspects of their grief in small amounts. As Rando (1993) has expressed it, "Respites and diversions permit distance and allow for replenishment, reconnection with other parts of life, and a renewed sense of control" (p. 47). Similarly, Shear (2010) has stated that "Coming to terms with the death is a process that works best if it is grappled with, set aside, and revisited" (p. 364). Approaching grief in manageable pieces is essential in treating traumatic bereavement, and is central to our treatment approach.

The Importance of Meaning

A major development in the treatment of grief is Neimeyer's work on meaning reconstruction following the death of a loved one (Holland et al., 2006; Holland & Neimeyer, 2010; Neimeyer, 2001; Neimeyer & Sands, 2011; Shear, Boelen, & Neimeyer, 2011). Unlike many accounts of the mourning process, Neimeyer has emphasized that grief is an idiosyncratic process in which people strive to make sense out of what has happened. Neimeyer and Sands (2011) have pointed out that this quest can occur at many levels, "from the practical (*How* did my loved one die?) through the relational (*Who* am I, now that I am no longer a spouse?) to the spiritual or existential (*Why* did God allow this to happen?)" (p. 11; emphasis in original). There is accumulating evidence that the effort to find meaning can play a constructive role in the mourning process (Holland & Neimeyer, 2010).

Much of our description of the impact of traumatic death has focused on how it robs our lives of meaning. We have drawn from Neimeyer's rich and thoughtful body of work to address how the traumatically bereaved are affected by their losses, as well as how issues surrounding meaning can be addressed with sensitivity and compassion.

Grief Treatment Effects

During the 1990s, there was a proliferation of opportunities for therapy for those mourning the loss of a loved one. This was reflected in the wide variety of workshops, professional conferences, and individual and group treatments offered in most communities (Neimeyer, 2000b). During this period, a new field called *grief counseling* was born. Generally speaking, grief counseling is based on the assumption that individuals must "work through" and accommodate their loss (see, e.g., Rando, 1993; Worden, 2009). Some practitioners have differentiated between *grief counseling* and *grief therapy*. For example, Worden (2009) has indicated that the goal in grief counseling is to facilitate the tasks of mourning, such as accepting the reality of the loss and processing the pain of grief. In contrast, he notes that grief therapy should be used when the survivor is experiencing feelings of grief that are more intense than usual, more prolonged, or both. Grief counseling or therapy typically includes such elements as helping a survivor to grasp the reality of what has happened; assisting her in identifying and expressing feelings; normalizing feelings that emerge; helping her to formulate a realistic appraisal of her relationship to her loved one; assisting her in learning to live without the deceased; and helping her to form a new identity and reengage with life (see Worden, 2009, for a more detailed discussion).

As Neimeyer (2000b) has indicated, it is widely assumed that grief counseling is "a firmly established, demonstrably effective service, which seems to have found a secure niche in the health care field" (p. 542). Has research in fact shown that this type of treatment is effective? In recent years, several reviews of grief treatment studies have appeared in the literature (e.g., Allumbough & Hoyt, 1999; Fortner & Neimeyer, summarized in Neimeyer, 2000b; Jordan & Neimeyer, 2003; Kato & Mann, 1999; Larson & Hoyt, 2007; Schut, Stroebe, van den Bout, & Terheggen, 2001; M. S. Stroebe et al., 2005). With one exception (Larson & Hoyt, 2007), these reviews have come to the same conclusion: that the scientific basis for the efficacy of counseling for grief and mourning is weak. The most comprehensive and methodologically rigorous review was conducted by Currier, Neimeyer, and Berman (2008). Overall, their analyses demonstrated that interventions had only a small effect when they assessed respondents at posttreatment and no significant effect at follow-up, which was on average about 36 weeks later.

Despite the absence of overall effects, Currier and colleagues (2008) noted that there was considerable variation in the impact of different treatments. They found that respondents' levels of distress strongly influenced the benefits derived from treatment. If the respondents were experiencing high distress, the results showed a clear benefit at both posttreatment and follow-up. Currier and colleagues indicated that effect sizes (a measure of clinical relevance) for respondents showing high distress compared favorably with the positive outcomes shown for psychotherapy in general.

Neimeyer and his colleagues have identified some additional factors that help to contextualize the findings from grief treatment studies. One important factor is the timing of the treatment. Jordan and Neimeyer (2003) found that interventions that were delivered shortly after the death had significantly smaller effect sizes than those delivered later. Jordan and Neimeyer have suggested that there may be a "critical window of time" (p. 774) when it is best to offer interventions—perhaps 6–18 months after the loss, "before problematic patterns of adjustment have become entrenched" (p. 774). These investigators have also emphasized that the types of counseling needed shortly after a loss may differ markedly from what is needed a year after the loss, or 10 years later, noting that therapists should attempt to customize the type of intervention to the particular points their clients have reached in the mourning trajectory.

Complicated Grief

One of the most influential and important lines of research on bereavement is that on complicated grief (abbreviated in this section as CG). Chief goals of this work involve identifying individuals who develop persistent and debilitating symptoms of grief, and examining the consequences of CG for subsequent physical and mental health. Researchers working in this area have been interested in developing effective treatments for those with CG. Finally, there has been increasing interest among researchers in getting CG classified as a mental disorder in the *Diagnostic and Statistical Manual of Mental Disorders* (DSM). (For a full discussion of CG and its implications for research and treatment of the bereaved, see Stroebe, Schut, & van den Bout, 2013.)

Since the 1960s, bereavement researchers have been interested in identifying individuals who maintain chronically high levels of grief symptoms that do not abate with time. However, there have been no standard guidelines to determine how therapists should diagnose and treat complications following bereavement. Researchers and clinicians have used a variety of terms to describe the mourning process of these individuals. Some of these terms include *atypical, neurotic, pathological, unresolved, chronic,* and *prolonged* grief (Prigerson, Frank, et al., 1995; Prigerson et al., 2009; Rando, 1993). As Rando has noted, different clinicians have used these terms in different ways, thus impeding communication not only among clinicians, but between clinicians and their clients.

There has been considerable interest in the development of a uniform set of criteria that could be used to diagnose CG (see, e.g., Horowitz et al., 1997), presumably in the interest of providing better treatment for mourners. Over the last 15 years, significant progress has been made in clarifying how CG should be conceptualized and measured. One way of conceptualizing CG has been proposed by Prigerson and her associates (e.g., Jacobs, Mazure, & Prigerson, 2000; Prigerson, Maciejewski, et al., 1995; Prigerson et al., 1999; for reviews, see Lichtenthal, Cruess, & Prigerson, 2004; Prigerson, Vanderwerker, & Maciejewski, 2008; Zhang et al., 2006). In a ground-breaking program of research, these investigators have focused on the development of diagnostic criteria to identify bereaved individuals who exhibit intense and prolonged distress and thus would be candidates for clinical intervention. Drawing from the opinions of experts as well as epidemiological and clinical research, Prigerson and colleagues have identified a unique pattern of symptoms that they call *prolonged grief disorder* (PGD).[1] They maintain that these symptoms are associated with enduring mental and physical health problems that are typically slow to resolve, and that can persist for years if left untreated.

Prigerson and colleagues (2009) have also developed a scale to measure PGD, and have devoted considerable effort to establishing its reliability and validity. To meet criteria for PGD, an individual must experience intense yearning or longing for the deceased, either daily or to a disabling degree. In addition, she must have five or more of the following symptoms, and these must be experienced daily, or to a disabling degree: feeling stunned, dazed, or shocked by the death; avoiding reminders of the reality of the loss; having trouble accepting the death; having difficulty trusting others; feeling bitterness or anger related to the loss; experiencing difficulty moving on with life; experiencing confusion about one's role in life or a diminished sense of self; feeling that life is unfulfilling, empty, or meaningless since the loss; and feeling numb (absence of emotion) since the loss. These symptoms must cause clinically significant impairment or dysfunction in social, occupational, or other important roles, and a diagnosis should not be made until at least 6 months have elapsed since the death.

Several other criteria sets have been proposed for CG (see Shear, Simon, et al., 2011, for a review). Shear, Simon, and colleagues (2011) identified three symptoms not included in Prigerson's criteria: suicidal thinking and behavior; rumination about the circumstances or consequences of the death; and physical and emotional activation when one is exposed to reminders. Except for these symptoms, there is considerable overlap between the two sets of criteria.

Virtually all of the empirical work on CG has focused on these two sets of criteria. However, it must be noted that there are other ways of conceptualizing CG. For instance, CG can be manifested in a variety of symptoms or syndromes, or as a diagnosable mental or physical disorder (e.g., PTSD, irritable bowel syndrome; Rando, 1993, 2013). Recently, a panel of experts identified several types of grief-related syndromes that, in their judgment, reflect CG and warrant further research and consideration. These included, but were not limited to, delayed grief, inhibited grief, and other forms of chronic grief that can be differentiated from PGD (Rando et al., 2012).

For the remainder of this section, the reader should be aware that when we are talking about CG, we are focusing on research that has been conducted primarily using PGD (or the

---

[1]More recently, Prigerson and colleagues (2009) have referred to complicated grief as *prolonged grief disorder* (PGD). The term *complicated grief* (CG) is more commonly used in the literature. For the purpose of clarity, we choose to use the latter term except when we are discussing the work of Prigerson's group.

Shear model), mentioned above. To the extent that a therapist is working with different forms of CG, the research cited below may be less applicable.

Research indicates that CG symptoms form a unified cluster and that they are distinct from depression, anxiety, or PTSD. For example, feeling sad and blue is characteristic of depression but not of CG, and hyperarousal is characteristic of PTSD but not of CG (Bonanno et al., 2007). Treatments for depression or PTSD are not effective for intense and prolonged grief symptoms. In fact, available evidence indicates that antidepressant medication has little impact on the symptoms associated with CG (Zhang et al., 2006). Consequently, if persons with CG symptoms are diagnosed with depression or PTSD rather than CG, they may not receive the treatment that is most appropriate. Moreover, until CG or a comparable diagnostic category is given formal recognition as a mental disorder in the DSM, clients with CG symptoms who do not meet criteria for another diagnosis may not receive insurance reimbursement for their treatment.[2]

With its focus on specific criteria for identifying those with PGD, Prigerson's program of research laid the groundwork for research on the physical and psychological ramifications of CG. Studies suggest that the prevalence of CG among individuals who have lost a loved one is between 10 and 20%. Symptoms of CG typically last for several years. They predict morbidity (e.g., suicidal thoughts and behaviors, incidence of cardiac events, high blood pressure), adverse health behaviors (e.g., increased alcohol consumption and use of tobacco), and impairments in the quality of life (e.g., loss of energy) (for reviews, see Boelen & Prigerson, 2013; Prigerson et al., 2009; Zhang et al., 2006). As a result, it is critically important that those with CG be diagnosed and treated. Interestingly, bereaved people with CG are significantly less likely to seek professional services

---

[2]There was considerable interest among bereavement researchers and practitioners in including CG as a diagnostic category in the DSM-5 (Boelen & Prigerson, 2013; Shear, Simon, et al., 2011). As Boelen and Prigerson (2013) noted, this would have given formal recognition to the significant minority of bereaved individuals who struggle with persistent and debilitating symptoms of grief. It would also have encouraged research on effective interventions and provided a foundation for insurance reimbursement for treatment.

Both the Prigerson and Shear groups gave evidence for inclusion of a diagnosis of either PGD or CG in DSM-5. Despite the strong empirical support in favor of these two approaches, neither was ultimately selected. Instead, the DSM-5 Work Group developed a third criteria set to assess problematic grief reactions, which they have labeled *persistent complex bereavement disorder* (PCBD). The criteria set selected by the Work Group drew several items from the scales developed by Prigerson and by Shear. PCBD also included new items. In addition, it utilizes a different time frame than that of Prigerson or Shear: The condition is diagnosed only if at least 12 months have passed since the death, whereas Prigerson and Shear adopt a 6-month criterion. The criteria set developed by the DSM-5 Work Group also provides the possibility of specifying "with traumatic bereavement," which refers to a death that occurred under traumatic circumstances and adds "persistent distressing preoccupations regarding the traumatic nature of the death" (American Psychiatric Association, 2013, p. 790) to the grief symptoms in the diagnosis. The DSM Work Group decided to include the PCBD criteria for problematic grief in the Conditions for Further Study of the DMS-5, concluding that additional research was necessary.

As Boelen and Prigerson (2013) have noted, there is no empirical evidence that the diagnostic categories developed by the Work Group are reliable and valid. In addition to problems with the approach as a whole, Boelen and Prigerson have identified specific features of the new approach that they regard as problematic. They cite several studies suggesting that a 12-month time frame would result in missed cases of dysfunctional grief, and would also delay the provision of treatment for those who are suffering at 6 months postloss. Moreover, they emphasize that none of the research findings regarding the prevalence, risk factors, and treatment of dysfunctional grief are directly applicable to this new disorder.

By developing a new criteria set not based on research, and then referring the diagnosis for further study, the American Psychiatric Association DSM-5 Work Group has delayed the recognition of a condition that has been well researched by two established groups. In our judgment, this will impede the development of treatment for CG.

than bereaved persons without CG. People with CG may have difficulty mobilizing themselves to go into treatment. Alternatively, they may also avoid treatment because they believe it would be unbearably painful to focus on the loss. Even those who are interested in receiving treatment may have difficulty getting the help they need. Shear, Simon, and colleagues (2011) interviewed over 200 individuals seeking help for CG about their previous treatment experiences. According to these investigators, many patients had "been on treatment seeking odysseys for years" (p. 106). Shear, Simon, and colleagues reported that 85% of their respondents had previously sought treatment for grief, and that many had made multiple attempts to get help.

What is the relation between CG and traumatic bereavement? Both focus on individuals who are unable to move forward, to accept the reality of their loved ones' deaths, or to reinvest in the future. Among the traumatically bereaved, circumstances surrounding the loss (e.g., whether it was sudden or untimely) are critically important. Such characteristics of the loss are not essential risk factors for CG. Instead, researchers posit that vulnerability to CG is rooted primarily in threats to secure attachment. As Zhang and colleagues (2006) have noted, CG "is fundamentally an attachment disturbance" (p. 1195). Most of the other risk factors for CG that are discussed in the literature include person-related factors, such as a family history of mood or anxiety disorders, childhood abuse and neglect, childhood separation anxiety, insecure attachment, and marital closeness (see Shear, Simon, et al., 2011, and Zhang et al., 2006, for reviews).

Despite this focus on person-related variables, researchers have noted increasingly that the circumstances surrounding the death indeed constitute an important risk factor for the development of CG. For example, Shear, Boelen, and Neimeyer (2011) emphasized that CG is more likely to occur among those who experience an "untimely, unexpected, violent or seemingly preventable death" (p. 140). Thus, at this time, it appears that some thinking about CG is placing greater emphasis on the circumstances under which the loss occurs. In fact, some investigators have maintained that CG has two components: *separation distress*, assessed by such factors as yearning and considered the core of CG; and *traumatic distress*, assessed by such factors as feeling shocked or stunned by what has happened (Holland & Neimeyer, 2011).

Yet the traumatically bereaved population faces issues that are not typically encountered by those with CG. Because of the traumatic circumstances under which the death occurred, most survivors of traumatic bereavement will be preoccupied with the issues raised in Chapter 3, such as difficulty accepting the loss, grappling with meaning, questioning their faith, struggling with issues of guilt and blame, and preoccupation with their loved ones' possible suffering. It is critically important that these issues be thoroughly addressed during the course of the treatment. In many instances, this has not been the case in the research on CG or its treatment. Of course, some people with CG will struggle with these issues as well, but in our reading of the literature, they are not as predominant among those with CG as within the traumatic bereavement population. These clients have lost loved ones in deeply shocking ways. The traumatically bereaved population is, by definition, dealing with trauma in addition to grief. This is why our treatment places great emphasis on developing clients' internal and external resources to support trauma processing and facilitate mourning.

TREATMENT FOR PTSD

In contrast to the research on treatments for grief, there is a substantial body of research demonstrating the efficacy of several treatments for PTSD. Given the prevalence of PTSD symptoms among survivors of sudden, traumatic death, this body of work has important implications for the treatment of traumatically bereaved persons. Of course, there are many other reactions to traumatic events besides PTSD symptoms. Elements of complex trauma, such as dissociation, somatization, and affect lability, are also very significant among survivors of traumatic death. Because a traumatic death is a sudden (Type I) rather than a chronic (Type II) stressor (see Terr, 1995, for more on this distinction), however, we focus on PTSD rather than complex trauma responses. We use *PTSD* at times, and *trauma* at other times, to refer to the traumatic stress element within traumatic bereavement.

Below, we first summarize the evidence for PTSD treatment effects among trauma survivors. We then focus our attention on three treatments for PTSD that are particularly relevant to the treatment of traumatic bereavement. Two of these treatments—one developed by Edna Foa and one developed by Patricia Resick—were originally designed to treat survivors of rape (for reviews, see Cahill, Rothbaum, Resick, & Follette, 2009; Riggs, Cahill, & Foa, 2006; Shipherd, Street, & Resick, 2006). The third treatment was developed by Marylene Cloitre for adult survivors of childhood sexual abuse (for a review, see Cloitre & Rosenberg, 2006).

PTSD Treatment Effects

A large number of randomized studies have been conducted to evaluate various treatments for PTSD. Over time, these studies have become increasingly rigorous and methodologically sophisticated. Most of the treatments evaluated in these studies have involved some type of CBT. Several different types of CBT programs have been tested empirically. *Prolonged exposure* (PE; Foa & Rothbaum, 1998) involves imaginal exposure to the traumatic memory and behavioral exposure to reminders of the traumatic event. *Cognitive processing therapy* (CPT; Resick & Schnicke, 1993) involves challenging distorted beliefs and includes a form of PE. In some studies, elements of these treatments have been implemented individually; in others, they have been combined. For example, Cloitre and colleagues (2002) combined an initial phase of training in self-regulation with a second phase that involved exposure.

It should be noted that these studies have not focused specifically on survivors of traumatic death. Many of the treatments were developed for survivors of sexual assault or for war veterans. Some have focused on survivors of a broad array of traumatic experiences, including the deaths of loved ones (see Foa, Keane, Friedman, & Cohen, 2009, for a review). It is our belief that the results of these studies will generalize to those facing the sudden, traumatic death of a loved one. Consequently, we discuss them in some detail.

As treatment research on PTSD has continued to accumulate, a number of meta-analyses have appeared in the literature. Some have focused on the broad array of CBT treatments that are available. For example, Bradley, Greene, Russ, Dutra, and Westen (2005) conducted a meta-analysis of randomized treatment studies for PTSD. The authors reviewed 26 studies focusing on a wide array of traumatic stressors, including violent crime, combat, accidents, rape, and childhood sexual abuse. The vast majority of studies involved some form of CBT (including eye movement desensitization and reprocessing [EMDR]).[3] These treatments were compared with

---

[3]Investigators have begun to explore the application of EMDR to grief. Solomon and Rando (2007) have delineated how EMDR can be utilized within a comprehensive framework for the treatment of grief and mourning. They emphasized that EMDR is not a shortcut to resolution of trauma or movement through the processes of mourning. Clinical observations indicated to Solomon and Rando that a client receiving EMDR goes through the same mourning processes, but perhaps more efficiently because obstacles to successful integration and movement can be processed more efficiently. Solomon and Rando offer specific guidelines for using EMDR within each of the six "R" processes in order to promote adaptive assimilation of the loss of a loved one.

control conditions, some of which involved supportive counseling and some of which were wait-list controls. In examining pre- to posttreatment change among those who received some form of CBT, the authors found a large effect size for these treatments, and a far smaller effect size for supportive or wait-list controls. At the conclusion of the treatment, 67% of those who completed one of the CBT treatment programs no longer met the criteria for PTSD. Bradley and colleagues concluded that based on these results, the treatments produced "substantial improvement for patients with PTSD" (p. 223). Several other reviews have drawn similar conclusions about the efficacy of CBT for PTSD, including the expert consensus guidelines on the treatment of PTSD (Foa, Davidson, & Frances, 1999); the practice guidelines from the International Society for Traumatic Stress Studies (ISTSS; Foa et al., 2009), and a narrative review completed by Harvey, Bryant, and Tarrier (2003). Taken together, these reviews, and the studies on which they are based, provide overwhelming evidence for the efficacy of CBT for PTSD.

This body of work has a great deal to offer those who are treating survivors of traumatic death. We believe that three types of PTSD treatments are critically important: offering PE; challenging distorted beliefs about the traumatic event; and strengthening clients' personal resources (e.g., helping them identify and regulate their feelings) prior to exposure. Below, we first review the evidence in support of these treatment types. Next, we describe how we have drawn from these treatments in developing our treatment approach for traumatic bereavement.

Types of Treatment for PTSD

Prolonged Exposure

Foa and her associates (e.g., Foa, Dancu, et al., 1999; Foa, Zoellner, Feeny, Hembree, & Alvarez-Conrad, 2002) have been involved in a program of research to assess the efficacy of PE in the treatment of rape survivors. The term *exposure therapy* refers to "a treatment strategy for reducing anxiety that involves confronting situations, activities, thoughts, and memories that are feared and avoided even though they are not inherently harmful" (Riggs et al., 2006, p. 65). PE is a treatment involving four components: (1) psychoeducation about trauma and PTSD; (2) breathing retraining; (3) *in vivo* (meaning "in life") exposure to the trauma-related situations that the client fears and avoids; and (4) imaginal exposure that involves repeatedly reviewing memories of the traumatic event. In many studies, each client is asked to make a tape recording of her account of the rape and to listen to it between sessions (for a more detailed description, see Foa & Rothbaum, 1998).

Studies conducted by Foa and her colleagues have provided consistent evidence that PE is a powerful treatment for survivors of rape (for a review, see Riggs et al., 2006). For example, Foa and colleagues (2002) compared PE alone to PE combined with cognitive restructuring and a wait-list control condition. Results showed that both treatment conditions were highly effective in reducing PTSD, as well as alleviating depression and anxiety, in comparison with the wait-list control. Since these studies have been conducted, PE, either alone or in combination with other CBT approaches, has been found to be effective for a wide variety of populations, including survivors of motor vehicle accidents (Blanchard et al., 2003), domestic violence (Aderka, Gillihan, McLean, & Foa, 2013; Kubany, Hill, & Owens, 2003), and physical assault (Foa, Dancu, et al., 1999; Foa et al., 2002).

Powers, Halpern, Ferenschak, Gillihan, and Foa (2010) conducted a meta-analytic review of studies using PE to treat PTSD. Their goal was to determine the effectiveness of PE in comparison to control conditions (wait-list or "psychological placebo"). Analyses showed a large effect of PE in comparison to controls at the conclusion of the study, and a medium to large effect at follow-up. The average PE-treated patient fared better than 86% of patients in control conditions. Powers and colleagues concluded that "PE is a highly effective treatment for PTSD that confers lasting benefits across a wide range of outcomes" (p. 639).

In a narrative review of studies using PE, Sharpless and Barber (2011) concluded that there is more evidence in favor of using PE to treat PTSD than using any other treatment. These investigators further note that PE is one of only two therapies selected by the Department of Veterans Affairs (VA) and the U.S. military for widespread dissemination. Sharpless and Barber point out that the effectiveness of this treatment has been replicated across gender and types of traumatic events.

Cognitive Processing Therapy

A second treatment that has implications for treating traumatically bereaved clients is CPT, developed by Resick and Schnicke (1992, 1993) for the treatment of rape survivors. The PE component of their treatment involves writing accounts of the rape, including thoughts, feelings, and sensory details, and reading the account daily and in session. However, Resick and Schnicke maintain that PE alone may be insufficient to deal with the powerful emotions that rape survivors sometimes experience. One emotion that is quite prevalent among these survivors is guilt. Resick and Schnicke (1993) believe that emotions like guilt and the related self-blame may benefit from a more direct and focused intervention targeting the distorted beliefs that maintain them. Hence CPT combines PE with cognitive therapy. Clients focus on distorted beliefs that underlie guilt and self-blame. They work with the therapist to complete several exercises, such as "faulty thinking pattern" sheets, in order to challenge these erroneous beliefs.

In developing CPT, Resick and Schnicke (1996) drew from the work of Pearlman and colleagues (McCann & Pearlman, 1990b; Pearlman & Saakvitne, 1995), mentioned in earlier chapters, in identifying disrupted beliefs or schemas (safety, trust, control, esteem, and intimacy) particularly sensitive to trauma. They conducted a randomized study in which they compared CPT with the best available empirically tested treatment, which was PE, and a minimal-attention wait-list condition. The target population in this study was female survivors of rape. The findings indicated that both treatments were highly effective and were superior to the control condition. Results of the two therapies were similar, except that CPT produced better scores on some of the scales measuring guilt. It should be noted, however, that far more research has been conducted on the efficacy of PE than on CPT. In their review, Sharpless and Barber (2011) state that the treatment has very strong empirical support. These investigators also note that CPT is the other psychological treatment chosen to be utilized by the military and the VA.

Further Comments on PE and CPT

The treatments described above, PE and CPT, both involve exposure to reminders of the traumatic event. There is consistent evidence that exposure plays a critical role in reducing symptoms among individuals with PTSD. More studies support the use of exposure than any other treatment.

To summarize, there is a striking difference between the scientific literature on treatment for grief and treatment for PTSD. As discussed above, there is weak evidence that grief therapy, as it is practiced today, is effective overall in reducing symptoms (although there is stronger evidence of its effectiveness for highly distressed persons). In contrast, there is overwhelming evidence for the effectiveness for such treatments as PE and CPT for the treatment of PTSD. Taken together, the studies on the efficacy of PE and CPT demonstrate that in most cases, respondents improve on a variety of measures. For example, Resick and colleagues (2008) found that female survivors of interpersonal violence with PTSD showed marked improvement following CPT not only in PTSD, but in depression, anxiety, anger, guilt, shame, and cognitive distortions. There is also clear evidence that in many cases, these treatments result in enduring changes. For example, Resick, Williams, Suvak, Monson, and Gradus (2012) conducted a long-term follow-up of rape victims with extensive histories of trauma, who were previously treated with CPT or PE. These respondents were assessed 5–10 years after the original study. They showed lasting changes in PTSD and related symptoms.

In the past few years, books have been written for clinicians who wish to integrate these evidence-based treatments for PTSD into their practice (see, e.g., Foa, Hembree, & Rothbaum, 2007; Foa et al., 2009). The latter book focuses specifically on the use of PE, and provides specific and detailed suggestions about how to implement it. Nevertheless, many investigators have commented that despite overwhelming evidence of its effectiveness, practicing clinicians rarely implement exposure-based treatments (see Cahill, Foa, Hembree, Marshall, & Nacash, 2006, for a more detailed discussion). Becker, Zayfert, and Anderson (2004) reported that only 17% of the sample of 207 psychologists they interviewed reported using exposure treatment for PTSD. These researchers note several possible reasons why clinicians may be reluctant to use exposure. Some may be concerned about patient dropout rates. In a study of the efficacy of PE in a clinical practice, the treatment completion rate was only 28% (Zayfert et al., 2005). This rate encompassed patients electing not to start the therapy, as well as those dropping out prematurely. Some therapists may fear the intensity of emotions that exposure can generate. Others may be concerned that such treatments may exacerbate symptoms and possibly retraumatize the clients. As one therapist indicated while treating a woman who had been brutally attacked and then raped, "I was overwhelmed by her feelings of profound anger and shame as she recounted what happened. My initial impulse was to steer her away from her painful feelings and disturbing memories. I thought that if she continued to describe the incident, it might make her feel worse, that she might have a flashback or something. And to be honest, I had a hard time staying with her as she continued her graphic description of what happened."

Research by Foa and colleagues (2002) has demonstrated that only a small minority of respondents show an exacerbation of symptoms, and that these respondents are nonetheless likely to experience treatment gains. Moreover, many potential clients prefer exposure over medication. When asked to choose among treatments for PTSD or when asked to rank-order their preferences, clients rate exposure therapy as one of the most preferred treatment options (Jaeger, Echiverri, Zoellner, Post, & Feeny, 2010).

Strengthening Self Capacities

As described earlier, PE and CPT play a central role in our treatment for traumatic bereavement. Our approach is also designed to strengthen peoples' self capacities so that they will be able to tolerate exposure work. A third important program of research has provided clear evidence that strengthening self capacities is critically important in treating trauma (Cloitre et al., 2002). This program, developed for survivors of childhood sexual abuse, has two phases. The initial phase focuses on *skills training in affect and interpersonal regulation* (STAIR). For example, the therapist teaches the client to identify and label his feelings, use positive self-statements, and identify and challenge maladaptive cognitions. The second phase of this treatment, the exposure phase, was adapted from Foa's PE treatment for PTSD in rape survivors (Foa, Rothbaum, Riggs, & Murdock, 1991). Cloitre and her associates (2002) reasoned that the first phase, STAIR, would strengthen the development of the therapeutic relationship and facilitate clients' ability to tolerate and benefit from PE.

Cloitre and colleagues (2002) conducted a study that provided clear support for their ideas. The study focused on women who were sexually abused as children. Compared to wait-list controls, women who completed the treatment program showed a dramatic drop in PTSD symptoms. At the end of the treatment, 75% of the respondents no longer met criteria for PTSD. Clients in the treatment condition showed improvements in many different areas, including affect regulation skills and interpersonal problems. Similarly impressive results were obtained in a more recent study (Cloitre et al., 2010). These investigators compared STAIR followed by PE to two control conditions: supportive counseling followed by PE, and skills training followed by PE. They found that the STAIR/PE group was more likely to achieve sustained and complete PTSD remission relative to the other conditions. In this study, dropout rate was lowest among respondents who were in the treatment that combined skills training and PE. Respondents in the two control groups were more likely to drop out of the study. This study provides compelling evidence that including STAIR as part of the treatment enables survivors to derive maximum benefit from exposure work. This work has additional relevance to those in the traumatically bereaved population who demonstrate difficulties with affect regulation.

INTEGRATING GRIEF AND TRAUMA TREATMENT RESEARCH

It is evident that a treatment is needed for traumatic bereavement that integrates elements from both grief and trauma therapies. What are the implications of the research reviewed above for that treatment? Although the overall findings from the literature on treatment following the death of a loved one are disappointing, there is a clear indication that grief treatments focused on people who are highly distressed are likely to be helpful. Unfortunately, prior research on treatment for grief provides little guidance regarding the elements of treatment that should be included or how these should be implemented. In contrast, the treatment research on PTSD has identified many specific treatment components that are effective in alleviating PTSD symptoms. Until recently, however, these treatments have not been evaluated among respondents coping with sudden, traumatic death.

The fields of trauma and grief, for the most part, have developed independently of one another (see, e.g., Brom & Kleber, 2000; Figley, 1998; Figley, Bride, & Mazza, 1997; Malkinson, Rubin, & Witztum, 2000). People from both fields have commented on the separation of these two disciplines. According to Brom and Kleber (2000), for example, trauma and grief research have much to offer one another, but this cross-fertilization has not occurred. They indicated that neither field has benefited from the existing body of empirical research in the other.

A few authors in each field have recognized the importance of drawing from work on both trauma and loss in treating survivors of sudden, traumatic death. Pioneers in the integration of these two fields include Eth and Pynoos (1985, 1994), Green and colleagues (2000), Nader (1997), and Lindy (1986) in traumatology; and Raphael (1986), Redmond (1989), Rynearson (2001), Rynearson and McCreery (1993), and Shear and colleagues (2005) in grief. Green and colleagues (2000) was one of the first people to emphasize that the mode of death is a critically important issue in determining the psychological ramifications of the loss. Rynearson (2001; Rynearson & McCreery, 1993) has focused on the recurrent images of the unfolding horror that typically accompany deaths by homicide, and has argued that these may be misinterpreted as pathological grief. Raphael (1983; Raphael & Martinek, 1997) has described how the circumstances surrounding the death influence the nature of the bereavement response and dictate the type of treatment approach that may be most effective. In addition, she has discussed the disturbing images that often accompany a traumatic death, and has stressed the importance of integrating these images within grief therapy.

Despite these and other contributions, little headway has been made in the development of theoretical or clinical approaches that integrate research on trauma and grief. As Stroebe, Schut, and Finkenauer (2001) concluded over a decade ago, "Much work still needs to be done to pinpoint the exact differences and similarities between trauma, bereavement, and traumatic bereavement" (p. 198). According to Neria and Litz (2004), the phenomenology, clinical symptoms, clinical needs, and risk factors associated with traumatic death have yet to be studied systematically. As Brom and Kleber (2000) have observed, "In clinical practice, we still encounter therapists who consider themselves fit to treat only one of the fields of extreme distress (i.e., bereavement or trauma) and not others" (p. 60). These investigators also emphasize that even therapists who draw from both treatment approaches often assume that grief processing and trauma processing are separate, and thus implement them sequentially rather than integrating them.

The research on complicated grief, reviewed earlier in this chapter, emphasizes the importance of developing interventions for mourners who are at high risk for a poor outcome. In a landmark study, Shear and her associates (Shear & Frank, 2006; Shear et al., 2005) did just that. They drew from research on trauma, as well as from their expertise on grief, to develop a multifaceted treatment for people with complicated grief. They compared this intervention, which they call *complicated grief therapy* (CGT), to a more standard treatment for depression (interpersonal therapy). Shear and colleagues' treatment starts with a phase designed to strengthen the therapeutic alliance and explore current and past relationships, including the relationship with the deceased. The client also tells the story of the death in this phase. In addition, this phase focuses on helping the client to understand the mourning process. Drawing from the dual-process model of loss described earlier in this chapter (see, e.g., Stroebe & Schut, 1999), the therapist explains that grief typically oscillates between two distinct processes: thinking about the death and its ramifications; and avoiding or distracting oneself from grief and focusing on thoughts or activities that are restorative. The therapist explains that the restorative process involves work on future goals. The clients are asked to identify things they would like to be doing if they were no longer grieving, and to meet one or more of these goals each week.

Next, there is a middle phase, which includes imaginal exposure and cognitive processing. In this phase, the therapist gives the client exercises to help in confronting avoided situations. The client is also asked to tell her story into a tape recorder and play it back during the week, and to participate in an imaginal conversation with the deceased. Work on the client's goals continues during this period.

In the third and final phase of treatment, the therapist and client discuss plans for reinforcing treatment gains and continuing progress. The therapist assists the client in developing concrete plans for reaching her goals. The client is also encouraged to reengage in meaningful relationships. Therapist and client also discuss the client's feelings about ending the treatment. The average length of the treatment is 19 weeks.

Shear and colleagues' study revealed that although both the CGT and interpersonal therapy groups showed improvement in symptoms, there was a higher response rate and a faster time to response for those in the CGT group. This study suggests that integrating treatment elements developed to target symptoms of grief with those designed to address PTSD is highly effective in treating complicated grief. (For a more detailed discussion of treatments for complicated grief, including an updated version of Shear and colleagues' CGT, see Shear, Boelen, & Neimeyer, 2011.)

Similar findings have been obtained by a number of investigators who drew from the PTSD treatment literature to develop a treatment for complicated grief (see, e.g., Boelen, 2006; Boelen, de Keijser, van den Hout, & van den Bout, 2007; Boelen et al., 2006; for a review, see Boelen, van den Hout, & van den Bout, 2013; Wagner, Knaevelsrud, & Maercker, 2006). In each of these studies, the authors developed a treatment that used exposure and cognitive processing. In fact, in a recent meta-analysis of 14 randomized controlled studies of treatment for complicated grief, the treatments were found to be effective. The authors maintain that during the follow-up period, the positive effect of the interventions actually increased (Wittouck, Autreve, Jaegere, Portzky, & van Heeringen, 2011).

In an innovative approach to combining grief treatment with exposure-based and cognitive processing elements, Wagner and colleagues (2006) developed a treatment for complicated grief that was designed to be offered on the Internet. Bereaved individuals were randomly assigned to a treatment group or to a wait-list control condition. The intervention had three components. The first component involved deliberate exposure to bereavement cues. Respondents were asked to write about the circumstances of the death, and to express their thoughts about the event in as much detail as possible. The second component focused on cognitive restructuring. Participants were given exercises to help them develop new perspectives on the death and how it came about. They were taught how to question biased automatic thinking, such as guilt or self-blame. In the third phase, each participant was asked to write a letter to the deceased, and also to describe plans for coping with the loss at the present time and in the future. Participants in the treatment group showed significantly greater improvement on symptoms of intrusion, avoidance, maladaptive behavior, and general psychopathology. These improvements were maintained at follow-up, 3 months after loss. Kersting, Kroker, Schlicht, Baust, and Wagner (2011) obtained similar results in a study of parents who had lost a child during pregnancy. (For a review of Internet-based interventions for traumatic stress–related mental health problems, see Amstadter, Broman-Fulks, Zinzow, Ruggiero, & Cercone, 2009; Wagner, 2013.) As these interventions become more widely available, they may constitute a good alternative for mourners who cannot afford, or for other reasons do not have access to, psychotherapy.

Taken together, these studies provide strong evidence that two elements from the PTSD literature, PE and CPT, can play a central role in the treatment of complicated grief. We certainly believe that they will be effective with traumatic bereavement clients. As noted above, however, the treatment would be more effective for these clients if two additional elements were included. The first entails augmenting the clients' personal resources. The second involves including content that has direct relevance for survivors of sudden, traumatic loss, but not necessarily for clients with complicated grief. This would include discussion of the themes that are prevalent among these survivors, such as struggling with guilt or self-blame, or feeling betrayed by God, difficulty accepting the loss, grappling with meaning, and preoccupation with the deceased's suffering (see Chapter 3).

CLINICAL INTEGRATION

Because Harriet was putting so much energy into avoiding painful reminders of Gwen, she was unable to live in the present. This precluded opportunities to process her grief, engage with life, and move forward in ways that might ultimately prove fulfilling. Her children sensed how much she missed their other mom; their hearts broke for her, adding to their own grief. Partly in order to relieve her own heartbreak over losing two parents—which was how it felt to her—the oldest daughter, Amy, begged her mother to see a psychologist. After several requests, Harriet agreed. Amy accompanied her to the first session and was surprised when the psychologist invited both of them in. He asked who wanted to start, and Amy jumped in.

"My mom's been through a lot after witnessing Gwen's death, which was really traumatic for her. Now, over a year later, she seems frozen by her own grief—by the grief she's keeping in and not sharing with anyone," said Amy to the psychologist. "Can you help her?"

"What do you think of this, Harriet?" asked Dr. Joyce Lake.

"I think Amy's always had a way with words. *Frozen* is right. And *traumatic* is right also. My daughter can explain how I feel better than I can," Harriet sighed.

"Can you tell me a bit about Gwen?" Joyce addressed this question to Harriet.

"She was my light." Harriet, seemingly surprised and clearly moved, was happy to answer. "I mean that almost literally. My world had been dark before I met her. I was isolated and withdrawn. I had a difficult upbringing—an abusive father—and Gwen showed me I could enjoy life. She was really funny. And very social: always meeting people and happy to strike up a conversation. I'm having a hard time surviving without her."

"Well, you're doing well in here." Joyce smiled at both women, noting their resemblance to one another. Harriet sighed again, but this time she was experiencing the first whisper of relief she had felt in months.

In the next session, which Amy again attended with her mom, Joyce noted, "We've just begun talking, and already you have touched on some important themes. It seems possible that you may be suffering from *traumatic bereavement*. This is a term that describes the aftermath of losing a person you love in a traumatic way. A traumatic death is usually untimely and unexpected, as Gwen's was, and such deaths are often marked by other traumatic elements. In your case, these included feeling powerless while you waited for help to arrive, watching the paramedics swoop in to work on your partner in your own home, hearing Gwen gasping for breath—as you described to me when we first spoke by phone. When you're dealing with grief *plus* traumatic stress, your resources are likely to be used up. Without resources, it's hard to process the trauma, and the inability to process trauma gets in the way of mourning. The result is often a feeling of being really stuck—or frozen, as Amy so aptly described in our last session."

"I recently put our house on the market," said Harriet slowly. "I'm hoping that might help me to unfreeze, but I don't know. It's hard to have any hope that anything will work."

Joyce heard Harriet's hesitancy within this comment, as well as a possible question underneath the hesitancy: "Can you help me?" Joyce decided to address this. "Selling the house may help. It may not. If you decide to work with me, one of the things I'll talk a lot about is *adaptation*." Joyce stressed this word. "As human beings, we are constantly adapting to our circumstances in a way that allows us to meet our needs. For example, maybe Amy doesn't like to work, but she might love to spend money." (As Joyce said this, Amy and Harriet smiled for the first time since they had come in.) "She therefore decides to work part-time so she can spend some money. It's a compromise. Maybe the compromise works well; maybe it doesn't. One of the things we would do together is to explore how you're adapting to Gwen's death and ask how well these adaptations are working. If they're not working well, we'll see if we can add some more choices. We could look at whether selling the house would be a useful adaptation. Can I give you another example?"

Harriet nodded yes.

"My guess is that withdrawing from friends isn't helping very much. It seems as though it's difficult to be social without Gwen by your side, but I think some part of you does want the satisfaction that comes from being with friends. Gwen gave this to you: an opening up of your social life. Remember, she turned the light on? She *was* the light. One way of honoring both her and you would be to learn to do this for yourself. You depended on Gwen for this, and research shows us that depending on a spouse in such a way makes it more difficult when she's gone. It makes sense, right? I think you might be able to adapt and do this for yourself."

Amy looked at her mom, who looked back at her. Each saw the reflection of a tear in the other's eye. Joyce understood something that Harriet did not have words for, and with that, an alliance was beginning to form.

CONCLUDING REMARKS

Joyce knew that helping Harriet to adapt to her partner's death would require an integration of interventions. She knew she would need to complete some exposure work with Harriet, and in preparing to do so, she hoped to discover any beliefs Harriet held that might prove to be maladaptive. Harriet's belief that she couldn't be social without Gwen—a belief that Joyce questioned—appeared in their first session together. Throughout their work, they would discover and address others; they would move through the sometimes difficult process of exposure; and they would concretely explore the "R" processes of mourning—all in an attempt to assist Harriet to accommodate Gwen's death so that she could reinvest in life.

Throughout this chapter, we have pointed to research supporting specific interventions and approaches to treating both grief and traumatic stress. From our review of this research, and from our own theoretical knowledge and clinical experience, we have concluded that integrating treatment elements targeting grief (facilitating mourning) with those targeting traumatic stress (processing trauma), while shoring up a person's coping strategies and support (building resources), is the most effective means of helping those suffering from traumatic bereavement. We now turn our attention to designing and implementing such a treatment approach.

PART IV

GUIDELINES FOR IMPLEMENTING THE TREATMENT APPROACH

CHAPTER 8

Client Assessment

Barbara entered the therapist's waiting room nervously. She walked with a limp—a continuous reminder of the car accident that had injured her 4 years ago and killed her daughter, Janie. Their car had been hit from behind by a sleep-deprived truck driver. As Barbara took a seat, she noticed that her hands were shaking, her heart pounding, and her thoughts racing. This anxious state was not new to Barbara; neither was seeking help. With the support of Alcoholics Anonymous (AA), Barbara had been sober for 7 years prior to Janie's death. After the accident, she stepped up her program of recovery, attending meetings at least three times per week. Still, not a single day passed when Barbara didn't struggle against the urge to drink. She had relapsed twice in the time since the accident.

Barbara had sought out other support as well. She attended a support group for bereaved parents for about 3 months. She met with a therapist for another few months. She also spent time online in a chat room for people who had lost children. Although she received some help from each of these sources of support, the accident that stole her daughter still haunted and debilitated her, and left her wishing that she rather than Janie had died. Barbara spoke this wish aloud once she was seated across from Donald, her new therapist: "Why couldn't it have been me who died that day? How can I go on living knowing that Janie is gone forever?" She added in a whisper, "Janie would have turned 16 next month."

There are many reasons to conduct a thorough assessment of every client entering psychotherapy. Assessment is of even greater importance with a population as vulnerable as those who may be experiencing traumatic bereavement. Careful evaluation will allow you as the therapist to ensure that this is the right treatment approach for a particular client at this time, facilitate the formulation of a treatment plan, and yield the diagnosis or diagnoses required for insurance payment. Given the possibility (as for all mourners) of past trauma, past loss, mental health issues, or a troubled or very dependent relationship with the deceased, those experiencing traumatic bereavement may present with a complicated combination of problems. Beyond these issues, sudden, traumatic death produces a host of challenging symptoms and responses even in individuals who have no history of trauma, loss, or excessive dependence on their loved ones. It is imperative to understand both the client's resources and the client's needs in order to apply the treatment effectively. The more care that goes into the assessment and planning phase, the more the client will feel hopeful, safe, and understood, and the greater the likelihood of a successful treatment will be. In addition, a careful assessment will equip you to adapt as new information or problems arise, crises erupt, the client develops new skills, and so forth.

There is an ethical imperative to understand the client's needs before proceeding with this treatment. Without adequate information about who this client is, how he manages memories and feelings, and what resources he possesses for dealing with distress, there is a genuine risk of endangering the client. Without such a foundation, the treatment may retraumatize the client; solidify the client's avoidance; shame or humiliate him; or use his valuable therapy time, money, and motivation to no avail. It can be difficult for people to go to psychotherapy for the first time, and if their first experience is a failed therapy, they may never return. In addition, it is essential that clients have adequate resources to support the challenging work of this treatment approach. Assessment is vital to these concerns.

This chapter provides an overview of areas for assessment with traumatically bereaved clients. We do not address in depth general assessment issues that any therapist would consider, such as the client's safety and the fit between the client and therapist. We encourage you to spend time on assessment with each client, addressing the issues identified below in whatever style best suits your client's clinical needs and your own expertise. Throughout the assessment process, your clinical judgment is your best tool for gathering, interpreting, and using the information you collect.

An additional important role of assessment is in measuring progress. Such assessment can provide feedback to both you and the client about whether and how the client is progressing. This can help shape subsequent treatment and provide hope to the client. In addition, if the client should leave the treatment before it is complete, midcourse assessments may provide some clues about the reasons.

APPROPRIATENESS OF THIS TREATMENT APPROACH FOR A PARTICULAR CLIENT

This integrated approach is designed for people who have experienced the sudden, traumatic death of a loved one. By this, we mean a death that occurs suddenly and is characterized by one or more of the risk factors described in Chapter 5 (e.g., it was untimely, it is viewed as preventable). The death must overwhelm the person's capacity to manage her thoughts, feelings, and behavioral responses to the death and related losses. The treatment can help a person with one or more of the following indicators:

- The person needs to process *both* trauma and grief.
  - Trauma, as evidenced by symptoms of PTSD (such as intrusive thoughts, avoidance of reminders of the event, cognitive and mood alterations, and physiological hyperarousal) or other trauma responses (such as dissociation, loss of meaning, affect dysregulation, somatization, impaired concentration, and disrupted relationships—complex trauma adaptations that have been described by Pelcovitz et al., 1997, and Courtois & Ford, 2009).
  - Grief, as evidenced by such symptoms as shock, sadness, yearning for the deceased, difficulty accepting the loss, avoidance of reminders of the loss, anger, feeling numb or empty inside, and suicidal thoughts (for further information about grief symptoms, see Prigerson et al., 2009; Rando, 1993; Shear, Simon, et al., 2011; Worden, 2009).

- The person feels stalled or stuck and is having difficulty fulfilling role obligations (e.g., as parent, as worker) or moving forward with life (e.g., making friends, pursuing new interests; see Prigerson et al., 2009).

- The person is experiencing relentless, debilitating automatic thoughts or disrupted cognitive schemas, which can be assessed with the Trauma and Attachment Belief Scale (Pearlman, 2003), for example.

Readiness for This Treatment Approach

This treatment approach requires clients to participate actively in the processes of mourning a traumatic death. It requires that clients engage with trauma material, identify and challenge problematic cognitions that interfere with mourning, and connect with internal experiences that can include a host of very challenging feelings.

As is the case in all therapies, decisions regarding appropriateness and fit of a particular approach are both clinical and ethical in nature. You must consider whether a particular client has the ability both to participate in and to benefit from the treatment. One of the advantages of this treatment approach is that even if you decide that the treatment approach as a whole is inappropriate for a given client, you can utilize certain aspects of it effectively. For example, Dr. Hogarth decided to use only the resource-building interventions and activities, with an emphasis on self capacities work, with his client, Ms. Lestor, who reported dissociation (e.g., persistent inability to recall activities performed within a given day, difficulty paying attention to time, lack of connection between thoughts and feelings) during the intake process. The treatment approach requires engagement with trauma material, and effective engagement requires an ability to stay grounded in one's internal experience (i.e., the opposite of dissociation). Dr. Hogarth concluded that Ms. Lestor would not be able to participate in the treatment at this time, that she would not be likely to benefit from it, and that it might actually lead to increased dissociation. However, he felt that a focus on building self capacities could greatly help this client, and that with such help, she might become an appropriate candidate for other aspects of the treatment in time.

As a second example, Dr. Hogarth was contacted by Mr. Waters, whose best friend had been murdered within the past few weeks. At the end of their initial session, Dr. Hogarth concluded that Mr. Waters was not a candidate for this treatment. Recall that the treatment is designed for survivors who are stuck in the process of mourning—in other words, unable to engage actively in one or more of the essential tasks of mourning. This young man was still experiencing some shock over this sudden death. Mr. Waters was grieving, but had not yet moved into a process of actively attempting to accommodate this loss (i.e., mourning). Furthermore, he was not yet aware of the various secondary losses he would experience, including how this death would violate his assumptive world. Launching into this treatment approach with Mr. Waters at this time would have been premature. However, he did benefit from a supportive therapeutic relationship and from psychoeducation about grief, mourning, and trauma—both important elements of this treatment approach. Four months after his friend's death, Mr. Waters's initial grief subsided, although he had unsuccessfully attempted to accommodate the loss. He found himself haunted by the traumatic circumstances of the death, stuck in self-blame, and overwhelmed with rage. At this time, Dr. Hogarth determined that the treatment approach as a whole might benefit him.

As a third example, Ms. Arnold, an employed mother with three children, lost her wife, Jennifer, in an automobile accident. About 6 months later, she went to see a therapist, Ms.

Rodriguez, who thought that she seemed to be an appropriate candidate for this treatment approach. In the assessment process, Ms. Arnold demonstrated an ability to tolerate strong affect (she stated that she cried often, but was usually able to calm herself and minimally continue to fulfill her responsibilities as worker and mother). She reported being unable to remember Jennifer without being consumed by memories of the accident; and spoke of experiencing overwhelming self-blame. In other words, she demonstrated the sort of distress targeted by the treatment, and at least the minimum capacities needed to engage with the treatment interventions. However, she canceled the first therapy session and arrived 15 minutes late for the next one. As she and her therapist talked, it became clear that Ms. Arnold had very little support in taking care of her three young children, and thus that child care issues were already interfering with the treatment in the opening sessions. Ms. Rodriguez decided to modify the treatment approach and to address the need for increased social support as a prerequisite for moving into any exposure work. As it turned out, Ms. Arnold was harboring some problematic beliefs about asking for help, which prevented her from seeking the support she would need to move forward in mourning Jennifer's death. A focus on augmenting social support, and using cognitive processing to address obstacles to this, were effective adaptations of the treatment approach for this particular client.

During this same time period, Ms. Rodriguez was deciding whether to use this treatment approach with Mr. Hyun, a 42-year-old man whose wife had died in a fire at her office building a year earlier. Mr. Hyun was having great difficulty parenting his teenage son and daughter, due to symptoms of severe depression. Since his wife's death, he was also experiencing insomnia, symptoms of PTSD, and constant exhaustion that interfered with even simple daily tasks. During his initial session with Ms. Rodriguez, Mr. Hyun reported feeling guilty about his inability to be more present for his son and daughter, and his tone and language suggested severe self-criticism about the state he was in. Ms. Rodriguez had two specific concerns in her assessment of Mr. Hyun: (1) Did he have the physical energy needed to attend appointments, engage with independent activities, and participate within sessions? (2) If Mr. Hyun were to feel worse before he felt better within the therapy, would he be able to continue so as to experience the lifting of symptoms that Ms. Rodriguez believed was possible for him? She concluded that this treatment approach offered the potential for Mr. Hyun to feel better; she thought carefully about how to maximize the likelihood of his success in therapy; and she sketched out a treatment plan that heavily emphasized resource building, both initially and throughout the treatment. She believed that her supportive connection with Mr. Hyun would help to contain his anxiety as he confronted painful memories of his wife's death through exposure work, which would in turn help to alleviate the PTSD symptoms. She also knew that she would target his self-criticism with cognitive restructuring techniques, believing that this would diminish his depression. Finally, Ms. Rodriguez referred Mr. Hyun for a medication consultation, in order to establish whether an antidepressant and/or a temporary sleep aid might be appropriate.

As this last example illustrates, it is not necessarily the severity of symptoms that rules out a person as a candidate for this treatment. Rather, the guiding question is whether the supports available within the treatment will enable the client to engage in the tasks of mourning and exposure while remaining grounded in his experience.

The rationale for each of the treatment elements provided in Chapters 10, 11, and 12, along with the material presented in the remainder of this chapter, will help you think through the questions of whether a survivor can participate actively in this treatment and whether it can address her distress effectively. With regard to the former, one of the main concerns involves the client's ability to tolerate exposure work. Clients who are currently living in a dangerous situation (such as a violent relationship), abusing substances, or experiencing extreme dissociation need to work with you or with other clinicians or agencies to address those concerns before pursuing the exposure activities outlined in this treatment. Clients who are mildly dissociative or emotionally numb may benefit from a stronger emphasis on the strategies for coping with emotion and other resource-building strategies described in Chapter 10. A foundational assumption of this treatment approach is that a client will only be able to address and process painful thoughts, feelings, and memories if she has the internal and interpersonal capacities, stability, and coping strategies to do so fully and consciously. The approach is designed to assess, build, and utilize the resources required to engage in processing work. Clinical judgment and the art of psychotherapy come into play as you assess your clients' needs for resource development.

When an individual's current status, behaviors, or needs seem to be in conflict with the treatment (e.g., the client is actively overusing alcohol, in the midst of a work-related crisis, or unable to use the written handout materials because of limited English literacy or for other reasons), you should use your judgment about whether to adapt the treatment and proceed, or to abandon it and try a different approach. It is crucial to provide the client with a thorough description of what the therapy entails, including both the opportunity to learn and practice new coping strategies and the rationale and process of exposure. This therapy is a collaborative process, and the client's thoughts and feelings about his readiness to engage in all the aspects of this work are the most important sources of information to consider in designing your therapy approach. Clients often respond to the description of aspects of the therapy (from examining thoughts about the loss to engaging in imaginal exposure) with a mixture of anxiety and an intuitive understanding that avoiding thoughts and feelings associated with the loss does not alleviate them. The natural reluctance to confront those thoughts and feelings highlights the role of psychoeducation about avoidance. You can base the decision about how to proceed on your assessment of the client's resources (including typical coping behaviors and use of social support) and a thorough evaluation of current risk potential (including history of suicidal or other potentially dangerous behavior).

PROGRESSION THROUGH THE SIX "R" PROCESSES

Because the treatment will foster movement through Rando's (1993) six "R" processes, you will also need to understand where each client is in that journey at the outset of treatment. We refer you to Rando's (1993) volume *Treatment of Complicated Mourning*—particularly the appendix containing the Grief and Mourning Status Interview and Inventory (GAMSII), and Chapter 6 of that book, which provides guidance in using the GAMSII. Part III of the GAMSII is a structured interview designed specifically to assess the client's mourning processes to date and to identify areas that need to be addressed in treatment. Some of the issues addressed in this comprehensive inventory include the following:

- Circumstances surrounding the death
- Nature and meaning of what has been lost
- The mourner's reactions to the death

- Changes in the mourner's life since the death
- The mourner's relationship to the deceased
- The mourner's self-assessment of how well she is coping with the loss
- The mourner's comprehension of the mourning processes and her expectations regarding the mourning process

In addition to assessing the client's mourning processes, the GAMSII can assess relevant demographic information (Part I) and provide a comprehensive evaluation of the client's history, mental status, and selected premorbid personality characteristics (Part II). Rando (1993) has granted permission for therapists to reproduce the GAMSII for clinical use.

RESOURCES

Both a sudden, traumatic death and this treatment approach, particularly the exposure component, are likely to elicit strong affect. For this reason, supportive resources (self capacities or feelings skills; social support; coping skills; the ability to manage bereavement-specific issues; values and goals; and meaning and spirituality) constitute the foundation for the treatment. In this and all trauma treatment, it is important to balance support with challenge, helping the client to stay in the so-called "therapeutic window" (Briere, 1996a; Briere & Scott, 2006)—that place where more challenge would be too much, and less would not be enough. Thus a very early task is to assess these resources, which must precede and accompany any exposure work.

To assess how the client has coped with stress and distress until now, you can use questionnaires such as the Inner Experience Questionnaire (Brock, Pearlman, & Varra, 2006) or the Inventory of Altered Self-Capacities (Briere & Runtz, 2002) as well as conversations with the client. For example, you can ask (as well as generally listen for) what the client does when he is very upset or how he brings himself out of a state of numbness. Praising positive strategies and exploring potentially destructive ones are ongoing processes that may continue throughout the treatment.

Certain coping strategies may be problematic for anyone. These include immersion in potentially addictive behaviors, such as excessive physical exercise, drinking, shopping, gambling, sexual activity, eating, and Internet use; they also include engagement in destructive activities, such as aggression against oneself or others or risk-taking behaviors. In the context of treatment for traumatic bereavement, additional potentially problematic coping activities include those that promote unhealthy or immoderate avoidance of memories or feelings about the deceased, and withdrawal from people or constructive activities. Some of the behaviors mentioned above, such as alcohol use, may lead to emotional numbing—a form of avoidance.

Individuals may use other activities that are not inherently destructive to avoid feelings. These may include using work or exercise to distract themselves from memories or feelings. Avoidance is not problematic when individuals use it consciously, in a balanced way, to take a needed break from confronting memories or feelings; in such cases, it might better be termed *distraction* than *avoidance*. It can be useful to discuss the difference between distraction, a healthy coping strategy in which a client exercises conscious choice to manage or dose pain, and avoidance, which is often automatic and does not include returning to challenging thoughts or feelings. It is important to explore and understand both the activity *and* the ways the individual uses it. The aim is to help the client find a balance between support and exposure—in other words, to keep moving back to the therapeutic window, where there is enough challenge for growth but not so much that the client's anxiety precludes that growth. Table 8.1 provides guidelines for assessing a client's resources.

TRAUMA AND LOSS HISTORY AND PROCESSING

It can be useful to acknowledge that the treatment will focus on one particular traumatic death, but can accommodate other losses in a client's history. It is important to assess a client's entire trauma history because processing one loss may trigger thoughts and emotions related to another. The therapy can address the primary loss and then other losses the client identifies as less traumatic, using the same techniques. Note, however, that asking a new client to list all of the painful, traumatic things he has ever experienced can overload his self capacities. As Najavits (2002) has indicated, eliciting a full trauma history can be like conducting an exposure therapy session without any preparation or safeguards. Clinical skill is needed to obtain this history in a way that is sensitive to the client's ability and willingness to share this material. Such skill will also help to manage the affect that may emerge in the telling or its aftermath (Pearlman & McCann, 1994). This task is sometimes easier in the context of asking the client to name major life events or experiences, traumatic and otherwise. For example, you might ask the client whether there is anything he would like you to know at this time about past traumatic experiences (Najavits, 2002).

It is important to determine whether any traumatic event from the past stands out as more problematic now than the sudden death. If another loss is more significant than the target loss, the client will have difficulty focusing and working effectively on the target loss. If prior losses are continuing to exert a powerful impact on the client, you and the client can create a plan to address those losses after the target loss has begun to feel less overwhelming. Working on automatic thoughts and issues related to one loss may generalize to other losses, and it may make processing of another loss less painful. Understanding the client's trauma history enables you to address issues related to all the traumatic events in the client's life, and it may help the work on the sudden, traumatic death generalize to other losses even before they are addressed directly. It is also important to assess how the client has processed other traumatic events, as this may alert you both to potential resources and to possible obstacles.

With all of this in mind, you can consider the following questions. If the client has experienced prior traumatic events, you can obtain valuable information by following up with the question "What helped you cope at that time?"

1. Are there any other traumatic experiences the client would like to let you know about (other than the target death)?

2. What has been going on in the client's life since the death? (probing for subsequent losses or traumatic experiences not directly related to the target death, e.g., job loss)

3. Does some other traumatic event stand out as more powerful than the current (target) death?

4. (If the client reports other traumatic experiences) Has she received treatment related to these experiences? Has she told anyone about the violence, victimization, abuse, or traumatic loss or had the opportunity to think, write, or express or process feelings about it?

TABLE 8.1. Guide to Assessing a Client's Resources

I. Self capacities

    A. Signs of difficulties in self capacities: depression, anxiety, avoidance of affect, easily becoming overwhelmed, problematic behaviors (self-injury, substance overuse, dissociation, etc.). Most people coming for treatment will demonstrate or report trouble with self capacities, which the treatment can enhance.

    B. Questions to explore:

        1. How does the client respond to his own strong affect?

        2. Will he be able to maintain or regain his position within the therapeutic window in the face of strong affect? If so, how?

        3. Can he maintain or regain connection with his inner experience (feelings, thoughts, and needs) in the face of strong affect? If so, how?

        4. Can he manage the necessary tasks of his daily life? What strategies does he use when this is difficult?

    C. The Inner Experience Questionnaire (Brock et al., 2006) and the Inventory of Altered Self-Capacities (Briere & Runtz, 2002) can provide systematic evaluations of self capacities.

II. Social support

    A. Signs of social support difficulties: discomfort in the presence of others, a persistent feeling that others' remarks or behaviors are insensitive; increased conflict with one or more members of the social network; social withdrawal or isolation.

    B. Questions to explore:

        1. What type of support does the client need?

        2. Are there needs for social support that are not being met?

        3. Who is in the network? How available are they? Are they helpful? If so, in what specific ways?

        4. Who is not helpful?

        5. Who is damaging or hurtful and in what ways?

        6. Can the client identify any potential additional support providers?

III. Coping skills

    A. Signs of coping difficulties: use of destructive coping strategies such as substance abuse, compulsive or addictive behaviors; inability to self-regulate affect and/or bodily states.

    B. Questions to explore:

        1. What coping strategies is the client currently using?

        2. How are these coping strategies useful?

        3. How are these coping strategies problematic?

        4. What has been helpful in the past?

        5. What obstacles can the client identify to using previously helpful coping strategies?

IV. Bereavement-specific issues (these are events and experiences related to the loss, dealing with the deceased person's belongings, anniversaries, and holidays, that can trigger trauma or grief reactions).

    A. Which bereavement-specific issues does the client identify as problematic?

    B. How has the client managed these issues to date?

V. Meaning and spirituality

    A. Is the client struggling to make sense of or find meaning in what happened?

    B. Does the client feel that life has no meaning without the deceased?

    C. (For a client who believes in God) In dealing with the loss, does the client feel supported, abandoned, or betrayed by God?

    D. (For a client who attended religious services prior to the death) Has the loss affected the client's participation in his faith community?

VI. Values and goals

    A. If you ask the client what matters most to him at this point, is he able to articulate any values that guide her behavior?

    B. If you ask the client whether he has any goals at the present time, is he able to articulate future goals?

Of course, it is important to keep in mind that events are defined as traumatic by those who experience them, and that people react in myriad ways to events, so you should not assume that any particular event requires processing.

In Table 8.2, we list many other considerations for deciding whether to use this treatment with a given client. Note that the treatment can help with some of these issues, so they are not necessarily exclusionary criteria. Rather, they are important considerations in deciding whether the client can engage in the treatment, and if so, whether and how the treatment ought to be tailored to fit this particular client's needs. You can think of these not as red flags that should stop you in your tracks, but rather yellow ones that call attention to an issue so as to encourage

---

TABLE 8.2. Considerations for Deciding Whether to Use This Treatment Approach with a Particular Client

1. Very recent loss. That is, the loss occurred so recently that the survivor is still in a state of total shock, and his natural coping responses have not had time to launch.

2. Problematic reality testing (e.g., a woman whose husband has died is unable to comprehend that her husband is not alive, that she and her children and other loved ones are not doomed to early deaths, and that your intention is to help her).

3. Problematic or questionable judgment regarding safety of self or others (e.g., dependent children). For example, the survivor is leaving his young children unattended, or is engaging in risky behaviors such as very fast driving or excessive alcohol consumption.

4. Difficulty maintaining continuity in life and between sessions, such that engaging in this treatment might overload the client rather than helping her manage her life challenges. For example, the client's degree of disorganization makes it difficult for her to get her children to school, pay her bills, go to work, or to find someone to help her to do these essential life tasks).

5. Persistent inability to recall what happened in the last session, despite your reminders.

6. Anything that interferes with the person's ability to participate actively in the treatment. Examples:
   a. Lack of physical or emotional safety, and inability at present to enter into a treatment in which the client could let down protective psychological barriers in order to yield to the demands of treatment.
   b. Limited memory of material related to the deceased or the loss. The treatment will require the client to engage in actively recalling the loss, as well as his relationship with the person who died.
   c. Psychosis, disabling depression, or other serious, uncontrolled mental health problems.
   d. Dissociation, active substance abuse, or self-injury that the person can't control.
   e. Active suicidal ideation (although the treatment can address hopelessness and despair).
   f. Absence of adequate English language literacy (resulting in inability to use the handouts); however, you can read handouts to the client and/or share the currently relevant points in session to overcome this potential obstacle.
   g. Inability to come to appointments regularly (e.g., lack of child care, health issues, lack of transportation, ambivalence).
   h. Violent behavior.
   i. Financial problems that might prohibit the client from attending sessions or focusing on processing the loss.
   j. Genuine lack of time to do this work.
   k. Client's self-described lack of interest in moving forward (e.g., the survivor has come to treatment only because someone else insisted he do so).
   l. Inability to participate and collaborate (e.g., the client wants you to "administer" the treatment).
   m. Other current life circumstances that would make focus on a specific traumatic death difficult (e.g., impending active military duty; active primary relationship distress [not related to the target loss]; job loss; or serious, ongoing physical health problems, such as diabetes or cancer).

further thought about treatment fit and design. Once you have addressed these issues, you can turn your attention to planning and conducting the treatment.

CLINICAL INTEGRATION

Donald looked down at his notes as he waited for Barbara to arrive. They had met once already, and in today's session he wanted to discuss the appropriateness of this treatment approach for Barbara. Donald's highest priority in moving forward with Barbara was to support her sobriety, and his concern was whether the tasks of the treatment might jeopardize it. He decided to present this concern to Barbara directly.

Once Barbara arrived, Donald introduced his thoughts and concerns. "I want to spend some time today discussing the appropriateness of this treatment approach for you. I know that you have sought support and therapeutic intervention in various ways over the past 4 years, and that you continue to experience symptoms of trauma, depression, acute grief, and a strong urge to drink. I think I can help you find further relief, and I think you are a good candidate for the specific treatment approach we've discussed. You've demonstrated psychological insight about your situation; an ability to draw on resources available to you, including AA; willingness and even determination to seek help; and the capacity to experience difficult feelings in here with me. As you know, this is a challenging treatment: It involves reviewing Janie's death in detail, and engaging with your memories, feelings, and thoughts about her death and the car accident more generally—all in an active and planned way. Before we dive in, I want to explore my concern for your sobriety. You have done such a good job maintaining your sobriety, and . . ."

"I've relapsed twice," Barbara interrupted with a tone of self-reproach.

"Yes, you did. And each and every other day of each and every other year since Janie's death, you have maintained your sobriety. Relapse can be part of recovery, right? You sounded harsh toward yourself just now?"

Donald presented this as a question, which Barbara then attempted to answer. "I've been told that before, especially in relation to Janie's death. My sister tells me that I expected myself to prevent her death, and that this was just not possible."

"I agree with your sister, and the thoughts and expectations that you hold related to your role as a mother are one of the elements this treatment approach can address. I'm wondering if you judge yourself according to unrealistic standards and then criticize yourself accordingly. If so, this could be feeding into the depression you experience. A potential dilemma for us is this: In order to elicit these thoughts and expectations so that we can examine them, we need to engage with the details of the accident, details of Janie's death, and details of your grief. I imagine that you'll want to move—maybe even run—away from some of these details and feelings. In other words, it will be difficult to engage with this material. I will help you do so. This treatment is designed to help you do so. There are supports in place. I can talk more about these today and in the future, but before I do, I'd like to ask you: What do you think you'll need throughout this treatment in order to assist you in maintaining your sobriety?"

"I know I'll need to keep my schedule of at least three AA meetings per week, and I know I need to continue the recovery work I've been doing with my sponsor," Barbara replied.

"Good. One of your strengths, which will help you in this therapy, is that you have a strong awareness of the support you need. Now let me ask you this: What do you know about your most recent relapse? When you look back on it, were there warning signs or steps that might have led to your decision to drink?"

"It was 5 days after Janie's birthday, about 3 years after her death. The day was excruciatingly painful, but I got through it. I spent time at her gravesite, attended an AA meeting, and fought the urge to drink. The day was horrible, though, and even though I did everything I thought I should do, nothing felt better. In fact, the feelings of grief were worse than ever that day. I thought it was supposed to get easier with time. It wasn't easier, and I felt as though I were being punished for not protecting Janie and for not doing enough to somehow make myself better."

"I hear some harsh thoughts again," Donald noted.

"Yeah. It's easy for me to blame myself. One day at a time had been helping me up until then, but after Janie's birthday that year, I began projecting into the future— thinking that it would never get easier, and that everything I was doing to stay sober and to grieve wasn't helping. The symptoms I told you about were at their worst around that time, too. I wasn't sleeping, and the flashbacks to the accident were more frequent."

As Barbara spoke, Donald was making notes about a few things. He jotted down what he heard to be several problematic beliefs: Barbara's beliefs that her pain was evidence of punishment; that somehow she was solely responsible for "making herself better," as if this were purely a matter of will; and that she should have saved her daughter. He also noted what seemed to be her openness to examining these beliefs. Finally, Donald jotted down a note about Barbara's knowledge of some specific strategies for maintaining her sobriety, as well as some potential warning signs of an increased vulnerability to drinking, which included worsening trauma symptoms. He wondered whether she had addressed *her* traumatic experience of the accident, apart from Janie's death, and noted that as a question as well. He also made a mental note of his feeling that they were developing a rapport; Donald believed they could be direct with one another as concerns arose throughout their work together. Although Barbara's history of alcoholism presented a concern for Donald, he believed that her strengths and resources, the tools offered by the treatment, and the therapeutic relationship could together offer the support needed to usher Barbara through the treatment while she maintained sobriety.

CONCLUDING REMARKS

Within this chapter, we have offered a framework for assessing the appropriateness of this treatment approach for any given individual. This framework can act as a foundation that will support you as you make decisions and judgment calls based on your own clinical experience and knowledge. Donald's assessment of Barbara offers one example of thinking through the appropriateness of the treatment for a particular client. In this example, the therapist honed in on a history of alcoholism as a potential risk factor for this client. In response to his concern, Donald assessed the resources Barbara had utilized successfully to aid her recovery to date; signs of increased vulnerability to drinking, based on past relapses; and what Barbara knew about what she would need to prevent a relapse. Donald also took note of those strengths and resources that made Barbara a good candidate for the treatment approach more generally, noting that her long-term experience in AA had probably contributed to the development of these strengths.

While assessing treatment fit, Donald also noted targets for intervention. He identified certain problematic beliefs that might be contributing to Barbara's distress, and wondered about her experience of the accident apart from her daughter's death. Barbara had also faced death that day, and he hadn't heard her talk about this piece of the experience. Throughout the assessment, Donald was listening for strengths, vulnerabilities, places Barbara might be stuck, and targets for intervention. Together, these elements would help him to tailor the treatment approach to Barbara's specific needs.

Thoughtful evaluation of a survivor's vulnerabilities—including her trauma and loss history, as well as her resources and strengths—will help you to determine the appropriateness of this treatment approach for a particular client. A thorough assessment will also help you to assess where a client is in terms of the six "R" processes of mourning, where she may be stuck in processing the trauma, and where she may need added support for building resources. Such an assessment, in turn, will help you to craft a specific treatment plan and to assess the client's progress along the way. Of course, the tasks of assessment and evaluation continue throughout the treatment, so that you and your client can make adjustments as needed.

CHAPTER 9

Implementation Issues

Shantal sat at her kitchen table with a cup of coffee, wondering whether she would make it to her therapy appointment later in the day. She'd had a bad panic attack that morning and didn't feel up to going. Shantal contemplated asking her friend, Jan, to drive her there if she were still feeling out of it by the afternoon. "I probably should go, and I probably shouldn't be drinking coffee," she thought to herself as she took the next sip.

Shantal was a self-described survivor. She grew up in a single-parent home, in poverty. She was raped at the age of 17. She suffered the loss of several family members, including her mother and a younger sibling. She divorced soon after she had her youngest son. But her faith had remained strong through all of her experiences of trauma and grief. This, along with good friends and children she loved, carried her through. Shantal was the kind of woman who knew how to put one foot in front of the other and did exactly that through a series of profoundly difficult experiences.

The loss of her youngest son was different. Nothing could have prepared her for the anguish she felt watching her 7-year-old son, Tyler, die from a bullet wound in their front yard. While playing ball with his older sister, he was caught in the crossfire of a gang shooting. The mental pictures of that day were as vivid for Shantal now as they were on the day of the shooting 2 years ago. Although the shock of her son's tragic death had worn off, the pain was now more intense than it had been in the initial months after the shooting. In fact, Shantal sometimes wished for the shock and numbness that first characterized her grief and traumatic stress. The memories, panic, sleeplessness, emptiness, and pain that now lived in her heart seemed too much to bear.

In this chapter, we discuss both general psychotherapy issues (e.g., therapeutic relationship, therapy frame, and termination) as they apply to working with this population. We also discuss issues that are specific to this treatment approach (e.g., using independent activities and designing a treatment plan to meet each client's needs).

GENERAL PSYCHOTHERAPY ISSUES

Therapeutic Relationship

Clients must participate actively in this treatment approach: They must engage in resource-building activities both during and between sessions, as well as challenging their own thoughts, beliefs, and behaviors. From the beginning of the treatment, it is important to set the expectation for a collaborative relationship with the client. As in any psychotherapy relationship, the client is the expert on her own experience. Pearlman and Saakvitne (1995) have described the ideal therapeutic relationship with a trauma survivor client as one in which you as the therapist provide information about the common effects of traumatic events, help the client develop self capacities, are genuine and present emotionally, focus on development of the therapeutic relationship, and openly invite the client to process transference. These principles apply equally to the relationship with a traumatically bereaved client, since such clients constitute a subset of the trauma survivor population.

A collaborative relationship empowers the client to face his fears and do the difficult work of processing the loss. Such a relationship is based on respect, information, connection, and hope, as described in *Risking Connection* (Saakvitne et al., 2000). As the therapist, you can provide *respect* by acknowledging the client's experience as valid, attending closely to his needs and concerns about both the content and process of the treatment, offering a collaborative approach, participating in the treatment with honesty and integrity, and maintaining the treatment frame. You can provide *information* about sudden, traumatic death and traumatic bereavement, as well as about paths to adaptation to the new reality. The handouts in the Appendix and on this book's website supplement (*www.guilford.com/pearlman-materials*) can be used for this purpose. *Connection* refers to the sense of partnership between you and the client; the connection the client will make with his own feeling states, his past relationship with the deceased, and his future without her; and with a supportive community that he will access or develop in this treatment. You can provide *hope* by encouraging the client to engage fully in the treatment process, giving feedback on progress and successes, guiding the client to create a meaningful future, and maintaining your own belief that the client can continue to move forward through the mourning process. These treatment relationship elements are central to any effective psychotherapy, and are essential for psychotherapy with a traumatically bereaved client.

Developing a therapeutic relationship with the client requires sensitivity to the nature of the client's attachment to the deceased significant other. For example, it would be wrong to assume that a client will have few challenging issues to address because she was no longer married to her deceased ex-husband. Such an assumption will probably diminish the empathic connection to the client and result in missing important readjustment needs.

Sensitivity to the nature of the attachment includes considering how you will refer to the deceased. The issue of which term to use can be resolved by using the deceased's name, by referring to the specific relationship (e.g., "child," "spouse," etc.), or simply by asking the client her preference. Referring to the person as "the deceased" may sound too formal to the client. In addition, the use of such an impersonal term may reinforce the client in avoiding the emotions related to the loss. Of course, you will need to use clinical judgment to adjust the tone of the therapy to suit the actual relationship between the client and the deceased.

Therapy Frame

The chaos that sudden, traumatic death creates in people's lives can leave them feeling disoriented and lost. Establishing the frame of therapy and maintaining boundaries help to create the sense of safety and support necessary for clients to engage in this treatment. You can begin setting the frame for the therapy in the first session by discussing the nature, goals, and process of therapy (Handouts 1, Sudden, Traumatic Death and Traumatic Bereavement, and

2, Orientation to the Treatment, can be useful for the client to take away, but will not replace a discussion of these issues with the client); the roles of, and expectations for, you and the client; meeting time; length and frequency of sessions; and appropriate types and frequency of contact. Additional important frame issues to discuss—such as financial responsibility for the therapy and the involvement, if any, of third parties (e.g., insurers, family members, collateral treaters, consultants to the treatment)—will be included in a standard written form that the client will sign if you are requesting consent to consult or include others in the treatment and also merit discussion. A collaborative, respectful decision-making process about the treatment frame helps a client to feel empowered, hopeful, and safe, and provides an open invitation to express feelings, concerns, and needs related to the therapy (Pearlman & Courtois, 2005; Pearlman & Saakvitne, 1995; Wilson, Friedman, & Lindy, 2002).

As the therapist, your role is to provide information, guidance, and skills. It is important to practice the techniques developed through independent activity assignments with clients until they can do them on their own. You may talk about theory and research during sessions because it is important that clients understand why they are doing what they are doing. Understanding the ideas behind the work increases the likelihood that clients will be able to apply their new skills in novel situations in the future. Moreover, for traumatically bereaved clients in particular, understanding the nature of the treatment helps to restore a lost sense of control.

Boundaries

It is important to manage boundaries in a way that conveys respect and security for both parties and creates a warm, supportive environment for the client. A sense of safety and warmth may seem difficult to maintain in a therapy that focuses on something as distressing as sudden, traumatic death. Survivors may be concerned that their thoughts, feelings, or accounts of their experiences will upset you. As described in Chapter 3, for example, survivors of deaths that were caused by others often experience rage toward the perpetrators, as well as fantasies about ways to make them suffer. Clients need to understand that they will not overwhelm you with their stories or their distress.

Clinical judgment must be your guide in countertransference disclosures. If you express shock, horror, or some other distress reactions (e.g., crying) in response to a client's account of a death, the client may feel ashamed or may conclude that you are not strong enough to deal with the situation. Yet if you show no response to the account, the client may not feel understood or supported, or may experience you as cold or distant. Generally, a mild but warmly concerned verbal response is a good starting point ("I'm so sorry this happened to [your loved one]. How truly terrible"). You can gauge the appropriate intensity of your remarks by using the client's language and responses as a guide. Part of the art of psychotherapy is to balance the expression of your authentic responses with what you deem best for the client at any moment.

You may struggle with the urge to overextend yourself in order to protect a client from further loss or to attempt to "make up for" the loss. You might feel compelled to provide sessions at times you don't typically work because the client tends to experience more loneliness or distress at those times (e.g., evenings or weekends), or to have frequent or lengthy phone or e-mail contacts with clients between sessions. In order to maintain the necessary balance between strength and empathy, to protect the therapeutic relationship, to convey respect for and faith in the client's ability to function, and to prevent burnout and minimize vicarious trauma, it is essential to establish and maintain good boundaries. These boundaries are guidelines that prevent a client from becoming excessively dependent on you as the therapist, and prevent you from doing more for the client than is therapeutic. These guidelines should be shared (and, as appropriate, developed) with the client in the first session of therapy, and later as the need arises. For example, during a difficult exposure period, one client began phoning her therapist regularly between sessions. The therapist talked with the client about her possible need for more support. Together, they agreed that the client could attempt to elicit support from family members and close friends, and that they would meet twice a week during the remainder of the exposure work. (More detailed information on frame and boundaries in psychotherapies with survivors of traumatic events can be found in Courtois, 2010; Pearlman & Saakvitne, 1995; and Saakvitne et al., 2000.)

Documentation and Informed Consent

Careful documentation of therapy is a legal requirement, a therapy tool, and an ethical issue. Traumatically bereaved clients often have legal involvements, and their therapists' notes may be required in legal proceedings. These considerations necessitate careful note taking and documentation of attributions of guilt and blame, as well as the risk of harm to self or others. Depending on a client's wishes and the possibility of legal involvement, you may choose to keep the copies of the Automatic Thought Record (Handout 13) the client completes, or allow the client to keep them. You should be aware of relevant statutes governing note taking, and ensure that your notes and records meet state/provincial and professional ethics guidelines. At the same time, you must take care not to misrepresent the client in the record. As described previously, many survivors of sudden, traumatic loss blame themselves for their loved ones' deaths. It is important to note in the client's record that self-blaming thoughts are distorted thoughts. Poorly worded or misrepresented descriptions of a client's self-blame could be used against her in a court case. One resource for therapists whose clients may have court involvements is Barsky's *Clinicians in Court* (2012).

Our approach focuses heavily on helping clients challenge their thoughts. Clients' choices of words and specific phrasing often reveal their underlying distorted beliefs. Clients may not be far enough in moving through the six "R" processes to be ready to challenge their negative thoughts. You may wish to make verbatim notes of such clients' words, in order to challenge later the thoughts they convey. Early in therapy, you may notice a distorted thought in a client's independent activity writing, but choose not to address it because either another thought/issue takes precedence or the client does not yet have the skills to challenge it. Writing down and keeping a list of automatic thoughts, or saving independent activity assignments, will make it possible to go back to these at a later point in therapy. For example, you may address self-blame-related automatic thoughts before addressing thoughts about God or spirituality, but you will want to keep a record of these latter thoughts for later reference. You may also want to refer in sessions to past independent activities as a way of showing the progress the client has made.

Because this therapy is a collaborative relationship between you and the client, it may be helpful to explain to the client how you take notes, and to show the client the form or format you use. Clients may worry about what you are writing about them, or may feel intimidated by what they imagine is a process that only you understand. Making these methods transparent allows a client to feel more in control of the therapy—control that was absent at the time of the loss.

Clients may feel reassured by a discussion of your specific policy on note taking, as well as of the relevant law on confidentiality, which varies from state to state. Traumatized clients may feel safer knowing that you will not share any information about them without their consent unless they are in danger of hurting themselves or someone else, or unless they report child or elder abuse (in addition to whatever legal statutes specify in each state). This discussion is also a way to acknowledge to the client that traumatically bereaved clients do sometimes think of hurting or killing themselves and that you will try to help him with these issues.

Independent Activities

Independent activities are a critically important component of our treatment approach. These activities are designed to be completed between sessions. We have developed them to expand the work performed during the sessions, and to facilitate resource building, trauma processing, and mourning. Independent activities give clients the opportunity to practice the desired behaviors on a regular basis.

Such activities have been a core feature of CBT since its inception. Although this approach is employed among practitioners of many theoretical orientations, the use of independent activities is highest among cognitive-behavioral therapists. In one study, it was reported that therapists using CBT approaches used homework in an average of 66% of their sessions (Kazantzis & Deane, 1999). In a second study focusing on 827 American Psychological Association members who practice CBT, 68% reported using homework (Kazantzis, Deane, Ronan, & L'Abate, 2005).

The most widely used term for independent activities is *homework*. Over time, an increasing number of practitioners have moved away from this label, arguing that for most people it has negative connotations. As Kazantzis and colleagues (2005) put it, this term "evokes a powerful dynamic in which patients are completing it for the therapists rather than for themselves" (p. 218). Consequently, a number of alternative terms have emerged in the treatment literature, such as *home practice, personal practice, self-help assignments, between-session activities*, and *independent activities* (Kazantzis et al., 2005; Tompkins, 2004). The last of these is the term we use in this book.

Independent activities have been studied more than any other process in CBT (see Kazantzis, Whittington, & Dattilio, 2010, for a review). A meta-analysis conducted by Kazantzis and colleagues (2010) provided empirical support for the use of such activities. The results, based on a review of 44 studies, provided clear evidence that independent activities enhance therapy outcomes. Their findings suggest that 62% of patients improve when receiving therapy with independent activities, whereas only 38% improve if receiving therapy without such activities. As these authors emphasize, their findings demonstrate that treatments that include such activities as a main component "produce superior treatment effects to those that do not" (p. 153).

There are numerous benefits to using independent activities (for an excellent discussion of this issue, see Tompkins, 2004, or Kazantzis et al., 2005). First, by providing clients with additional opportunities to practice specific skills, these activities can facilitate learning key components of the treatment and accelerate the pace of doing so. In a sense, these assignments provide the opportunity for clients to transfer the skills they have learned in therapy to everyday situations. Second, independent activities provide an opportunity for clients to test the validity of their underlying assumptions and beliefs. Third, these activities also enable clients "to collect information regarding their thoughts, moods, physiology and behaviors in different situations" (Kazantzis et al., 2005, p. 2). Fourth, since these between-session assignments are carried out in a variety of different settings, they can help clients generalize what they have learned. Fifth, using independent activities can help clients gain confidence in their ability to deal with their problems without the assistance of a therapist. Sixth, the handouts assigning independent activities (and other handouts associated with the treatment) constitute a permanent record of the issues that have been addressed, and can be utilized as a resource as needed in the future. Seventh, independent activities provide the opportunity for clients to work on issues that cannot be addressed fully in sessions. For example, a client whose child died in a motor vehicle crash may find that she is paralyzed by anxiety whenever she attempts to drive a car. This issue can best be addressed by exposure activities that involve driving. Such activities are particularly helpful in combating avoidance. Eighth, independent activities allow clients to take responsibility for their treatment gains, which can be empowering. Finally, as Kazantzis and colleagues (2005) have noted, independent activities provide a structure and rhythm across sessions that is beneficial to many clients.

Some practitioners regard independent activities as a way of extending the treatment beyond the end of therapy. As Kazantzis and Deane (1999) have indicated, the pressures of managed care have often resulted in fewer sessions being reimbursed. Independent activities enable a client to obtain maximal benefit from the sessions available. Tompkins (2004) asserts that independent activities allow a client to practice skills that would take many months to learn if she could only practice once per week in her therapy session. Experts agree that independent activities constitute a cornerstone of CBT. These activities should therefore not be regarded as "add-on" or adjunctive procedures, but rather as a crucial aspect of the treatment (Kazantzis et al., 2005).

Termination

Typically, clients who engage in this treatment will not have had an opportunity to say goodbye to their deceased loved ones. This can result in a fear that others will leave or die before they have been able to say goodbye. Even clients who previously had the ability to end relationships constructively may face challenges in doing so after a sudden death. As a result, they may end relationships abruptly in order to feel a sense of control over endings, or may avoid intimate connections in order to try to protect themselves from the pain of endings. It is valuable to help each client realize that while all relationships eventually end, they need not all end traumatically. We strongly recommend that you begin processing the client's feelings about the ending of this therapy during the early sessions, and that you revisit the topic frequently. This is especially important for a survivor of sudden, traumatic death, who may experience the termination of treatment as another abandonment. Although the focus on the ending may feel unfamiliar, it provides an opportunity for the client to acclimate to the fact that this treatment will end. It also gives both parties an opportunity to reflect on progress.

The two of you can approach the termination of therapy as an example of an anticipated, planned, and mutual end to a relationship instead of another wrenching loss. Since the therapy is designed to foster the client's increasing confidence in his own resources, including his social support network, his reliance on you as the therapist should decrease over time. The main goal of discussions about termination should be to process the client's feelings about the losses inherent in finishing therapy, as well as the different experiences of planned or expected versus unexpected losses. A planned loss (such as the ending of a therapy relationship or sending a child off to college) or an expected loss (such as losing a loved one after a lengthy illness) offers the opportunity to conclude unfinished conversations, to reflect on the relationship, and to say goodbye. None of these important processes can take place when the death of a loved one is sudden.

In initial termination discussions, you can educate the client about common reactions to ending therapy. (You can also give Handout S2, Ending Therapy, to the client.[1]) You may discuss the difference between the end of this relationship and the end of the relationship with the deceased, focusing on the planned nature of this ending. Later termination discussions may include talking about the feelings that the prospect of ending raises for the client. You can also prepare the client for using the new skills learned in therapy to cope with potentially distressing experiences in the future, such as anniversaries related to the death. In addition, it will be useful to discuss signs indicating that the client might need to return to therapy (with you or another therapist) in the future.

The ending of treatment need not signal the end of the client's internalized relationship with the lost loved one. In other words, we all hold our relationships in our hearts and minds, and they can remain important and sustaining even when we no longer have contact with the other party. Yet a client may hold this fear, implicitly or explicitly, and may need to discuss it with you. For example, the client may fear that this therapy is the only relationship in which she is able to talk about the deceased, her memories of him, and her feelings about him and about the death. If you encounter strong reluctance in the client to ending the treatment, this may be a dimension to explore.

Of course, not every client will decide to complete the treatment. In some cases, the treatment may begin to feel too challenging to the client. Alternatively, the client may feel that he is making inadequate progress, or that the treatment model or your therapeutic style is simply not a good fit with his personal style and/or needs. Another possibility is that the client will leave treatment soon after he begins to feel better. What is a "premature" termination in this treatment model? If the client leaves the treatment without starting or resuming movement along the six "R" processes of mourning, we consider this a premature ending. If the client announces his intention to leave the treatment before it is complete, you should discuss the client's reasons for leaving. First, you will want to ascertain whether the client has made the decision to leave, or whether this is only the client's way of expressing some dissatisfaction with the treatment or with your therapeutic style. If the latter, you can discuss ways of addressing the client's concerns. If the former, you should address the ending as a potential loss (even leaving a relationship one is ready to end represents a change with inherent loss).

Of course, it is possible that a client will decide her needs have been met before you consider the treatment to be finished, and yet the termination is not "premature." The client may, for example, have strengthened her resources enough to address the trauma and may now feel that she is on a clear path to move through the remaining mourning processes. She may feel prepared to do that work on her own. She may feel that her work is complete and she is no longer feeling stuck or plagued by problems related to trauma and grief. In any of these instances, it is your job to enter into a positive ending process with her, as described below, unless you feel she is avoiding work that remains to be done. Even if you disagree with the client's decision, a positive ending is important so that the client does not take away a sense of failure, but rather leaves with an understanding of what she has gained and what may remain to be done.

Once the client has announced a decision to leave and you have accepted this decision, the client's focus may shift to positive or valued aspects of the treatment relationship. In any case, this ending will be planned, and thus different from the loss of the deceased. The client is

---

[1]Note that numbers for handouts provided *only* on this book's website supplement (*www.guilford.com/ pearlman-materials*) begin with S (S1, S2, etc.).

choosing when and how to end, and there is an opportunity to reflect on the relationship and to say goodbye, even if it must be done in that session. In the course of this discussion, additional reasons for ending (such as the client's wanting to be in control of this ending process) may emerge, and these can provide opportunities for reflection and reconsideration.

If you are moving toward ending the treatment for any reason, we strongly recommend a planned ending. This means that you discuss ending, the feelings the ending raises for the client, the advantages and disadvantages of ending at this point, and the value of not ending abruptly in light of the client's previous sudden loss of a loved one. Ideally, you will discuss in one or more subsequent sessions what the client has gained from the treatment, what expectations were not met, what remains to be addressed, and the client's need for further treatment (related to this loss or not) with referrals to other therapists (if either you or the client feels that it would not be optimal to continue together and that further treatment is warranted). You can also invite a mutual expression of positive feelings for each other (e.g., you can express appreciations of each other's strengths and contributions to the treatment process, and talk about ways you will remember each other), as well as a discussion of possible signs that the client might want to seek therapy in the future, if she is not doing so at this time. We discuss possible countertransference responses to therapy termination in Chapter 14.

DESIGNING THE TREATMENT PLAN

Together, you will develop a treatment plan. This plan will be based on the client's unique manifestation of traumatic bereavement, as well as his resources (e.g., his adaptations, needs, goals, and strengths) and your clinical knowledge and judgment. Together, you will also develop the content of specific sessions. This is where the art of therapy takes place, reflecting some combination of spontaneity and careful planning. The 25-session sample treatment plan offered on this book's website supplement (*www.guilford.com/pearlman-materials*) outlines a framework within which you and the client can design your approach. You can use the sample treatment plan as a foundation, drawing from, tweaking, and building upon it. It is based on a pilot study that provided information about how the elements of the treatment approach can be integrated to serve the goals of the therapy.

Ideally, you will sketch out a clear vision for the treatment in the first few weeks of meeting with the client, and develop working plan after the third or fourth session. For example, a client with a history of self-injurious behavior may need more sessions devoted to building self capacities and coping resources in the beginning of therapy. Someone with little social support may need a greater emphasis on building and accessing a social network. People with few problems in a specific area may be able to skip many of the independent activities in that area and focus their efforts elsewhere. The assessment process will reveal much about a client's strengths (self capacities, coping skills, social support) and challenges (including distressing beliefs and other signs of trauma and grief). Of course, you can and should revisit and revise this plan as needed along the way. This preparation can be time-consuming, but will require less time as you become familiar with the treatment elements and the process of matching them to clients' needs. Appropriate planning and preparation will facilitate the smooth development of individual sessions, as well as the whole of the treatment. We strongly recommend that you read the handouts presented in the Appendix and on the website supplement as you begin treatment with each new client. It may be useful to review this material again along the way to remind yourself of available resources.

Maintaining a structured approach facilitates the completion of many activities within a moderate time frame. Again, you may want to use the sample treatment plan mentioned above. This is a plan for moving through all three of the core treatment components (resource building, trauma processing, and facilitating mourning). If so, you will have to stay on task in order to finish each session in 45 minutes and to finish the entire treatment in 25 sessions. Although it will be challenging at times, the structure offers many other advantages. It can provide a level of confidence for both you and the client. As a result of your or the client's preferences or the client's resources (e.g., time; child care; or financial constraints, including limitations in the number of visits covered by the insurance plan), you may choose to modify the treatment, selecting and prioritizing those elements that best address the client's needs.

Whether or not you use the structured treatment plan, the use of handouts gives the client a sense of active participation in the treatment and concrete tools to use outside treatment sessions. The use of Handout 13, the Automatic Thought Record, for exploring cognitions ensures that each belief receives detailed attention. The structure also helps to manage potential avoidance.

Alternatively, you can use the session topics and subtopics listed in Table 1.2 to help design a treatment plan for a particular client. You should review this plan frequently to adapt the treatment plan to the client's evolving needs. Once you identify the topics and subtopics you plan to address with your client, you can refer to Table 9.1 to identify the relevant handouts to use.

It is only over the course of working with a particular client that you will gain a clearer understanding of how much material you can cover in a session and what the client is able to do between sessions. In addition, a client's capacities, resources, and needs may become more apparent after the initial assessment, as you begin working together. Thus one aspect of treatment planning that may need adjusting over time involves the amount of work that can be accomplished in a given session, as well as its intensity. This should be regulated to keep the client within the *therapeutic window* (Briere, 1996a, 2002), which, as noted in Chapter 8, is the place where there is enough challenge for growth and enough comfort to be able to engage in the work. You must remain aware of the tension between overwhelming the client (which would indicate the need to build more resources or reduce the amount of material in, between, or across sessions) and collaborating in (often unconscious) avoidance of trauma material. When in doubt, it makes sense to invite the client to reflect on this dynamic tension along with you, in order to build the working alliance and include the client in modifying the plan to meet her goals.

While a thorough assessment is important at the outset of any psychotherapy relationship, it is crucial when only a few sessions are available. For clients who are struggling with acute trauma symptoms, sessions should focus on (1) building coping skills; (2) providing psychoeducation about other resource-building activities (particularly developing social support), even if trauma and mourning work cannot take place in this round of treatment; and (3) providing resources that the client can draw upon during and after the treatment. Many clients will present for treatment with coping skills that are more than adequate to allow them to move forward with the trauma and mourning work. Often 9–12 sessions are adequate to pursue trauma and mourning work if the client has strong coping skills. Many survivors of sudden, traumatic losses have spent years honing their coping skills and building resources (including social support), but have never had the opportunity to speak candidly about their losses. Thus, no clients can complete trauma work in a relatively short period of time. In addition, you should help the client to think creatively about how to finance therapy, offering solutions such as 9–12 weekly sessions followed by bimonthly sessions.

TABLE 9.1. Handouts by Treatment Element

<u>Sudden, traumatic death</u>

Handout 1   Sudden, Traumatic Death and Traumatic Bereavement
Handout 27   Guilt, Regret, and Sudden, Traumatic Death
Handout 28   Anger and Sudden, Traumatic Death

<u>Self capacities</u>

Handout 8   Feelings Skills
Handout 27   Guilt, Regret, and Sudden, Traumatic Death
Handout 28   Anger and Sudden, Traumatic Death

<u>Coping strategies</u>

Handout 7   Breathing Retraining
Handout 18   The Importance of Enhancing Social Support
Handout 19   Building Social Support

<u>Social support</u>

Handout 18   The Importance of Enhancing Social Support
Handout 19   Building Social Support

<u>Bereavement-specific issues</u>

Handout S5   Bereavement-Specific Issues
Handout S6   Getting through the Holidays: Advice from the Bereaved

<u>Meaning and spirituality</u>

Handout 31   Spirituality

<u>Values and goals</u>

Handout 21   Values
Handout S1   Personal Goal Setting

<u>Cognitive processing</u>

Handout 5   Exploring the Impact of the Death
Handout 8   Feelings Skills
Handout 9   A Model for Change
Handout 10   What Are Automatic Thoughts?
Handout 11   Identifying Automatic Thoughts Worksheet
Handout 12   Sample Automatic Thought Record
Handout 13   Automatic Thought Record
Handout 14   Challenging Questions Worksheet
Handout 26   Account of Your Relationship with Your Significant Other[a]
Handout 29   Letter to Your Significant Other[a]
Handout 30   Exploring the Meaning of the Loss[a]
Handout S8   Continuing Your Relationship with Your Significant Other[a]
Handout 32   Final Impact Statement

<u>Imaginal exposure</u>

Handout 7   Breathing Retraining (for use before or after the exposure only)
Handout 16   First Account of the Death
Handout 20   Second Account of the Death
Handout 22   Third Account of the Death

(continued)

TABLE 9.1. *(continued)*

In vivo exposure

Handout 13	Automatic Thought Record
Handout 25	Fear and Avoidance Hierarchy Form

Mourning

Handout 5	Exploring the Impact of the Death
Handout 6	The Six "R" Processes of Mourning
Handout 17	Secondary Losses
Handout 24	Positive and Negative Aspects of Your Relationship with Your Significant Other
Handout S4	Review of Your Relationship
Handout S7	Your Assumptive World
Handout 30	Exploring the Meaning of the Loss[a]
Handout S8	Continuing Your Relationship with Your Significant Other[a]

[a]These handouts also include an emotional processing aspect.

The handouts in the Appendix and on the website supplement can be valuable resources, although it is important not to overwhelm the client with too much information. It can be useful to review the list of all handouts at the beginning of the Appendix with the client and together identify a small number that you and the client believe might be useful. Alternatively, you may choose to make this selection yourself, based on the treatment plan. However, it is best to offer clients exposure exercise handouts, such as Handouts 5 (Exploring the Impact of the Death), 15 (Processing the Loss), and 16 (First Account of the Death), during a period when they are scheduled to attend at least weekly sessions. These handouts invite them to engage in exposure work that raises strong feelings. During this process, they may benefit from reassurance, encouragement, and support from you. The activities we describe in a full treatment plan can be used in a shorter treatment, with the caveat that exposure work requires adequate support and self capacities for the client. If you have not addressed support activities during an abbreviated treatment, it may be worthwhile to provide the psychoeducational handouts related to resource building, such as Handouts 4 (Self-Care), 6 (The Six "R" Processes of Mourning), and 8 (Feelings Skills).

If the client can only attend a small number of sessions and chooses to schedule the individual sessions at 2- or 3-week intervals, it may be feasible to assign more independent activities, thereby increasing the benefit of treatment. However, we do not recommend this less frequent session scheduling if the client's symptoms are acute or if you are doing exposure work. Another option would be to meet for a block of sessions (perhaps 5 or 10), take a break for an interval to be decided by the two of you together, and then meet for another block of sessions. The client can use the interval to practice using her resources to manage challenging situations, and can bring back to the treatment her observations about what went well and where she needs further work.

If your assessment suggests that the client's self capacities and resources are strong, and if you are well versed in CBT and exposure techniques, you may be able to complete exposure work within 10 sessions. Clients will benefit most if they are committed to attending sessions at least once a week and to doing both self capacities work and exposure exercises between sessions.

Therapy will usually include planned breaks, such as vacations or other absences. It may also include unplanned breaks, such as those related to illness or family emergencies, that interfere with the regular schedule. Such breaks can be difficult for any distressed client, and moreso for those who are mourning traumatic losses. Ideally, you will notify your client of any planned absence several weeks in advance, and explore the client's feelings about the absence both beforehand and afterwards. Even client absences can create distress for a traumatically bereaved client because of the vulnerability that separation elicits. Anticipating such reactions, normalizing them, and planning for them with the client can assist her in managing them effectively. These breaks provide important opportunities to practice coping skills and build self capacities.

Structured Session Format

Table 9.2 presents the format of a typical structured session. Each session begins with *introductory activities*: setting the *session frame* (an introduction to the work that lies ahead), as well as a discussion of any *treatment frame issues* (such as appointment scheduling or payment). We

---

TABLE 9.2. Format of a Typical Session

I. Introduction

   A. *Session frame: Focus, topics, rationale.* The therapist briefly describes the focus of this session, lists the topics to be addressed (see Table 1.2 and/or the sample treatment plan on this book's website supplement), and discusses how these topics contribute to healthy accommodation of traumatic death (the rationale). (All sessions)

   B. *Treatment frame issues.* This is the opportunity to discuss issues such as scheduling, payment, and (toward the middle of treatment and in later sessions) termination. (Most sessions)

   C. *Brief review of independent activities.* Here the therapist checks in to see whether the client has completed the independent activities from the previous session. If not, the dyad explores the obstacles to completing the activities and what support the client may need in order to complete them. The dyad may complete in session any activities not completed in advance, using the framework below. (All sessions)

   D. *Psychoeducation.* This is a place to provide information about the topics and tasks of today's session. Material in the handouts can be useful to this process. (Most sessions)

II. Core treatment components

   A. *Resource building.* Here the dyad may discuss the client's progress in building self capacities, social support, and coping skills, as well as in addressing bereavement-specific issues, values and goals, and meaning and spirituality. (All sessions)

   B. *Processing the traumatic death.* This is the place to process exposure activity assignments, as well as to engage in exposure activities in session as indicated. (Most sessions)

   C. *Mourning.* This is the place in the session to discuss the "R" process that is the current focus. (Most sessions)

III. Wrap-up

   A. *Integration.* Here the dyad looks at big-picture issues, such as how the elements of the treatment fit together and how the death and secondary losses have affected the client's worldview, values, or other broad beliefs. (Most sessions)

   B. *Independent activities for next time.* Here the therapist proposes activities for the client to engage in between sessions, ideally one or more from each of the following two categories, and explains them to the client. (Most sessions)

     1. Resource building, trauma processing, and mourning activities

     2. Other activities (e.g., cognitive restructuring)

   C. *Handouts.* The therapist will give the client the handouts at the end of the sessions that include them. (Most sessions)

Note. The categories that should be included in all or most sessions are followed by "(All sessions)" or "(Most sessions)," respectively.

suggest that you then conduct a brief review of the *independent activities* assigned during the previous session. Some of these activities entail very brief reviews; others will require more time and will essentially amount to separate interventions within the session. Whether you review the more time-intensive activities at this initial stage of the session or later on is a judgment call; it depends on which other topics are planned for that session, as well as considerations described below. In either case, follow the activities check-in with *psychoeducation* related to the topic of the session. Attention then moves to some combination of the *core treatment components*: *resource building, trauma processing,* and *facilitating mourning.* The specific treatment interventions are described in Chapter 10 for resource building, Chapter 11 for trauma processing (both exposure and cognitive processing), and Chapter 12 for facilitating mourning. Earlier sessions within the treatment are likely to involve more resource building, whereas later sessions will involve a heavier emphasis on exposure and cognitive processing. Most sessions require some combination of both, and these interventions will take up the bulk of the session. The session focus can then shift to the *wrap-up*, which includes big-picture or *integration* issues such as the relation among the three core treatment components discussed below. Sessions end with the assignment of new *independent activities*, and distribution of relevant *handouts*.

A client's particular manifestation of traumatic bereavement, her unique needs, and your clinical judgment will all contribute to the way the intervention elements fit together in a given session. Within the template, we leave the specific content blank; you and the client will "fill in" this content. The list of session topics in Table 1.2, the list of handouts by treatment element in Table 9.1, and the detailed sample 25-session treatment plan described earlier and presented on the book's website supplement provide further information about what sort of content fills in the template, based on the needs of the client.

Introduction

Session Frame: Focus, Rationale, Overview, and Topics. An overview at the beginning of each session helps to structure the session and reduces the possibility that the client and you might unconsciously collude in avoiding difficult topics or otherwise get off track. We refer to this as the *session frame.* As an example, you might introduce a session as follows: "Today we will focus on how traumatic bereavement has two components: trauma and loss. This might give you a way of understanding your experience that will help." In just a few sentences, you introduce the focus of the session, along with the rationale for that focus. An overview of the session tasks and topics further frames the session: "Today we will review the independent activities from the last session, discuss traumatic bereavement, help you to begin to process your loss, and end with discussing assignments for next time." This is also the place to identify any planned in-session activities such as breathing retraining. Preparing for each session by planning a session overview will result in a smoother flow, as well as the opportunity to cover more territory.

Treatment Frame Issues. Treatment frame issues will be most salient at the outset and ending of treatment, although some, such as payment of fees and regular attendance at sessions, and process issues, such as the client's feelings about the therapy and your therapeutic style, may arise at any time along the way. At the beginning of treatment, you and the client will typically discuss the goals and topics the treatment will address, the importance of both parties' active participation, the value of independent activities, and so on. This is also the time to discuss both the inevitability of termination and any associated feelings. At times, either you or the client may see value in increasing the frequency or length of sessions. For example, it is often helpful to meet twice a week when the client is engaged in exposure work, and to plan for longer sessions when in-session exposure work is scheduled. Such issues form the content for this part of the session.

Brief Review of Independent Activities. After addressing any treatment frame issues, you should review the independent activities assigned in the previous session. Asking the client about the assignments reinforces the understanding that they constitute a valuable aspect of the therapy. If the activity relates to today's topic, you can review it with the client later in the session. If it represents a completion of the previous session's work or is part of the ongoing work of resource building, you can discuss it at the outset of the session. Briefly covering each activity that was assigned in the previous session before focusing on any specific activity can keep you from getting bogged down. Otherwise, you may become involved in a detailed discussion of some activities, and run out of time before discussing other activities or issues planned for the session. In-depth discussions of one assigned activity may also indicate that the client is avoiding other therapy material. The amount of time spent processing each type of assignment will depend on where the client is in the treatment.

If the client has not completed independent activities, you should learn why, and then address relevant issues. Clients often benefit from exploring their avoidance of independent activities in session. Many of the skills you teach and assign to your clients as independent activities can be used for processing avoidance of the assignments themselves. For example, you might ask a client to label and discuss emotions that arise when he is contemplating assignments. Clients might also benefit from completing Handout 13, the Automatic Thought Record, on a thought related to independent activities (e.g., "I will fail at this assignment and disappoint my therapist," or "This assignment will make me so anxious that I'll make a mistake at work and my boss will reprimand me").

Many clients require concrete plans for engaging in avoided activities. If a client is avoiding independent activities, you might look together at the client's schedule and decide when and how the activity could be done. (The client could try it again under different conditions, such as with the participation of a support person, or the two of you could do the task together in session.) If the client is avoiding cognitive restructuring activities or exposure assignments, you should help her to complete these activities within the session. These two types of activities are the most challenging for many clients because they often prompt strong emotions.

Clients sometimes avoid independent activities because they are too painful. If this is the case, you should make sure that you are not choosing an activity that is too difficult for a client at this point in treatment. Clients sometimes underestimate the difficulty of an activity or exposure assignment. They may need to choose an easier assignment or modify the activity to make it more likely that they will succeed. However, if the avoided activity is appropriate, remind the client of the exposure rationale (we present a summary of it here for your use; further details are available in Handout 15, Processing the Loss), and encourage the client to engage in all of the activities as fully as possible.

"One of the most important goals of this treatment is to help you react to your significant other's death in a way that fits who you are and that is acceptable to you. Once you have identified, felt, and accepted your thoughts, feelings, and memories, you will be able to respond to them with more choice and freedom, and your emotions will become more manageable. We avoid feelings and thoughts about loss because they are painful. Unfortunately, the pain usually finds its way into our lives in one way or another, as flashbacks, intrusive thoughts, intense distress, or nightmares. Avoidance just prolongs this pain. This treatment will help you to experience emotions in a safe environment, with a lot of support."

Psychoeducation. Providing information by using the handouts in the Appendix and on the book's website supplement will be an important part of addressing the day's topics and core components (see below). In sharing information, you should create opportunities for the client to ask questions and clarify points of confusion. Of course, such discussions can become another means of avoiding difficult feelings, so you must continually assess the potential value of further explanation and discussion.

Core Treatment Components

Building Resources. This work focuses on developing self capacities, building social support and coping skills, addressing bereavement-specific issues, and working on values and meaning. We discuss these resource-building processes in Chapter 10.

Processing the Traumatic Death. This is the place in the session for exposure work and related emotional and cognitive processing. Processing the traumatic death begins once the client has some feelings skills in place. This processing should remain a focus of most sessions after the first few. A client (and sometimes you as the therapist) may be tempted to avoid this crucial element of treatment because of the feelings it raises. See Chapter 11 for specific information on trauma processing.

Mourning. Here, you and the client will address each "R" process as it becomes the current focus of the work. Independent activities, including those used for resource building and trauma processing, can help the client continue her movement through the six "Rs." Chapter 12 provides detailed information about this aspect of the treatment.

Wrap-Up

Integration. This is a place to discuss worldview, assumptive world, values, and other broad beliefs that shape the client's response to the loss and subsequent adaptation. It is also a good place to discuss the relation among the resource-building activities, processing the traumatic loss, and moving through the six "R" processes. For example, at this point in a session that has included exposure work, you might reinforce the client for the work he has done. Remind him that by confronting the painful aspects of the death, he is making it possible to move to the next "R" process; this will help him to understand the connection between trauma processing and mourning.

Independent Activities. In this final segment of the session, you will introduce the independent activities for next time. These include (1) resource-building activities such as building and using social support, coping skills, and self-care; (2) trauma-processing activities, such as cognitive restructuring,[2] exposure, and writing assignments; (3) mourning-related activities, such as recollecting the deceased or reflecting upon his positive and negative qualities; and/ or (4) other activities that relate to the treatment more generally, such as reading informational handouts about sudden, traumatic death (Handout 1, Sudden, Traumatic Death and Traumatic Bereavement) or treatment termination (Handout S2, Ending Therapy).

Independent activities between sessions are essential to the success of this treatment. You should select assignments that will further the work in which the client is currently engaged and that will balance support and challenge. It is essential that the client understand each assignment, and that you review the previous session's assignments with the client as part of each session. You should familiarize yourself with the resources in this book (especially those described in Chapters 10, 11, and 12 and in the Appendix), in order to be prepared to draw upon them as needed during sessions. Once you are familiar with the various types of independent activities, you can tailor them to address particular issues the client is facing.

When deciding whether and how to assign additional independent activities, consider the time and effort involved, so as not to assign too many activities at once. Encourage the client to use supportive activities (such as breathing retraining, self-care activities, and other coping behaviors) after, but not while, engaging in a challenging activity (such as an imaginal or *in vivo* exposure). This process will reinforce the client in using the activities on his own between sessions. You may decide to leave certain issues to the client to address using newly learned skills once the major work of therapy has ended. For example, one man lost his sister in a helicopter crash. About a year after her death, he lost his job. Although he found a new job, this second loss had affected his self-esteem, identity, and sense of purpose. Because there were so many pressing issues to address with regard to his sister's death, the therapist and client decided that he would use tools from the treatment to work on issues related to the job loss after his work with the therapist had ended. You may want to encourage clients to revisit particular independent activity assignments on their own once treatment has ended.

It is often useful to refer back to and elaborate on particular handouts. Several of these are designed to be referred to repeatedly. For example, the client's list of secondary losses (see Handout 17, Secondary Losses) and the fear and avoidance hierarchy (see Handout 25, Fear and Avoidance Hierarchy Form) provide techniques and resources that can promote recovery. If you perceive a client to be struggling with an issue that you have addressed in the past, you may choose to revisit previous assignments. The session would end with giving the client the relevant handouts. It is a good idea to photocopy the blank handouts that are used frequently (such as Handout 13, the Automatic Thought Record) so that you have multiple copies to provide to the client. This will allow you to work on challenging automatic thoughts easily within sessions. Keep an extra packet of handouts available for each client, so that if the client forgets to bring in an independent activity assignment, loses a handout, or needs an extra copy, it is readily available.

The handouts provide crucial opportunities for the client to apply the principles that are introduced in the sessions. After selecting relevant handouts, you may want to identify additional handouts that guide the client to work with and apply that information to her situation. Some of the handouts are information sheets (such as Handouts 1, Sudden, Traumatic Death

---

[2]Cognitive restructuring can be useful for building resources, processing trauma, and mourning. We include it within processing trauma because this is where it is indispensable in the treatment.

and Traumatic Bereavement; 2, Orientation to the Treatment; 3, Treatment Goals and Tools; and 4, Self-Care). Others are assignments (such as Handout 5, Exploring the Impact of the Death). Still others (e.g., Handouts 11, Identifying Automatic Thoughts Worksheet, and 14, Challenging Questions Worksheet) are worksheets to be used in sessions or as part of independent activities. Some handouts cover topics relevant to the major theoretical and conceptual underpinnings of the treatment (e.g., Handout 1, Sudden, Traumatic Death and Traumatic Bereavement; Handout 6, The Six "R" Processes of Mourning; Handout 19, Building Social Support) and the core treatment components (e.g., Handout 15, Processing the Loss). Effective use of the handouts requires a ninth-grade level of English language literacy. For clients without that skill level, or for those who are too distressed to concentrate, it may be useful to read handouts together or to extract the points that are essential to the client at this time and review those with the client in session.

Several practitioners have suggested ways to increase the likelihood that clients will complete independent activities successfully (see, e.g., Kazantzis & Deane, 1999; Najavits, 2005; Tompkins, 2004). From the beginning, it should be emphasized that these activities constitute a fundamentally important part of the treatment, and that they are integral to its success. It may be helpful to mention that studies show clearly that cognitive and behavioral therapy is more likely to result in a positive outcome if independent activities are used (Kazantzis et al., 2010). It is important to provide a rationale to the client for independent activities. Continue talking with the client about the benefits listed above—for example, that these activities help to build skills more quickly and also help clients gain confidence in their abilities.

Tompkins (2004) suggests that in introducing a particular independent activity, you should clarify the relevance of the activity to what a client has worked on in that session, as well as to the client's treatment goals. Najavits (2005) recommends creating a higher meaning for the activities (which she terms *commitments*) that you ask the client to perform. For example, an independent activity might encourage the client to schedule a medical appointment. According to Najavits, the higher meaning might be the awareness that the client is taking care of her body, or that she is showing respect for her children (who depend on her), as well as for her own future.

Moreover, independent activities should be appropriate to the client's sociocultural context. Tompkins (2004) provides an example of an unemployed, single mother of four, suffering from depression, who was assigned the task of going to a movie with a friend. In the next session, the woman tearfully indicated that she was not able to complete the assignment because she could not afford to pay for child care and a movie.

Ideally, the therapist should make the independent activity collaborative and provide some degree of choice regarding the assignment. Tompkins (2004) suggests that making a simple statement like "Would you be willing to try this?" can enhance a client's motivation to engage in the activity.

Finally, the activity should be set up to minimize the likelihood that the client will fail. Tompkins (2004) provides several excellent suggestions for how to make independent activities what he calls a "no-lose proposition." For example, he suggests saying, "There is no such thing as an unsuccessful homework assignment because we learn something every time a homework assignment is tried. . . . If you have trouble completing the homework assignment, that's okay. We can figure out what got in the way so that you can complete it next time" (p. 29).

INTEGRATING THIS APPROACH INTO AN ONGOING TREATMENT

In the context of an ongoing treatment relationship, the two of you may realize that the client needs to work on a specific sudden, traumatic death. Alternatively, such a loss may occur while the client is in treatment for other reasons. You then may want to conduct an assessment as described in Chapter 8. This is especially true if certain areas have received little or no attention to date in your work together. The best approach is to draw on your evaluation of the client to determine what she needs at this time, and then to review the resources in Chapters 10, 11, and 12 and the Appendix and on the website supplement for possible relevance to your client's situation. This treatment approach will be most effective when it targets one specific loss; when you maintain the flow and order of sessions and topics described in Table 1.2 (even if you are using only a subset); and when the client has adequate resources to process the traumatic memories in order to move through the six "Rs."

In the midst of an ongoing treatment other than this one, you may decide to use the resource-building elements of the treatment when you hit a rough patch. For example, Bill, who had served in the military in Bosnia, came to therapy to address his PTSD related to that experience. It quickly became evident that he could benefit from work on self capacities, coping skills, and values. His therapist used the material in Chapter 10, as well as the relevant handouts in the Appendix and on the website supplement, to facilitate this work. As another example, Dr. Sullivan had been working with Yani to address a worsening of trauma symptoms, triggered by the death of an uncle who had sexually abused her as a child. At the 1-year anniversary of her uncle's death, a memorial service was held, and Yani became increasingly distressed. Dr. Sullivan, who was familiar with this treatment approach, practiced the technique of breathing retraining with Yani. She also collaborated with Yani to create a list of self-care activities within the session, and then asked Yani to engage with at least one of these activities per day in between their sessions.

When you are integrating this approach into a therapy that will continue after the traumatic bereavement work is complete (as opposed to using it as the whole treatment with a particular client), you may choose to reserve the termination material until you are ending the therapy. In this case, we strongly recommend weaving discussion of the ending of the treatment into the therapy along the way and providing adequate time to say goodbye, since this is such an important process for survivors of traumatic death.

CLINICAL INTEGRATION

Anticipating her session with Shantal later that afternoon, Patricia felt anxious. She acknowledged a very strong desire to help alleviate her client's suffering; Patricia found that she was easily able to empathize with Shantal whose son was killed 2 years earlier. In today's session, which was their third, she intended to lay out a treatment plan in more detail. She hoped that orienting Shantal to a specific plan for the treatment as a whole would be organizing for Shantal, thereby reducing her anxiety about the therapy. Because Shantal's life had been so chaotic for the past 2 years, Patricia wanted the treatment to serve as an antidote.

Her notes, written for a case consultation, read as follows:

> **Resources**: Strong faith; experiences surviving and moving through past trauma and grief (though trauma history could also be a vulnerability); ability to tolerate

strong affect; social support from friends & family; desire to be a good mother to her remaining children.

Mourning process: Traumatic imagery seems to prevent Shantal from remembering her son, Tyler, before the accident. Can't remember realistically. Shantal can't find comfort in celebrating Tyler's life—it's almost as though she can't access information and memories of his life prior to the death. She can only picture him with a bullet wound. Seems to believe that if pain diminishes, she will lose an attachment to Tyler.

Trauma processing: Has Shantal begun to process her own experience of the gruesome accident apart from Tyler's death? Her daughter watched it happen. Shantal heard the gunshot. She reports many trauma symptoms, including flashbacks and acute anxiety. Solid resources available to help get through exposure work while remaining grounded; however, anxiety and panic are very high at times. Explore Shantal's experience of anger.

Problematic beliefs: "I should have protected Tyler; I've failed as a mother; trauma follows me everywhere." All point to self-blame.

Patricia's notes continued on the next few pages. Many of her observations and questions would prove to be relevant over the next several months. She understood that what was important at this stage of therapy was a flexible treatment plan that took into account the particular ways in which Shantal was stuck along the path of mourning her son's death and processing her traumatic experience. Patricia picked up her pen and began to sketch out the following plan:

1. With possibility of criminal case, discuss note taking and potential limits to confidentiality with Shantal again—hard to take in everything first time around.

2. Work to maintain and solidify Shantal's current resources. Assign a resource-building activity for each week, with an emphasis on breathing retraining. Check in about coping—particularly self-care—at beginning of each session, keeping coping explicit and front & center. Spend next three sessions (Sessions 3–6) focused on self-care and social support.

3. Listen for problematic beliefs. Provide Shantal with psychoeducation about maladaptive beliefs and automatic thoughts. Ask her to keep a running list of automatic thoughts that arise between sessions, and do so with her within sessions. Use handouts for identifying and challenging beliefs. Introduce in about Session 6.

4. Explore Shantal's expectations of herself as a mother, both before and after the shooting. Explore her thoughts and feelings about her trauma history. Session 6 or 7—with intro to automatic thoughts.

5. Provide some psychoeducation about exposure work and rationale for this. Given Shantal's level of anxiety, start small and work up to more anxiety-provoking situations. Keep ratings of anxiety levels while doing any kind of exposure. Discuss the idea of a therapeutic window and stay within that. Introduce exposure in Session 7 or 8 (later than in the sample treatment; need to strengthen resources first), assuming Shantal demonstrates an ability to utilize resources, and as long as anxiety does not further intensify.

6. *As exposure activities progress, assess where Shantal is with each of the "R" processes. As of now, seems to be struggling to remember Tyler prior to his death—Recollect and reexperience the deceased and the relationship. Explore "Rs" as suggested in sample treatment plan.*

7. *As treatment progresses, ask Shantal to consider places in her life where she might reinvest some energy. Could build on values and goals work later in the therapy.*

8. *Throughout, be explicit about our relationship/connection and eventual termination; a part of Shantal is very sensitive to perceived abandonment, though it's difficult for her to acknowledge this.*

Patricia's plan was to use these notes as a starting point. She included more specific information for the next several sessions, with a plan to fill in more details for later sessions as they approached. She planned to invite Shantal to consider this plan with her, tweak it as necessary, and continue to assess how Shantal was adapting along the way.

CONCLUDING REMARKS

This chapter presents considerations for implementing this treatment approach for traumatic bereavement. Shantal's therapy offers an example of the ways in which assessment of strengths and vulnerabilities, clinical judgment, general psychotherapy issues, and attention to the various elements of our treatment approach can be woven together to assist those suffering from traumatic bereavement. Shantal's therapist, Patricia, ascertained that she had the resources available to engage effectively in exposure work, but she was also aware of the potential for Shantal's anxiety to be very high. The therapist therefore took her time with a thorough assessment in the first few therapy sessions and developed a working plan that would emphasize breathing retraining, self-care, social support, and other resource-building activities. Given what she had learned about Shantal thus far, Patricia also took note of specific considerations with regard to the implementation of other aspects of the treatment—addressing problematic beliefs and working with the "R" processes, for example. Given Shantal's trauma symptoms, Patricia was willing to slow down the therapy if needed, in order to ensure that Shantal's level of agitation stayed within the therapeutic window.

In addition to discussing specific considerations pertaining to implementation of the treatment approach, such as informed consent and termination, we have offered an overview of possible ways to structure the treatment. You will need to attend to the overall structure of the treatment, as well as to the structure of a given session. The sample treatment plan on the website supplement, and Table 9.2, aid in these respective tasks. It is our hope that the nuts and bolts provided here help you to visualize how these pieces might fit together within a given individual treatment. You may wish to come back to this chapter after digesting the information presented in the remainder of the text.

CHAPTER 10

Building Resources

Phyllis, in her mid-50s, first sought therapy about 18 months after losing her fiancé, who died only days after experiencing the first symptoms of meningitis. She had reconciled herself to living as a single woman until the day she met Alex, who changed her life. Their whirlwind courtship and eventual engagement were an unexpected delight for her. Then, one day shortly after their engagement, Alex developed a terrible headache and photosensitivity. When, at Phyllis's insistence, he phoned his primary care doctor, the on-call doctor told Alex it was "probably just the flu" and to call in a few days if he wasn't feeling better. Three days later, Alex was dead, from bacterial meningitis. At that point, Phyllis, in her own words, "lost it." Prior to Alex's death, Phyllis had usually been able to hold things together. A survivor of childhood abuse, she was already acquainted with the ramifications of trauma. Although she continued to experience some trauma symptoms as an adult, she worked hard to manage them in order to function effectively as a secretary at a social services agency. With the death of her fiancé, Phyllis's life seemed out of control. She felt as though she were going crazy, was unable to trust anyone, and reported an almost complete inability to manage her day-to-day affairs. She no longer went to the office. She spent most of her days in bed, withdrew from social activities, and visibly shook when she did interact with others. During her frequent crying bouts, Phyllis's sobs turned into gasps as she struggled to take in air. She experienced physical pain throughout her body and was unable to find relief through the many remedies suggested to her. Her grief, rage, and sense of betrayal consumed her. She almost never took advantage of the emotional or practical support her friends offered; she felt angry with everyone, including herself. She found little or no comfort in distractions such as reading, movies, or physical exercise on the rare occasions when she was able to attempt them.

This chapter provides guidance for doing resource-building work with clients.

SELF CAPACITIES

Self capacities (also referred to as *feelings skills*) are inner abilities that help people regulate internal states. Their presence or absence reflects the individual's attachment experiences (Bowlby, 1969). Over time, self capacities provide the foundation for managing strong feelings, maintaining a fundamental sense of worthiness, and allowing for an internalized connection to loving others.

People who have early traumatic experiences (including, e.g., abuse, neglect, and chronic exposure to violence) may not develop adequate self capacities to function comfortably in a complex world. And even those with well-developed self capacities may find them challenged by a sudden, traumatic loss. Because traumatic death can evoke strong emotions, feelings skills are a foundational part of this treatment. In order to confront the trauma and approach what they may have been avoiding, survivors need adequately developed (or restored) capacities for regulating their emotions and maintaining a positive sense of self. Specific skills to deal with strong, intense, and potentially overwhelming emotions will help these clients to experience their feelings more fully, with less discomfort, less fear, and lower risk of destabilization.

Three self capacities are essential to this internal stability: *inner connection* (which helps people to stay connected to positive images and memories of loved ones), *self-worth* (which helps people to maintain a generally positive and stable sense of their own value), and *affect management* skills (which help people to handle their strong feelings) (Pearlman, 1998; Saakvitne et al., 2000). We describe each of these abilities and discuss ways to build them below.

Developing Self Capacities

It is important to assess a client's self capacities as a way of gauging how to pace the exposure work, how much additional support the client will need, and where the client can seek respite through means other than avoidance. (See Chapter 8 and Brock and colleagues [2006] for information about assessing self capacities.) The approach to developing self capacities is the same for clients with and without attachment challenges. The difference is that the process is likely to take longer and include setbacks as an attachment-challenged client builds self capacities, uses them in difficult situations, and refines them over time. The *Risking Connection* trauma training curriculum (Saakvitne et al., 2000) highlights the development of self capacities in adults with childhood trauma histories.

Cultivating self capacities takes place in the context of the therapeutic relationship. The therapist–client relationship is both the container within which these capacities germinate and the major tool for growing them. The feelings skills exercises the client engages in between sessions (see Handout 8, Feelings Skills) guide her in connecting with her inner experience and reflecting on the results of that connection. For each feelings skill, the handout describes the skill area, discusses its importance, and offers exercises for its development. In this context, connecting with inner experience means, for example, that the client will allow herself to feel grief, guilt, anger, curiosity, surprise, and happiness, even if momentarily, and then notice (with your support as the therapist) that she endured these feelings. Your confidence, respect, and guidance reinforce the client's self-worth, inner connection with loving others, and affect management.

Engaging in the emotional processing work of this treatment (described in Chapter 11) is another way that self capacities develop. Clients learn by doing. Their experience may be "I was afraid of facing my feelings, but I was able to manage this strong feeling, and I did not get overwhelmed." Successfully completing exposure activities reinforces and enhances the client's self capacities (self-worth, in this case). The self capacities (either the existence of affect management, or perhaps at first just an understanding of it) can help him to approach and tackle exposure. In turn, successes with exposure activities (initially talking about the deceased and the loss, then eventually going into the world to confront what the client has avoided) build self capacities (affect management and self-worth), all within the support of the therapy relationship. The client's awareness of your compassion for the experience of traumatic bereavement and for his attempts to strengthen coping behaviors and social support helps him to create an internalized representation of the therapist (a "benign other") that he can draw on in challenging times. This internalization process takes place over time, through forming a therapeutic alliance in which you convey respect and hope, reflect the client's value, and reinforce his efforts to grow.

In addition to the exercises in Handout 8, we offer some specific suggestions for developing each self capacity in the following sections. You can select those exercises that seem best suited to each client's needs.

Inner Connection

As noted above, inner connection allows people to carry positive images and memories of their loved ones, even in the loved ones' absence. Inner connection is the internal representation of loving relationships, rather than the interpersonal connection people may receive through social support. It can be thought of as a dimension of *object constancy*—the ability to maintain a stable internal representation of self and other (Mahler, 1975). The ability to imagine words of love, comfort, or support from a compassionate relative, friend, or other figure reflects a strong sense of inner connection with loving others. This resource can help people through difficult times, guiding and supporting them to feel less lonely and afraid.

Developing Inner Connection. Encouraging survivors to be creative in thinking about who their "loving others" are can help them develop a sense of inner connection. A "loving other" may be a friend or family member, a former teacher or clergyperson, a pet or imaginary figure, a historical figure, or a fictional character with whom a client has developed a special internal relationship. The person doesn't have to be alive. Some clients will choose to use you, the therapist, as the important "other." Whoever the "loving other" may be, encourage the client to imagine the "other" in times of pain or struggle—for example, "Can you imagine what your grandmother would say?" One survivor found it soothing to draw pictures of her beloved cat, which she then looked at when she was feeling lonely and distraught while at work.

If thinking of the loved one whose death is the focus of this treatment does not cause too much distress, the client may use the deceased as the internalized loving other. When clients find that thinking about their loved ones brings up a lot of sadness, support them in allowing themselves to feel the sadness. Remind them that they can keep this person's love with them by recalling special moments and connections they shared. This is also good practice in increasing affect management and in addressing avoidance.

Self-Worth

Feeling worthy or deserving of life and good fortune, even under difficult circumstances, is a sign of positive self-worth. It arises from a secure base in childhood, which develops when adults consistently treat children with love, compassion, and respect. Ideally, over time, people internalize that positive regard and come to feel "good enough" about themselves. You can say to a client:

"Adequate self-worth doesn't mean never feeling bad about yourself, but it does mean that even when you feel bad, you know or can recall that you are still a reasonably good human being. When you do something you know is wrong, you may feel guilty about what you did, which is different from feeling as though you are a bad person."

Developing or maintaining self-worth can be challenging for people whose childhood experiences have included unsupportive or harsh interactions with caregivers; bullying by peers; or other experiences of neglect, abuse, or humiliation. It is common for these individuals to shift into self-blame or feelings of worthlessness when they encounter stressful life experiences. Such clients are likely to require additional resource building in this treatment, and they will also benefit from the cognitive work on automatic thoughts (described in Chapter 11).

Developing Self-Worth. Traumatically bereaved clients who struggle with feelings of worthlessness should be encouraged to associate with people who treat them with respect and bring out the best in them. Self-worth can be increased by activities designed to help survivors learn to treat themselves with respect and engage in actions that are consistent with their dignity. Such activities might include spending time (even in small amounts at first) doing things they are good at, such as baking, arranging flowers, or repairing a bicycle. As clients begin to reengage with others, they may experience increased self-worth through your calling their attention to their helpful, respectful, or compassionate behaviors. Helping to care for a young child and offering to pick up groceries for a neighbor are examples of time-limited strategies that can build or rebuild a client's sense of worth. Helping others is also a way of reengaging with the world and beginning to resume a life that includes something beyond grief and mourning. Some survivor clients are tremendously relieved when they realize they still have something to give to others.

Affect Management

Affect management (or *feelings management*) refers to the ways people experience and handle particularly challenging emotions. A person who has trouble experiencing anger, for example, may try not to feel it or may pretend it's not there. Some people become so skilled at burying strong emotions—both negative and positive—that they are not even aware that they are experiencing them. Without awareness of emotions, such individuals lack essential information for understanding themselves and others and for maintaining relationships.

Emotions—even strong ones—help people to stay connected to themselves, to others, and to the world. They provide the feedback that assists clients in navigating the interpersonal world. For example, consider a person who becomes angry with a friend who is unsupportive after a sudden, traumatic death. This anger can be a signal that the relationship isn't meeting his needs and that he should consider what is happening to determine how to handle the situation. People who are not connected to their emotions will miss the information these emotions convey.

There are four steps involved in feelings management, each of which is important throughout this treatment and beyond. The four steps are recognizing, tolerating, modulating, and integrating feelings.

Recognizing feelings means being able to sense an emotion as it arises in one's body, and to label or name it. A client may find this step to be easy, difficult, or somewhere in between.

She may also find that she is able to recognize some feelings or connect some bodily states to emotions more readily than others. It may be easy to recognize sadness, and more difficult to recognize anger (or vice versa), for example.

Tolerating feelings means being able to accept emotions as they arise. It entails being open to experiencing one's feelings as opposed to avoiding them. It also involves responding to emotions nonjudgmentally rather than trying to block, denigrate, or change them. Tolerating feelings can be difficult for those who have learned (usually early in life) that some emotions are "bad" or "wrong" and that they should be avoided. For some children, showing certain feelings may have resulted in negative consequences such as reprimands, punishment, or abuse from caregivers. Tolerating feelings may also be difficult if a client is afraid that emotions will take over, causing him to lose control or to harm himself or someone else. For example, feeling fatigue, confusion, or panic instead of rage may be a familiar way of operating. Addressing this issue in treatment can help the survivor to accept and process his rage. Finally, people who are accustomed to having a great deal of control over their emotions and who value a "rational" or unemotional stance in life may find it hard to accept or tolerate the full range of often powerful and fluctuating feelings that can accompany traumatic bereavement.

Modulating feelings entails being able to control the intensity of the emotion. It does not mean "not feeling." Rather, it means regulating emotions so one can accept, learn from, and move toward integrating them. The ability to modulate feelings results in a decrease in the fear and distress related to experiencing them. An additional benefit is the knowledge that one can influence the intensity of emotions rather than feeling controlled by them, which itself is empowering.

Clients need encouragement to sit with their feelings long enough to practice modulating them. The idea that people can modulate their emotions may surprise clients who have learned that emotions control people, rather than the other way around. Modulating feelings is a learned skill, and thus clients need to be provided with the necessary information and tools.

Once clients can recognize, tolerate, and modulate feelings, they can begin to learn from them and integrate them. *Integrating feelings* means interweaving emotions with their context. This means that an individual can become aware of a feeling state and link it to a bodily sensation, the events and experiences that preceded or gave rise to the feeling this time, past experiences of this feeling, and ways she has responded to it in the past. Integrating feelings also means incorporating them into the narrative or story of one's life, so that one can make sense of them within a broader framework of self-understanding. For example, a person may come to realize that when she is with someone who does not respect her, she gets a stomachache. Through reflection, she may understand that the stomachache is a sign of feelings of worthlessness. She may further link this to her childhood experiences of an older sibling diminishing her. Having a stomachache was a way to end the taunting because her mother would suggest she lie down in her room for a while to rest.

Developing Affect Management. Traumatically bereaved clients may feel that painful, unfamiliar emotions arise suddenly, without apparent context. It can be useful to invite such a client to develop a "thinking–feeling–doing" continuum. When the client reports being unable to understand the source of his feelings, you can suggest that the next time he is surprised (or overwhelmed) by a feeling state, he should write down what he remembers thinking, feeling, and doing just before he became aware of the emotion. Filling out this timeline backward (e.g., right before the feeling came up, the hour before, that morning, the night before) until the client reaches a possible point of origin for the feeling can provide a context for it. This demystification of emotions may help to reduce hypervigilance, because it helps clients feel greater control over their emotional states and thus better able to tolerate strong feelings when they arise.

The *Risking Connection* trauma training curriculum (Saakvitne et al., 2000) offers another type of feelings continuum: The therapist invites the client to develop a variety of names for related feelings states. This exercise helps the client differentiate feelings and their intensity; rather than simply "sad," the client might start at one end of the continuum with "desolate" and move through "despondent," "melancholy," "unhappy," and "blue" to "down." The significant connotation of each word is the client's; the order of intensity or level of distress implied by each word is less important than the client's observation that she can feel bad without being at the most intense end of her own continuum for that feeling state.

More generally, some research has suggested that resilience-building behaviors can increase affect management capacity by increasing hippocampal volume, decreasing amygdala activity and size, increasing serotonin and endorphin production, and activating the prefrontal cortex (Southwick, Litz, Charney, & Friedman, 2011). Relevant resilience-building behaviors include physical exercise and adequate sleep (McEwen & Gianaros, 2011; Pietrzak, Morgan, & Southwick, 2010), developing role competence and confidence (Johnson et al., 2011), practicing gratitude (e.g., Emmons & Mishra, 2011), and other activities discussed elsewhere in this chapter (e.g., meaning making, cognitive appraisal, and social support).

Developing role competence means enhancing one's ability to fulfill such roles as worker, parent, or student. Guiding clients to resources for learning needed skills can help with this. *Confidence* comes about in part through the therapist's attention to and reinforcement of what the client is doing well and questioning self-deprecation where appropriate (e.g., through the use of Handout 13, the Automatic Thought Record, as described in Chapter 11). Clients also gain confidence through successfully navigating tasks, including the tasks of the treatment.

COPING SKILLS

In this treatment approach, we view *coping skills* as activities and strategies that comfort, calm, soothe, or support an individual. Augmenting these skills contributes to the development of self capacities; the client learns to recognize that she has strategies for managing strong feelings, and this recognition in turn increases both her affect management and her sense of self-worth. We have identified a number of coping strategies we believe are particularly useful for clients with traumatic bereavement. We recommend engaging in self-care and pleasant activities (see Handout 4, Self-Care); breathing retraining (described in Handout 7, Breathing Retraining); using social support (see Handout 18, The Importance of Enhancing Social Support); and addressing automatic thoughts (see Handouts 10, What Are Automatic Thoughts?, and 11, Identifying Automatic Thoughts Worksheet). We offer multiple strategies because different clients prefer different strategies. We recommend that clients choose the coping strategies they prefer, as long as those strategies address the issues each client is facing.

In this section, we discuss two important aspects of helping clients to develop their coping skills: integrating coping skills into this treatment, and addressing obstacles to coping behavior. Again, the therapeutic relationship is the crucible for the client to practice, refine, and broaden his repertoire of coping skills. Your therapeutic encouragement and consistency in discussing coping skills will support this growth; in turn, this will promote the client's ability to do the challenging work of confronting the loss, thereby facilitating movement through the six "R" processes of mourning.

Most practitioners would agree that ultimately, survivors must relinquish the avoidance that enables them to evade distressing thoughts and feelings associated with the death (Shear, 2010). In treating survivors of traumatic bereavement, therapists sometimes try to break down clients' avoidance by forcing them to do something before they are ready. Part of the art of this treatment is guiding a client and supporting him through challenging experiences without colluding in problematic avoidance or coercing him. With practice, the use of a fear and avoidance hierarchy (see Handout 25, the Fear and Avoidance Hierarchy Form), and feedback from the client, you will develop the ability to tune in to each client's needs and to present exposure assignments that will help the client move forward through the "R" processes.

Integrating Coping Skills into the Treatment

We recommend assigning coping activities in every session. These activities support the client in his recovery process and help him develop both strategies and the habit of using them outside the therapy room. The best way to do this is by emphasizing the importance of coping skills at the outset of treatment, inviting the client to create a list of current strategies, and working on expanding the list together over time. Toward the end of each session, ask the client which coping strategy he would like to engage in, experiment with, or practice over the week ahead. As noted above, some therapists may be inclined to introduce coping strategies that focus exclusively on dealing with the loss. However, it is also important to introduce restoration-oriented coping strategies, such as doing new things, and meeting new people. You can introduce these strategies as part of the work with the client on values and goals, described in more detail below. At the beginning of each session, it is important to inquire about the coping behaviors the client has used since last time, to ask how things went, and to address any problems.

Addressing Obstacles to Coping Behavior

Clients may be reluctant to engage in certain coping activities, particularly self-care and pleasant activities. It can be helpful to acknowledge that such activities are important, even though they may require a client to push herself. Positive coping activities can create guilt about focusing attention on oneself or feeling good in the context of a significant other's death. The client (or her culture) may have explicit or implicit strictures about laughing, celebrating, or displaying positive emotions. In one case, a mother who lost an infant organized a birthday party for her 10-year-old. She felt hurt by the criticism she received that having a party was inappropriate during a period of mourning.

The client may believe (and it may be true) that others will disapprove if she attends to her own needs. In fact, many clients report that they had difficulty attending to their own needs even before the loss. These individuals may need to start with small attempts at self-care and pleasant activities. The therapy should explore beliefs related to self-care, coping, and pleasant activities, and use the cognitive processing techniques described in Chapter 11 to address them. For example, you and a client may agree that reaching out for social support by asking a friend to go to the gym with her would be a good thing to do. You may ask the client what thoughts come up for her as she thinks about doing this. The client might report something like "People at the gym will think I've forgotten my husband." You could ask, "What would that say about you as a person?" The client might say something like "I'm selfish." You and the client can then explore this belief—a possible instance of an automatic thought—by using Handout 13, the Automatic Thought Record.

Pain can be a way of staying connected to the deceased. The client may fear that enjoying life would be a betrayal of her deceased loved one or that she would lose touch with him. Again, automatic thoughts may come into play here, and you and your client can use the Automatic Thought Record to explore them as appropriate.

SOCIAL SUPPORT

Social support is one of the most frequently studied coping resources. It is usually defined as the emotional and physical comfort that people receive from those in their social network, including family members, friends, co-workers, and neighbors. Effective social support helps people to feel loved, cared for, valued, and understood. Social support reduces the impact of major life events or chronic strains on health and well-being (Thoits, 1995). Based on this knowledge, interventions designed to enhance social support have been developed for those experiencing a wide variety of stressful life events, including the sudden, traumatic loss of a loved one (e.g., Murphy, Lohan, Dimond, & Fan, 1998).

Empirical studies have provided mixed support for the idea that social support protects the bereaved from the deleterious effects of loss (W. Stroebe, Zech, Stroebe, & Abakoumkin, 2005). However, few studies have examined the effects of social support on survivors of sudden, traumatic death. In one of the few studies to assess social support in this context, Murphy, Johnson, Chung, and Beaton (2003) followed parents for 5 years after their child's death by accident, suicide, or homicide. Perceived social support was one of only two variables studied that predicted a decrease in PTSD symptoms over time. In a more recent review of risk factors for poor outcome following the violent death of a loved one, Hibberd and colleagues (2010) also concluded that social support protects survivors from the development of PTSD.

W. Stroebe, Stroebe, Abakoumkin, and Schut (2005) have found that a variable called *emotional loneliness* is critically important in understanding spousal loss. These authors indicate that, contrary to popular belief, social support does not influence emotional loneliness. Widows and widowers report that even when they are with other people, they still feel deeply lonely because they miss their spouses. These results are troubling because bereaved individuals usually exhibit high levels of emotional loneliness for years (van Baarsen et al., 1999). Consequently, attention should be focused specifically on emotional loneliness and its ramifications for a widowed client.

We believe that survivors of sudden, traumatic death will benefit from a full consideration of issues surrounding support. We provide specific strategies for improving support below.

Developing Social Support

Initially, it is important to provide a rationale to the client for increasing useful social support and staying connected to others. At this point, we recommend giving the client Handout 18, The Importance of Enhancing Social Support, which provides a list of reasons for strengthening a personal support network as discussed above. It can be useful to ask the client specifically whether he has found himself withdrawing from others. If so, you can go through the list of reasons for social withdrawal (see Handout 19, Building Social Support) and ask the client whether these are true in his case. It is important to validate the client's desire to withdraw from others who make hurtful comments, while also exploring how the client can deal with such comments when they occur.

Next, you should ask the client about his current support network. Handout 19 can serve as a guide in eliciting information from the client, as a reference for the client to help him to assess his support network, or both. You and the client should establish who is in the network, which network members provide effective support, which members were in the network prior to the loss but have backed away, and so forth. If the mourner has difficulty providing such information, you can mention broad categories of people and ask whether specific people in that category have been supportive or unsupportive. Such categories might include parents, siblings, friends, co-workers, neighbors, and members of the client's faith community.

Drawing from this conversation, the next step is to guide the client in making a list of the types of support that she needs now. Some clients may need tangible assistance. For example, a widow may need help with household projects such as shoveling snow. Although the mourner may be reluctant to request such help, you might mention than many people find it valuable and meaningful to be in a helping role. Another client may be in need of a good listener—a person who allows the mourner to express his thoughts and feelings, and who accepts these feelings without judgment. Still another client may benefit most from being around friends who convey their love and concern, or who are willing to invite the mourner to share their daily lives without needing to focus on the loss. Once the client generates the list, you should assist him in going through it to identify people who would be particularly appropriate for providing specific kinds of support. Next, you can work with the client to generate small goals that involve relating to others (e.g., the client might call an old friend to see a movie or go for a walk). You may want to identify one or two of these goals together to schedule as independent activities, perhaps as part of the values and goals work described below.

Alternatively, you and your client may plan exposure activities (discussed in more detail in Chapter 11). This approach suggests establishing a hierarchy for the list of goals involving social support, and then addressing them from the easiest to the more difficult. The client may have to create social events that fit into his hierarchy, rather than waiting for social opportunities to arise.

In generating the list of social support goals, both you and the client should try to identify barriers to seeking support. If the client is unable to carry out the goals you agreed upon during the previous session, a discussion of potential barriers may prove fruitful. For example, a woman may decide not to attend a social gathering because she believes that others don't really want to see her. If you so desire, you can add this situation to the client's hierarchy, then structure one or more exposure tasks to fit into the treatment at the appropriate juncture. You can also use Handout 11, the Identifying Automatic Thoughts Worksheet, to address underlying beliefs that impede the client's ability to seek social support.

You can use Handout 19, Building Social Support, to explore the kinds of social responses that others have made to the client and the feelings they elicited. You should validate the client's anger and frustration with those who provide unhelpful support. One mother who lost her child had difficulty spending time with her sister, who cried the entire time they were together. "I felt that I had to take care of her," said the mother. In such situations, it may be beneficial to encourage the client to minimize contact with unhelpful people.

You can help the client to educate potential supporters about traumatic bereavement and about the types of responses that she finds helpful. Shear has developed an innovative approach to creating more effective support (see, e.g., Shear, Boelen, & Neimeyer, 2011). The client is encouraged to invite a family member or friend to a session. The therapist discusses issues pertinent to support provision and also provides psychoeducation.

For clients who are particularly troubled by the insensitive comments of others, it is important to help them understand why others make such comments. It may be worthwhile to encourage clients gently to consider the situation from the potential supporters' point of view. You may wish to initiate a discussion about why others behave the way they do. Of course, most potential supporters have never experienced a loss of this sort, so they are simply not able to comprehend the human suffering that is unleashed. Moreover, for people who have not experienced a traumatic death, interacting with someone who has can evoke discomfort, anxiety, or fear. Such feelings may lead potential supporters to blurt out inept comments that inadvertently hurt the survivor. Others' painful remarks usually result from lack of information or social discomfort, and not simply callousness. In fact, some mourners have stated that prior to their loss, they would not have understood what survivors are dealing with, and that they would have been just as insensitive to survivors of traumatic loss as their supporters are to them (Dyregrov, 2003–2004).

Mourners also find it helpful to tell others what they believe to be important elements of their loved one's death. For example, one couple lost a son as a result of a motor vehicle crash. Following the crash, he was rushed to the hospital, but he had extensive brain damage. This couple wanted their closest friends to understand the difficulties they had in removing their son from life support. Sharing such information provides common ground, enhancing the likelihood that support attempts will be on target.

Overall, survivors stress the importance of relating to others with openness and honesty. Many advocate giving clear signals to others regarding the kinds of support that are useful and appreciated. As Dyregrov (2005–2006) has noted, "thereby the ineptitude of social support networks could be diminished, and well-intentioned initiatives that result in unhelpful or even harmful support could be avoided" (p. 356). Dyregrov's (2003–2004) respondents indicated that social network members who had themselves experienced sudden, traumatic deaths provided the most helpful responses (see also Lehman et al., 1987). These findings suggest that it may be worthwhile to ask a survivor whether anyone in his social network has experienced traumatic loss. Interactions with such an individual can be extremely effective in validating the client's concerns and providing assurance that his feelings and behaviors are normal. In our experience, even someone on the periphery of the network—for example, a colleague at work whom the survivor does not know very well—may be an excellent source of support if he has experienced a similar loss.

Some clients may benefit from attending a support group for individuals who have experienced similar losses. Such groups may be particularly valuable for those who have few social relationships. However, there are considerable differences in how such groups are run, and whether there is any involvement by knowledgeable professionals. Some groups base interventions on grief models that lack empirical support, such as stage models. We strongly advocate making referrals only to groups with which you are familiar.

In addition to the direct benefits that stem from effective support, supportive ties also provide a context for work on other important issues. A survivor who has been avoiding a certain activity, such as going to temple or church, has a better chance of addressing the problem if she has a network of friends who encourage her to go and offer to accompany her. Supportive relationships can also help survivors begin investing in the future by exposing them to new people, ideas, and activities.

Internet Support Resources

An increasingly important source of support for the bereaved is the Internet. As Stroebe, van der Houwen, and Schut (2008) have noted, there has been an explosion in the number and types of Internet resources that offer support for bereaved individuals. Many clients seek information or support over the Internet before coming to treatment. (For informative reviews of bereavement support services on the Internet, see Dominick et al., 2009–2010, and Sofka, Cupit, & Gilbert, 2012.) Sofka and colleagues (2012) argue that modern communication technology has had a profound influence on how we think about grief and how we attempt to come to terms with it.

There are two broad categories of Internet resources that, in our judgment, can provide support for bereaved individuals: sites providing information about grief or online support groups, and sites serving primarily to memorialize or pay tribute to the deceased. Because each of these categories has the potential to provide unique sources of support, we describe them separately below.

Information and Internet Support Groups

Most websites designed to deal with grief and loss provide information about the mourning process, message boards, books about grief and mourning, and chat rooms, which afford opportunities for online interaction with others who have experienced similar losses. Gilbert and Horsley (2011) offer a cogent discussion of the appeal of such websites: They are available around the clock; they offer anonymity; and they offer support that may, for a variety of reasons, be difficult for a survivor to find elsewhere. Gilbert and Horsley maintain that interactions over the Internet are particularly valuable for mourners who do not feel comfortable in social situations. They give the example of a person whose loved one committed suicide. As described earlier, such individuals often feel that others blame them for what happened or are unsympathetic. The Internet can serve as a refuge for such people, who say that for once they are welcomed and encouraged to share their feelings.

In our experience, online communication can also be especially valuable to a survivor who, because of the type of loss that occurred, will have few opportunities to interact with similar others. Certain types of losses may raise unique issues that are best supported by those whose losses are similar. For example, parents who lost their only child may find it more beneficial to interact with similarly bereaved parents, as some of their concerns are not the same as those of parents who have surviving children. In addition, mourners who are disenfranchised, such as some gays or lesbians who lose life partners, or people who have been divorced, may find support online that is not readily available elsewhere. The website GriefNet (*griefnet.org*) has over 50 different bereavement support groups. Many of these are quite narrowly focused, such as death resulting from medical errors, from a murder–suicide scenario, or from a drug overdose (Lynn & Rath, 2012).

As is the case for support groups, however, online chat rooms are often unmoderated. Most sites do their best to remove posts that seem likely to cause distress. Nonetheless, a survivor may encounter members who are highly critical of how he is coping with the loss, which could undermine his motivation to continue to seek support. It is important to explore the client's use of these types of support, in much the same way as you inquire about support from network members. This practice will allow you to assist the client in evaluating the positive and negative dimensions of all these resources. You should also monitor whether Internet use contributes to a client's isolation by decreasing face-to-face contacts (Stroebe, van der Houwen, & Schut, 2008).

Internet Memorialization

The Internet is also increasingly used to commemorate the deceased and to create memorials (Gilbert & Horsley, 2011). People contribute narratives about their relationship, as well as poems, artwork, photographs, music, or videos. An advantage of such memorials is that they allow the bereaved to "honor their dead in their own way and at their own time" (p. 368). A major trend in how people handle their grief today is the use of social networking sites, such as Facebook, MySpace, and Friendster. Given the role of these sites in facilitating social connection, it is perhaps not surprising that they play an increasingly influential role in coming to terms with the loss of a loved one. As Fearon (2012) has indicated, these sites provide a vehicle for survivors to connect with other mourners. This vehicle is particularly popular with young people, who have grown up with Internet use and are very comfortable with it.

By far the most influential of the social networking bereavement sites are the Memorial Groups established by Facebook. These groups are typically created by a friend of the deceased. In a qualitative study of Facebook Memorial Groups, Fearon (2011) has identified a variety of purposes that such a group can serve. The first is that members feel that they are part of a group—a group linked together by their connection to the deceased. This is particularly important for mourners who are isolated (socially, geographically, or both) and have little opportunity to interact with other mourners. As one member expressed it, "By visiting the site, I could see that I was not alone." Second, these groups provide an outlet for those who wish to memorialize the deceased and create a lasting testament to his life and identity. Heartfelt comments from friends can console survivors and demonstrate that the loved one had an impact on the lives of others. As one bereaved parent expressed it, "It was not until we read the comments on Facebook that we saw how many lives our son had touched."

A Facebook Memorial Group also creates a community where mourners can give and receive support. Nearly 90% of Fearon's (2012) respondents acknowledged that they used such a group to initiate or maintain a connection with other mourners. The group provides validation for the magnitude of the loss and for the distress resulting from it. In many cases, it appears that writing about one's feelings on a website has advantages over discussing them with people. As one group member indicated, "It is a way to share how much I am hurting without directly making someone feel uncomfortable" (quoted in Fearon, 2012, p. 67). Stroebe, van der Houwen, and Schut (2008) maintain that Internet memorialization may be particularly beneficial for disenfranchised grievers—that is, people who experience a loss that is not openly acknowledged or validated. For example, a woman may be confronted with the death of a man with whom she was having an extramarital affair. She may feel uncomfortable discussing this loss with anyone.

An important feature of these groups is their continuity over time. Mourners can continue to use a Memorial Group as long as they wish. As one mother indicated approximately a year after her daughter's death, "Every so often I go on the site so that I can reminisce about her life, and see if there are any new posts from her friends." Survivors can also use the site to share information about new events to honor the loved one, such as a candlelight vigil to be held on her birthday.

An intriguing feature of these Memorial Groups is that in many cases, mourners leave messages directed toward the deceased (Williams & Merten, 2009). In reviewing posts from the members of several groups, Fearon (2011) found that about half of the participants he studied regarded one or more posts as a direct communication to the deceased. Some participants remarked that they found it healing to talk to the deceased. One person stated, "When I post something on [his] wall it makes me feel like I'm actually connecting with him even though I know I'm not" (quoted in Fearon, 2011, p. 63). Others believed there was a chance that their remarks would be read by the person who died. As one Memorial Group member stated, "Who knows? Maybe there is a Facebook in Heaven that she is reading, and seeing everything we say" (quoted in Fearon, 2011, p. 78). Available evidence suggests that these messages are motivated by the wish to maintain a continued connection with the deceased. Stroebe, van der Houwen, and Schut (2008) have emphasized that despite the widespread use of memorial sites, it is unclear whether memorializing the deceased "helps people work through their grief and toward accepting that the loved one is gone, or whether it . . . causes people to get stuck in or fixate on grieving" (p. 560).

To maximize the benefits that can accrue to your clients and to minimize the risks, it is important to touch base with them about the use of Internet resources such as Memorial Groups. Clients will benefit from your openness to their seeking information and support on the Internet, and your willingness to consider and examine these resources collaboratively. Equally important is your exploration of how clients are perceiving and processing this information and support.

BEREAVEMENT-SPECIFIC ISSUES

As mourners attempt to move forward in dealing with the loss, it is common for them to encounter *bereavement-specific issues*. These are situations, events, or experiences that evoke powerful (and often unanticipated) feelings of acute grief. Bereavement-specific issues reawaken intense grief and trauma responses that may have diminished to some extent. In this section, we describe bereavement-specific issues and discuss ways to address and manage clients' reactions to them.

Rando (1993) has termed such an acute grief response a *subsequent temporary upsurge of grief* (STUG) reaction. Rando's term emphasizes the secondary and temporary nature of such a reaction; that is, it occurs after the initial period of intense grief has subsided and in response to a specific trigger. The term STUG indicates that the reaction represents an upsurge of something that had decreased in intensity or become dormant when the person encountered the triggering event. Some therapists use terms like *waves* or *spurts* of grief.

In the case of traumatic bereavement, bereavement-specific issues can evoke grief or trauma responses that were not anticipated. Fortunately, with treatment, these responses are likely to be less intense than, not to last as long as, and to come less frequently than the mourner's earlier (pretreatment) trauma responses to the same triggers.

The power of bereavement-specific issues lies in their ability to underscore the absence of the deceased, and often, to do so when one least expects it. Such bereavement-specific issues may occur long after a death. For example, Jane, whose husband had died 10 years earlier, experienced acute grief when her son received a prestigious award and her husband was not there to see it. Renaldo, whose wife had died on their honeymoon years earlier, had a nightmare of her death the night after he proposed marriage to another woman.

At times, the situation that precipitated an intense grief reaction is itself unexpected, as was the case when Sabrina ran into her deceased daughter's best friend at the hairdresser. On other occasions, the intensity of the grief or traumatic stress may be what is surprising. This was the case for Emmett, a widower who experienced panic attacks while at a conference with colleagues. Emmett had anticipated that the conference might be difficult for him, since many of his colleagues brought their partners along, but he never expected his responses to feel overwhelming and incapacitating.

It is common for these reactions to occur in social settings. For example, a woman whose son was killed may be approached by an acquaintance unaware of the death, who asks how her son is doing at college. In most cases, both parties may experience such encounters as awkward. The survivor is typically caught off guard and feels confused about how to respond. Following the encounter, she may experience feelings of humiliation because she believes she responded inappropriately. The intensity of the survivor's distress can lead her to question whether she has made any progress in dealing with the loss.

It is important for therapists and clients alike to know that strong responses to bereavement-specific issues are a normal part of the mourning process. As a clinician, you will be better able to assist clients if you recognize the types of situations that can trigger STUG and traumatic stress reactions along the path of mourning. In fact, a STUG or traumatic stress reaction after a period of relative calm may be the reason a client seeks treatment.

Rando's (1993) three-part categorization of triggers of STUG reactions can help both you and your clients to anticipate such situations. The first category includes *cyclic* events, such as anniversaries, holidays, seasonal changes, and repetitive rituals (e.g., an annual family vacation to the beach). Many survivors experience these occasions as relentless and brutal. Regarding her deceased child's birthday, one mother asked, "How could I observe the day this child entered the world without completely falling to pieces? Yet how could I not observe it?" (Mehren, 1997, p. 89). Another mother, who lost her 10-year-old son, stated, "Last year I took Johnny and his friends to a theme park for his birthday. This year, I spent his birthday at the cemetery." As another survivor indicated when discussing family occasions, "When we're all together, we're not all together" (Wolterstorff, 1987, p. 14). Mourners may also have difficulty with innocent questions from others about their holiday plans, such as "Will the family all be home for the holidays?"

Rando's (1993) second STUG category is *linear* events, which are events that occur as a function of reaching a particular age, time, or state. Unlike cyclic events, these are one-time occurrences. A major one occurs when the mourner reaches the age of the person who died, in cases in which that person was older than the mourner at the time of the death. In other cases, these events are associated with particular occasions, such as graduations and weddings. Such events can be agonizing for parents who have lost children before they have achieved this milestone. A single mother who had lost her teenage daughter was invited to the wedding of her niece. Since she and her niece were close, she decided to attend. She became so distraught at the ceremony that she quietly slipped out the back door so as not to call attention to herself. Before she could drive away, two members of the congregation came after her and tried to comfort her. This only made her feel worse. "I felt terrible about leaving in the middle of the service," she said, "but I had to get out of there."

Some linear events are associated with particular stages in life. For example, Amy and Joan were life partners who had planned to retire when they both turned 65. After Amy's death, Joan experienced intense distress when she turned 65 and had to face retirement alone. Another type of linear event is related to life crises, such as losing one's job or being diagnosed with a life-threatening illness. At such times, it is common for the mourner to experience intense yearning for the security and comfort the loved one would have provided.

Rando's (1993) third category is *stimulus-cued* precipitants, which are reactions to stimuli unrelated by time. Some of these are memory-based, as when a bereaved husband encounters a woman who is wearing the same cologne that his wife used to wear. In other cases, the event may serve as a powerful reminder of the person who died, as when "Daddy's Little Girl" is played at weddings.

In some cases, someone may ask the survivor a question that evokes thoughts of the person who died. For bereaved parents, some of the most excruciating precipitants of STUG reactions are questions about how many children they have. Should a parent mention that he had three children but that one has died, and endure a painful and awkward scene? Or should he simply answer by giving the number of children who are alive now? Mourners typically experience this as a no-win situation. As one woman who opted for the second approach explained, "In one cold syllable, that response invalidates your child's existence." Other questions pertaining to their children are also likely to be quite painful for bereaved parents. For example, an acquaintance who is unaware of the death may ask, "What are your children doing now?"

Stimulus-cued precipitants may have a higher likelihood of evoking trauma responses because of their unexpected nature. For example, a father who had lost his youngest son took his two surviving sons on a camping trip. He was pulling them up a hill in a wagon when a passer-by commented, "Aren't you glad you don't have three?"

Typical responses to traumatic death include feeling helpless and out of control. As a woman who lost a child expressed this feeling, "I'm not in charge and I know it" (quoted in Finkbeiner, 1996, p. 187). No matter where they go or what they do, survivors of traumatic bereavement never know when they will encounter painful reminders of their loss. STUG and reawakened traumatic stress reactions such as those described above contribute to these feelings. Furthermore, each successive experience of lack of control can reinforce a sense of helplessness, impeding trauma recovery.

The fear of encountering triggers of STUG reactions often discourages the traumatically bereaved from being actively engaged in the world. This fear reinforces the tendency to withdraw from others, which can keep the survivors stuck in their grief and can interfere with healing. Finally, as described previously, available studies suggest that survivors of sudden, traumatic death are less likely to receive effective support from family members and friends than those whose loved ones died from natural causes under circumstances that were not traumatic. Thus survivors of traumatic death are likely to experience STUG reactions against the backdrop of others' disapproval and insensitivity. In many cases, STUG reactions may fuel others' insensitivity. This is particularly the case when survivors show signs of distress in a public setting. Recall the example in Chapter 4 of Peggy, who had lost her infant son and was attending her sister's baby shower. She had reservations about going to the shower because she knew it would evoke feelings of sadness regarding her loss. Because she and her sister were very close, she decided to go. She was determined to keep her emotions under control, but she did become tearful from time to time. After the shower, she overheard her mother criticize her to a friend, stating that she was so focused on her own tragedy that she could not be happy for anyone else. Peggy felt angry at her mother and hurt by her comment. She also questioned whether she should have stayed home to protect herself and others from her obvious distress. Later, she wondered whether her pain was simply too much for her mother to bear.

Addressing Bereavement-Specific Issues

How should therapy address STUG reactions such as those described above? First, it is important to help clients normalize what is typically a painful and bewildering experience. Second, clients will benefit from understanding the types of situations that are most likely to trigger trauma or STUG reactions. Third, you can assist clients in developing strategies for dealing with their fear that a bereavement-specific issue may arise. Finally, you and your clients can discuss ways they can respond when they encounter such situations, including how to manage trauma or STUG responses.

In many cases, bereavement-specific issues may appear to be small and inconsequential. For example, a man whose wife has died may become distraught when someone phones the house asking for his wife. In addition, clients regard their reactions as diagnostic of how well they are coping. Clients may infer that they are not making "progress" in dealing with the death if they continue to be caught off guard by sudden, intense rushes of overwhelming sadness or anxiety. Such experiences may lead them to believe that the treatment is not working. Consequently, clients may lose interest or confidence in employing strategies to deal with their loss. If you can normalize these responses, clients may become less self-critical and willing to invest in the treatment. In addition to helping the client understand that these reactions are normal, it may be useful to remind him that healing from trauma and accommodating grief are not linear processes. In other words, the natural progression in treatment may include rough patches—days when the grief and trauma symptoms are stronger than they were days, weeks, or even months earlier.

Clients may not raise the issue of trauma or STUG reactions because they may feel ashamed that they are still experiencing such intense feelings, believe that their reactions reflect badly on their coping abilities, or worry that they are letting you down. Knowledge of each client's unique situation, as well as of possible bereavement-specific issues that most survivors face, will facilitate the process of eliciting and discussing the client's reactions (Handouts S5, Bereavement-Specific Issues, and S6, Getting through the Holidays: Advice from the Bereaved, available on the book's website supplement, will also be helpful in this regard.) Gentle probing about how the client felt during a recent potentially evocative event, such as a wedding or a funeral, may be productive. It is helpful for the therapist to be aware of situations that may increase the likelihood that a STUG reaction will occur. For example, people are likely to ask a pregnant woman whether she has other children (e.g., "Is this your first?"). This question may prompt a STUG reaction from a woman who has previously lost a child.

It is important to assess how the client's feelings about past STUG reactions or her fears that future ones may occur have affected her coping strategies. For example, is this issue reinforcing the survivor's tendency to withdraw from social encounters? Together, you and the client can work to develop coping strategies that will reduce the likelihood of the client experiencing future trauma or STUG reactions in a particular setting. For example, the two of you may decide together that the client would benefit from using breathing techniques to regulate emotional distress if she has such a reaction.

Drawing from your understanding of bereavement-specific issues, you can also assist clients in developing coping strategies to reduce the likelihood that a trauma or STUG reaction will occur. Because holidays raise a host of bereavement-specific issues, it can be useful to address them in advance. As noted above, a handout on this book's website supplement (Handout S6, Getting through the Holidays: Advice from the Bereaved) describes the dilemmas that clients typically face during holidays, as well as possible coping strategies. Similarly, you can work with clients to strategize how they can approach other potentially challenging upcoming events, including anniversaries, funerals, and commemorations of the anniversary of their loved one's death within their faith communities. Survivors will benefit from an open exploration of whether they should attend such events or not. For example, in helping a Jewish mourner decide whether to attend a commemoration of his loved one's death at the temple, it is important to explore ways to balance his natural wish to avoid painful reminders with the potential value of including himself in his community's commemoration practices. If he decides to participate, you can discuss ways he can proceed that will give him some sense of control. Such participation can provide an opportunity for growth when it is used as an exposure activity, as described in Chapter 11.

In some cases, clients experience a STUG or trauma reaction in a situation that they are likely to encounter again. This is the case for parents who have lost a child. As discussed previously, it is common for parents to be asked how many children they have, and this question typically evokes great distress. Clients' tendency to be critical of the way they responded can increase their distress. Many clients then live in fear that they will be asked this question again. These fears are exacerbated in situations where they will be meeting people for the first time, such as a luncheon for new parents at a surviving child's school.

Such a client may fear that the question will require an explanation about her child's death, or that she will cry while providing such an explanation. The client may have the automatic thought that crying in front of someone else at this point in the mourning process may make her look out of control. You and the client can explore this thought, examining how likely it is that someone would label crying while in such a situation as "out of control." If someone reacts negatively to a survivor in such a situation, you and the client can use Handout 13, the Automatic Thought Record, to address the issue of whether this is more of a reflection on the client or a possible indication of discomfort of the person who reacted to her crying. Alternatively or in addition, you may choose to deal with the same situation behaviorally. The intensity of STUG reactions may be driven in part by the client's concerns about how she appears to others. Responding naturally in social situations that tend to prompt STUG reactions will be more difficult at first, but will gradually become easier with practice. In this way, the client can use the idea of exposure to lessen her anxiety gradually about appearing distraught when she encounters traumatic stimuli. Reducing the anxiety related to how others perceive the survivor may help to decrease the impact of situations that provoke STUG reactions and trauma responses.

You and the client may choose to design role-play or exposure activities (described in Chapter 11) in which the client practices disclosing information about the loss to you, in order to prepare for this type of question. This type of exposure may also be pursued with the help of a supportive friend or family member. Preparation may require a joint session with the client and the support person in which you help the client to explain his concerns (e.g., "I'm afraid that people will be horrified if I cry when they ask me about what my children are doing now"). You may then coach the client and support person through a discussion or role play to help overcome this fear.

In addition to providing validation for the client's distress about bereavement-related challenges, you should praise attempts to deal with these issues even if they are not entirely successful. Clients may tend to focus only on how they behaved and felt in a situation, and may fail to acknowledge the role of the other people involved. At times it may be useful to validate a lack of social skills on the part of others, and to help clients process whether others' behavior is the norm. Such acknowledgments may give clients hope about pursuing future social situations and avoiding maladaptive coping strategies, such as spending most of their time at home to avoid trauma and STUG reactions.

In sharing their thoughts and feelings about bereavement-specific issues, mourners can both anticipate and decide how to respond to them, restoring an element of control. Through these processes, they may be able to develop principles to guide their behavior when they encounter new bereavement-specific issues. For example, a survivor may decide to respond to any threat to his composure by taking several deep breaths and then asking himself, "How do I want to respond to this situation?"

MEANING AND SPIRITUALITY

Following the traumatic deaths of loved ones, many survivors become engaged in an intense and prolonged struggle to make sense of what has happened. Beliefs that they have held for their entire lives—such as "God is loving and protects us from harm," or "If we lead a good life, we will be rewarded"—are typically shattered by such losses. Survivors are likely to feel confused, betrayed, and uncertain about their connection to God or their spirituality.

In recent years, there has been increasing interest in understanding the conditions under which people seek meaning and the ramifications of not being able to find it (Gamino & Sewell, 2004). Both researchers and clinicians have maintained that one of the most significant new developments in the field of bereavement is the recognition that grief is essentially a process of reconstructing a world of meaning and purpose—a world that has been called into question by the loss (Neimeyer & Sands, 2011; Stroebe & Schut, 2001a).

Over the past decade, studies have emerged that provide support for the importance of finding meaning. In one study, Currier and colleagues (2006) focused on a large sample of college students who had experienced the violent deaths of loved ones through accident, homicide, or suicide. They found that participants' ability to make sense of what happened accounted almost entirely for the relationship between the violence associated with the death and complicated grieving. According to these authors, "failure to find meaning in a loss is . . . a crucial pathway to complicated grief" (p. 403). Keesee, Currier, and Neimeyer (2008) obtained similar findings in a study of parents who lost a child. Parents who reported having made little or no sense out of their children's deaths experienced more intense grief.

Regardless of the benefits that it might confer, research has shown that finding meaning may be an unrealistic goal for many people who have experienced the sudden, traumatic death of loved ones. As we have described in Chapter 3, this was the case for survivors who experienced the traumatic loss of a spouse or child (Davis et al., 2000; Lehman et al., 1987; Murphy, Johnson, & Lohan, 2003b). Most mourners indicated that they searched for meaning, but relatively few were able to find it. When asked how they felt about this, most survivors reported that it was painful that they could not make sense of what happened. A significant minority of respondents indicated that they never searched for meaning. Some of these people had found meaning, but others had not. Those who were not preoccupied with the issue of meaning showed the best adjustment.

As discussed previously, there are many different ways of finding meaning in a loss. Lichtenthal, Currier, Neimeyer, and Keesee (2010) conducted a study designed to identify specific themes of meaning or sense making among parents who had lost children. The most common response, made by 44.9% of the parents, was that no sense could be made of these deaths. Other responses included viewing it as God's plan, or assuming that God knows what is best (17.9%); believing that a deceased child is safe in heaven and will be reunited with the parent (16%); and believing that suffering and death are inevitable (10.9%). Other ways of finding meaning included working to help others who had experienced similar losses; developing new goals or a new purpose; placing the loss in a spiritual context; or finding benefit or redeeming features in the deaths. Most experts believe that the search for meaning requires a certain amount of reflection on a mourner's part. However, many survivors of traumatic bereavement report that it is difficult to reflect on the meaning of their losses. Doing so evokes disturbing thoughts about the loved one and his death.

Many mourners report that those in their social environment are uncomfortable with discussions about meaning. As one woman expressed it, "I was outraged that God took my beautiful and brilliant daughter, who had dedicated her life to serving others, instead of one of the rapists, murderers, or thugs who populate society. But no one wants to listen to an incensed mother who is raging at the fates." People may be more likely to make progress in dealing with issues of meaning with the aid of a therapist than on their own. It is also important to avoid assuming that a client is struggling with issues related to meaning, or to push her to do so.

Addressing Meaning and Spirituality

As a therapist, what can you do to help? We recommend taking a nuanced approach, listening for indications that the client is struggling with issues of meaning, and validating his feelings. Clients may find Handout 31, Spirituality, useful to this work.

Robert Neimeyer and his associates (Neimeyer, 2000a, 2001, 2012; Neimeyer, Burke, Mackay, & van Dyke Stringer, 2010) have suggested that therapists can facilitate meaning making by assisting clients in a process they call *narrative repair*. They maintain that if life is viewed as a story or narrative, tragic loss can be regarded as disrupting the coherence and continuity of the narrative. According to Neimeyer, such a loss "can occasion profound shifts in our sense of who we are as whole facets of our past that were shared with the deceased slip away from us forever" (1998, p. 90). Disruption of the narrative requires a survivor to envision major changes in the plot so that her story can move forward. It is also important for her to envision changes in her own identity—ideally, ones that capitalize on her strengths and encourage contemplation of moving forward without her loved one. In this narrative repair approach to treatment, a therapist's role is to guide survivors of sudden, traumatic loss through a process of accepting and processing the loss and challenging and refining their beliefs about the loss and its meaning. Neimeyer, Harris, Winokuer, and Thornton (2011) recommend employing such means as clinically guided journaling, poetic writing, and graphic recounting to help survivors arrive at an account or "repaired" narrative of the loss that renders their lives, their loved ones' lives, and the deaths meaningful. Neimeyer and Sands (2011) list several resources that describe these methods in more detail.

Another approach is to assist clients gently in widening their perspective on finding meaning. For example, you might ask your client to indicate what the death of the loved one means to her (Gamino, Hogan, & Sewell, 2002). In most cases, broad and general questions of this sort are more likely to result in a productive discussion of these issues than asking clients directly whether they have been able to find meaning in the loved one's death.

It can be beneficial for a client to shift from searching for meaning in the loss to searching for meaning in his life. We agree with Neimeyer (1998) that in most cases, it is helpful to focus on how the loss has affected the bereaved person's identity. It is important to recognize that such meanings do not have to be cosmic or spiritual. Neimeyer cites the case of one bereaved mother, a social activist, who came to believe that the world was imperfect and that everyone had pain in his life. However, she believed that her task was to ameliorate this pain whenever possible through involvement and advocacy. Clients may wish to honor their loved ones by carrying on their charity work, setting up a memorial scholarship, or working to prevent the types of events that caused the death. Validating clients' desire to be involved in such activities can facilitate the healing process (Lewis & Hoy, 2011).

Ancillary treatments may help clients deal with issues pertaining to meaning. Murphy, Johnson, and Lohan (2003b) studied the predictors of finding meaning 5 years after the death of a child by accident, suicide, or homicide. They found that parents who attended a support group were four times more likely to find meaning than parents who did not. It is not clear how support group attendance facilitates parents' search for meaning. Perhaps parents benefit from exposure to people who have dealt with the issue of meaning in different ways. Spiritual beliefs also facilitated finding meaning. Murphy and colleagues found spirituality to be the second most important factor predicting who would find meaning.

In an excellent discussion of this topic, Tedeschi and Calhoun (2006) have recommended encouraging the exploration of spiritual issues:

> Bereaved clients can find it to be a great relief when clinicians are open to all kinds of ideas and experiences in relation to the death of a loved one, and the spiritual and religious concerns this raises. For example: Is there an afterlife? If so, is it like the traditional versions of it that I might have been taught about? Is my deceased loved one aware of my thoughts, feelings, and actions now? Can we communicate with each other? Will I recognize them in the afterlife? Did God plan their death? Is their death God's punishment for me? If they weren't baptized, are they in heaven? Could they be reincarnated? (p. 112)

Tedeschi and Calhoun suggest that instead of offering answers to such questions, "[therapists should] regard themselves as companions on the journey through grief's unfamiliar territory. On this journey, it is useful for clinicians to assist clients in developing beliefs that provide some comfort in the midst of the distress that is death" (2006, p. 112). Such beliefs may include the notion that the deceased is at peace.

You and your client can also discuss spirituality as a potential resource. A client's spiritual beliefs are a significant aspect of his assumptive world, which is related to the search for meaning. The term *spirituality* refers to those aspects of a person's life in which he connects with something beyond himself and beyond interpersonal relationships. This may include a connection with God, nature, history, humanity, beauty, awe, wonder, and so forth. A sense of spirituality can be a source of sustenance in difficult times, and traumatic loss often disrupts it (McCann & Pearlman, 1990b). Addressing spiritual disruptions can help the survivor to articulate the effects of the death on his spiritual beliefs (which may or may not include a belief in God). It can also normalize spiritual disruption following a sudden, traumatic death. Finally, this work can introduce the idea of redirected, renewed, or newly developed spirituality as a potential resource.

You may invite a client to express current feelings about spiritual connection. Some of these may be healing (i.e., the belief that the loved one is no longer suffering), while others may be deeply disturbing (i.e., the belief that God is no longer worthy of the mourner's faith). You may wish to explore the disruption to these connections as a potential secondary loss. If a client has strong negative responses to talking about spirituality or does not connect with the concept of spirituality, then it is appropriate to discuss his worldview more generally. For example, clients may find it easier to talk about what gives their lives meaning or what they do to restore themselves when they feel depleted. Of course, it may also be important to explore the client's reluctance to discuss spirituality. In addition, it may be useful to make a distinction between spirituality and religion. A person can have an active spiritual life that sustains him without any connection to organized religion.

In virtually all of the studies that have focused on finding meaning in traumatic death, a subset of respondents concluded that the search for meaning was fruitless. As one mourner expressed it, "The meaning is that there is no meaning. Some things that happen just don't make sense." A clinician who believes that finding meaning is central to the mourning process may suggest possible meanings to a client, or impose his own desire to create meaning onto a client who sees her experience as meaningless. Such a dynamic can create an empathic disconnection (McCann & Pearlman, 1990b), set the client up for failure, decrease the client's motivation to collaborate in the treatment, and dishonor the client's experience. As clinicians, we all need to respect bereaved survivors' existential crises, searches for meaning, recognition of meaning-lessness, and the places they inhabit as they move through these experiences. Although it is important to normalize the difficulties of the search, we should not impose our preconceptions about the necessity of finding meaning or what constitutes recovery. Some clients may not wish or need to engage in such a quest for meaning.

VALUES AND PERSONAL GOAL SETTING

We use the word *values* to refer to people's fundamental principles or standards, or what they want their lives to stand for (Hayes, 2004). *Goals* are steps that people take in the direction of their values. Sudden, traumatic death often brings about a profound change in a mourner's values and wreaks havoc with goals for the future. As one father expressed it,

> I will never be the same person as before the loss of my child. Then a new era started. What was of great importance before does not matter now. At work, I am listening to what my colleagues define as problems in their private lives, but it is nothing. Therefore, I rather choose to withdraw or to leave the room. My scale of values is turned upside down. (quoted in Dyregrov et al., 2003, p. 158)

Values and goals both reflect and provide a sense of purpose and meaning. People's values also convey how they define themselves and how they relate to others. As the quotation above illustrates, traumatic events often derail the fundamental goals that guide a person's behavior.

Disruption of survivors' goal-seeking behavior can occur for many reasons. The sudden, traumatic death of a loved one provides incontrovertible evidence that everything can change in an instant. Many people feel that in such a capricious world, there is no point in working toward long-term goals. When asked about goals, a traumatically bereaved survivor's typical response is something like this: "At this point, I don't have long-term goals. My only goal is to get through the day."

Survivors may abandon the pursuit of goals because their goals and those of the deceased were intertwined. As one woman explained after the death of her spouse, "We had bought a recreational vehicle, and our dream was to visit every state in the country. Every night we pored over maps to plan our trip. When my husband died, this dream died along with him."

The purpose of values work with traumatically bereaved clients is to help them regain a sense of purpose and direction in their lives by identifying what matters to them most at this point. Values work helps people choose to move forward in a meaningful direction and become engaged in activities they view as worthwhile. It can also propel forward movement in a client who seems to be stuck in the mourning process. For all of these reasons, values work can be extremely useful for survivors of traumatic death.

This book's approach to values and goals is drawn from *acceptance and commitment therapy* (ACT), which was pioneered by Steven Hayes in the mid-1990s (see Hayes, 2004). This evidence-based intervention uses strategies based on acceptance of one's difficulties, mindfulness, commitment, and behavioral change. This approach is part of the "third wave" of interventions within CBT (Hayes, 2004; Zettle, 2007). Those working within an ACT framework have applied ideas on goals and values to a wide variety of problems, including depression, anxiety, addictions, and chronic pain. Although we are not aware of any ACT work focusing on grief, the approach has been used effectively with individuals who have PTSD (Walser & Westrup, 2007).

A major tenet of ACT is commitment to and action toward living a life consistent with one's values (Eifert & Forsyth, 2005). Within the ACT framework, values are chosen life directions. As Hayes (2005) describes them, "values are vitalizing, uplifting and empowering. They are not another . . . measurement to fail against" (p. 155). The therapist helps survivors of traumatic experiences to "embrace living in ways that are meaningful and value driven" (Walser & Westrup, 2007, p. 3). The goal is for clients to stop living in reaction to negative experiences and to start living according to what is important to them.

Our integrated treatment approach also draws from the work of Katherine Shear and her colleagues (Shear & Frank, 2006; Shear et al., 2005). These investigators have used work on personal goals as part of their treatment program for complicated grief, described in Chapter 7. Therapists ask clients to identify things they would like to do if they were no longer grieving. The therapists then work with the clients to come up with specific steps the clients can take to reach these goals, and monitor progress toward the goals. According to Shear and Frank (2006), "We were surprised to find that many people with complicated grief do harbor such goals. Even in earlier sessions, an individual's affect becomes noticeably more positive as he or she focuses full attention on the discussion of personal goals" (p. 297). In addition, Shear and Frank emphasize that such work conveys to a client that the therapist has confidence in his ability to recover. It also conveys that it is perfectly acceptable—in fact, desirable—for the client to be experiencing less grief. Finally, it illustrates that the therapist considers the life of the mourner to be important apart from his grief and loss.

Addressing Values and Goals

It is important to provide a rationale for working on values and goals. We recommend discussing how the traumatic death of a loved one can drain a survivor's life of purpose, meaning, and vitality, and how focusing on goals and values will help the client to move forward in the mourning process. For clients who are not yet ready to engage in this work, activity scheduling, described in Chapter 11, is a good alternative.

To facilitate this focus, we have drawn from the work of Hayes (2005) to develop two handouts. The first is Handout 21, Values, which is located in the Appendix. The second, Handout S1, Personal Goal Setting, is on the book's website (*www.guilford.com/pearlman-materials*). Both handouts are designed to help clients clarify and prioritize their values. Both guide the client through the process of developing goals that are consonant with their values, and identifying action steps that will help them reach their goals. Handout 21 provides a more comprehensive analysis of how to develop goals and action plans. It also addresses how to overcome barriers that may keep us from reaching our goals.

After providing a rationale for this work, it may be beneficial for you and your client to review Handout 21 in session. Drawing from this material, you should help a client understand the difference between values and goals. "Maintaining good health" is an example of a value, whereas "exercising three times per week" and "not eating fast food" are goals. Next, you and your client can explore what value she would like to work on at this time. Then she develops one or more goals that will move her in the direction of the value she has identified. The next task is for the client to identify specific steps or actions that she will need to complete in order to reach her goal. If her goal is "making new friends," an action plan might include "invite a colleague out for coffee" or "accept the dinner invitation that I received from my neighbors." You can explain that the main reason many people don't reach their goals is that they do not have an action plan. Such a plan will help the client to move forward step by step. We encourage you to assign Handout 21 to your client as homework. This will help her consolidate the information reviewed in session.

Focusing clients' attention on what matters most now can also facilitate the process of goal and activity selection. In her work with homicide survivors, Armour (2003) has used this approach extensively. She has maintained that if survivors can engage in activities reflecting what is important to them now, they are more likely to find meaning in the loved one's death. In working with traumatically bereaved clients, we have found this approach to be very effective. One woman who had lost her older son decided that what mattered now was to be the best possible mother to her surviving son. "I arranged a sleepover for my son, and cooked him his favorite dinner. It made me feel good," she said. A woman whose partner had died decided that what was now most important was staying healthy so that she could raise their children. "I had canceled my two previously scheduled mammograms, but this time I kept my appointment," she said. "I was proud of myself."

Keep in mind that clients may not feel ready to pursue their own goals. They may feel that their most important goals were shattered with the loved one's death. They may also feel that pursuing something that would be positive for them is disloyal to the lost loved one. In these cases, it can be helpful to frame the values and goal-setting work as a way of minimizing the encroachment of trauma and grief into their lives. Clients may also be unable to move forward with their goals because of avoidance. You should address these barriers to making progress on goals on a regular basis. Both cognitive processing and the exposure approach described in Chapter 11 can be applied usefully to this realm as well. Finally, as Armour (2006) has indicated, it is important to help survivors celebrate their movement forward "by recognizing the myriad of small but important decisions they make daily to prevail rather than despair" (p. 83).

It is common for a client to make an action plan but be unable to carry it out. If this occurs, it can be useful to discuss barriers that may have interfered with the client's successful completion of the tasks he identified. For example, the client's fear that someone may ask him how he is doing may keep him from reaching his goal of getting together with others.

Values and goals work may confer two additional benefits. First, there is often an increase in positive affect. As discussed earlier, positive emotions can play an important role in the coping process. They can also provide a psychological break or respite from grief, allowing mourners to replenish their resources; they are also reinforcing in and of themselves. Both these factors in turn promote more effective coping and problem solving. Second, focusing on goals and values often helps to alleviate a client's struggles with finding meaning in the loss. It is not clear whether such work facilitates finding meaning or whether it renders the search less important;

this may differ from one person to the next. It appears that positive feelings and less distress about meaning are by-products of working on values and goals. The more the client engages in work with values and goals, the more these processes will come into play, and this in turn will facilitate additional work on these issues. Taken together, these processes can result in an upward spiral of well-being, and can help the client to begin living a more vital and purposeful life.

CLINICAL INTEGRATION

Phyllis sought therapy on the advice of her sister. She wanted to feel better, and she had to return to work, but she didn't know how to help herself. Upon meeting Phyllis, Dr. Santiago Gonzales immediately observed how overwhelmed she seemed. Phyllis tried to be open and to stay in control of her emotions as she spoke with Dr. Gonzales, but she could barely get her words out. She spent most of the first session shaking and sobbing. At the end of the first session, she told Dr. Gonzales that she was afraid that he, too, would let her down, as Alex's doctor had.

Dr. Gonzales knew they would need to strengthen and rebuild Phyllis's self capacities as well as her social support—two resources that had been easier for her to access before Alex's death. He knew, too, that they would eventually have to address Phyllis's disrupted trust schemas. He thought he would introduce the Automatic Thought Record and Challenging Questions Worksheet once they had shored up her emotional regulation and social support a bit. He reasoned that if this early work went well, Phyllis might have more confidence in him—and herself—for the trauma processing ahead.

When they met for their fourth session, Dr. Gonzales asked, "So how did you do with your breathing retraining and social support activities since our last session?"

"It went OK," answered Phyllis. "I asked my friend Mary to go to the attorney's office with me last week. I've been so consumed with the decision of whether to pursue a lawsuit against the doctor that exercises almost fell off my radar. But then I thought to myself, 'Why not use them for support when I meet the attorney to discuss the case?' And this is what I did. I called Mary and asked her to come, and I practiced the breathing retraining on my way there while Mary drove."

"And how did it go?"

"It was strange for me to ask Mary for support. Part of me thought that she would not follow through. Still, it was mostly OK."

"That's good to hear, Phyllis. You said it was 'mostly OK.' Can you say more about what 'mostly OK' means to you?" Dr. Gonzales wanted Phyllis to reflect on how she was doing and to articulate this for herself.

"Well, first of all, Mary showed up, which meant a lot to me. Also, I was able to get through the meeting without breaking down. In general, I'm doing better than I was when I first came here. I'm going through my day without feeling so overwhelmed. It's as though I'm beginning to trust myself again. I feel less suffocated by my anger. I think the breathing retraining activity is helping with this. I've been practicing this exercise every morning. I'm learning to breathe through my tears. I used to cry and lose my breath as I was crying. Now when I cry, I'm aware of also breathing. It makes me feel like I'm beginning to have some control over my feelings.

"Also, when Mary and I went for coffee afterward, I was able to acknowledge that I'm still angry, I still can't trust people, and I'm still struggling but I'm not getting stuck there. I could say those things, and then also ask her how she was doing and be genuinely interested in that. I could sort of leave my own pain for a while, which I wasn't able to do before. Mary really understands; she doesn't pressure me to not be angry or to depend on her too much, you know what I mean?" Dr. Gonzales nodded. "Because she lets me be angry, I can also then calm down. It sounds weird, but I'm learning that the less I fight my feelings, the more I'm able to handle them. Mary seemed to help me with that just by being her supportive, accepting self."

"I'm curious about what made you decide to call upon Mary in particular for support with your legal consultation," said Dr. Gonzales.

"I actually spent time thinking about several people I could ask to come with me. Mary has been so consistent and reliable in the face of my grief and anger during the past year and a half. As I thought about this, I realized that part of what keeps me from socializing and asking for support is a fear of being disappointed. I think I'm afraid of trusting too much, being let down, then going into a rage. When I thought about Mary, this fear wasn't as strong."

"That's a very important awareness, Phyllis," said Dr. Gonzales. Phyllis had just expressed many important things; he was taking his time to sort through them, deciding where to move next. "You've just expressed many significant developments and insights," he began. "First, I want to point out how you knew what you needed with regard to social support. Somewhere within yourself, you knew that Mary could be a support to you. It sounds as though you felt that support, maybe a bit of calmness, even as you brought her to mind—before the two of you actually met. That's an example of the feelings skill we talked about: drawing on internalized, positive others. And the breathing practice seems to be helping you to tolerate and manage your strongest feelings—another skill we've discussed. I think you've had those skills and abilities for a long time, but you forgot how to use them or something got in the way of using them. My hope and my guess is that the more you practice using these skills, the easier they'll be for you to use, and that you'll then feel more comfortable going out and accepting support from others. Can you see how all of these elements that we've been discussing fit together?"

Phyllis nodded.

"You mentioned a fear of being disappointed. And of losing control. This is a good place to introduce another element of the treatment approach we've been using. It's the element of maladaptive beliefs and automatic thoughts. The thought 'Others will disappoint me, and then I'll lose control of my anger' is a good example of a thought that may get in the way of your mourning. Are you ready to shift to a discussion of automatic thoughts?" asked Dr. Gonzales.

"As ready as I'll ever be," said Phyllis.

CONCLUDING REMARKS

Building and solidifying resources are crucial aspects of this overall treatment approach. Phyllis is a good example of an overwhelmed survivor in need of a lot of attention to resource building. As a childhood trauma survivor, Phyllis was vulnerable to the disruption of self capacities that her fiancé's death evoked. Fortunately, Dr. Gonzales recognized this and prioritized this aspect of the treatment, front-loading the treatment with resource building. As their work progressed and he introduced other elements, resource building remained central and was integrated throughout the treatment. This heavy emphasis won't always be the case, as some clients will need less of this, but all clients ought to receive some attention to solidifying resources.

The example of Phyllis and Dr. Gonzales also demonstrates the importance of the treatment alliance as a container for building self capacities, trust of others (and therefore ability to use social support), and other resources such as breathing retraining and coping skills. Notice Dr. Gonzales's tone as he spoke to Phyllis; it was encouraging, respectful, and collaborative. Finally, Phyllis showed us how the ability to access various resources increased her self-confidence, which positively affected her self-worth and enhanced her capacity to continue with the work of moving through traumatic bereavement. Supportive resources are particularly important in challenging times and situations, such as when there is legal involvement. As Phyllis's ability to utilize various resources grew, she and Dr. Gonzales might wish to focus on setting some goals for her future—yet another resource-building strategy discussed within this chapter.

CHAPTER 11

Processing Trauma

Larry grew up in a working-class family on the outskirts of the city. His family struggled financially throughout much of his childhood. As the oldest of six children, Larry often felt a sense of parental responsibility toward his younger siblings. He was especially protective of his two youngest brothers. By the time they were of middle school age, gang violence had become more widespread in and around their neighborhood. Larry somehow felt responsible for making sure they would "make it"—for ensuring that neither brother would become another sad statistic, and instead that both would have careers and start families of their own. Motivated by his desire to support his siblings, Larry worked hard to establish a career. He also married his high school sweetheart and had two daughters.

Lawrence senior was an alcoholic who became verbally abusive toward his sons when he drank, and Larry junior seemed to get the worst of it. His father often told him that he was "good for nothing" and wouldn't "amount to anything." Larry used this as motivation to do just the opposite in order to prove his father wrong: to be successful, and to do so within his father's field of work. Lawrence was an ironworker, and his son followed in his footsteps, proving his own skill, work ethic, and eventual managerial skills. At the time Larry married, he landed a high-paying job as a construction manager. Twenty years later, he was still with this company. He had remained married and had one teenage daughter. His older daughter had died 5 years earlier while on vacation in the Bahamas. Her unexpected death crushed Larry's spirit. He did everything possible to meet the responsibilities of his job and his family. But he could not shake the feeling that life as he knew it was over.

Trauma processing is one of the three core treatment components (resource building, trauma processing, and mourning) of this approach. Trauma processing occurs on both a cognitive and an emotional level. Clients learn different techniques for both types of processing, which can be very useful when applied together. In this chapter, we discuss the application of trauma processing to traumatic bereavement.

Cognitive and behavioral theories for alleviating traumatic bereavement inform our treatment approach.[1] Challenging depressive and anxiety-provoking automatic thoughts, and pursuing behavioral activities that expose clients to avoided stimuli, can help in several ways. These processes can help survivors to stop negative cycles of thoughts, moods, and behaviors; process

---

[1] If you are trained in EMDR, you may wish to use that approach to trauma processing as an alternative to the approach we describe here.

traumatic memories; break anxiety-provoking behavioral associations; fight against the apathy and isolation that were triggered by the death; create meaning from traumatic death; and reengage in their lives.

Behavioral techniques, in the form of exposure to feared stimuli or the behavioral experiments of activity scheduling, allow traumatically bereaved survivors to experience their feelings and to gain corrective information from the world. Clients are often too afraid of their feelings to do the processing necessary to move forward. Avoiding powerful emotions can consume all of their time and energy, and can keep the survivors stuck in their mourning process. Facing anxiety-provoking situations reduces fear and engenders feelings of pride and hope that things can change. Allowing themselves to experience the feelings stirred up by facing reminders of traumatic death helps survivors to *habituate* to their emotions—that is, to tolerate the affect until it decreases. Purposely delving into their emotions, by confronting feared situations or by describing their memories in detail, allows clients to reengage in life.

The cognitive element of cognitive-behavioral theory posits that people can learn to monitor their own thought processes and identify related negative emotions and behaviors. They can then learn to challenge the damaging automatic thoughts they identify, thereby lessening the impact of these thoughts on mood, behavior, and physical reactions. A sudden, traumatic death will generally prompt painful thoughts about oneself, the loved one, the relationship, and the world. This therapy approach teaches clients methods for recognizing, challenging, and restructuring the thoughts that cause them distress. Therapists work with clients to identify, challenge, and then modify the thoughts, beliefs, and interpretations that may have become habitual and that may inhibit the process of mourning the loss. Repeatedly challenging negative automatic thoughts gradually decreases their frequency and reduces the power of the beliefs at their root. For example, using the tools described later in this chapter, a traumatically bereaved survivor may be able to identify the belief that he doesn't deserve to live because he "allowed" his sister to kill herself. The work on challenging this automatic thought will help him to understand the links among this thought, his depressed mood, and his social avoidance. It will provide him with the opportunity to assess realistically his role in the suicide and the opportunities he had to intervene.

In this treatment approach, as is the case in CBT more generally, cognitive and behavioral techniques work together. When clients become aware of the distressing schemas underlying their automatic thoughts, strong emotions can surface because of the close link between thoughts and feelings. Being aware of the thought that "Loved ones always abandon me," for example, may evoke emotions associated with a previous abandonment, as well as the vulnerability associated with the need to trust in others. This kind of situation then allows you and the client to address the overgeneralized thought, the need for trust, and the associated emotions. Likewise, facing a feared situation such as cleaning out the closet of a deceased child is likely to evoke strong feelings of grief and may elicit maladaptive schemas as well: "I should have bought her that dress she really wanted," or "I should have never let him drive that night." In other words, thoughts, emotions, and behaviors relate to each other in a complex matrix, and addressing one aspect of the matrix is likely to bring the others into focus as well. This integrated treatment approach intervenes in all three facets of this matrix—thoughts, emotions, and behaviors—with the awareness that each aspect relates to the others.

As described in Chapter 7, several different versions of CBT have demonstrated effectiveness in the treatment of PTSD (Blanchard et al., 1996; Foa & Rothbaum, 1998; Resick & Schnicke, 1993). PE, both alone and with the addition of cognitive techniques such as CPT, is a highly effective treatment for PTSD (Foa et al., 2005, 2009; Hollon, Stewart, & Strunk, 2006; Rauch et al., 2009). Moreover, Shear and colleagues (2005) recently demonstrated the effectiveness of CBT for complicated grief as assessed by the Prolonged Grief Disorder Scale (Prigerson, Maciejewski, et al., 1995).

In this chapter, we describe cognitive processing interventions, emotional processing interventions, and behavioral interventions. As stated above, these techniques are intended to be utilized in ways that complement one another. The art of implementing this treatment approach requires an awareness of these interrelationships. In utilizing the techniques for processing sudden, traumatic death on both the cognitive and emotional levels, you can help survivors to reengage with life and once again seek fulfillment of their needs, even in the absence of their deceased loved ones.

COGNITIVE PROCESSING INTERVENTIONS

Cognitive work is very helpful in reducing distress. Learning to identify automatic thoughts or problematic beliefs is the first step toward decreasing their power over moods and behavior. Once a client learns to identify the thoughts, his goal is to consider them carefully and decide whether they really make sense. Like exposure, cognitive work requires patience, courage, and concentration. If clients understand the rationale for the cognitive techniques, they will be more likely to put in the necessary effort. We therefore recommend reviewing Handout 9, A Model for Change, with each client, as it describes the rationale for the cognitive work. Clients begin by identifying their distressing thoughts related to the death by using the Identifying Automatic Thoughts exercise (described in Handout 10, What Are Automatic Thoughts?, and Handout 11, the Identifying Automatic Thoughts Worksheet). They then learn to challenge these thoughts and to reframe or replace them as appropriate. We detail the process of identifying and challenging distressing automatic thoughts below.

Identifying Automatic Thoughts

Identifying distressing automatic thoughts takes practice because they are so "second nature" that many people don't realize they have them. Problematic automatic thoughts tend to be extreme and are often quite harsh. They often contain thinking errors such as all-or-nothing thinking, discounting the positive, catastrophizing (predicting a negative future), and overgeneralizations. "I'm a failure as a parent," "People always abandon me," and "God never loved me" are examples. People tend to believe them because they have repeated them in their minds so often. Such automatic thoughts often express problematic schemas about the self, others, and the world that were developed early in life and that are then reinforced in the wake of a traumatic experience. To help clients recognize automatic thoughts, we suggest reviewing Handout 10, What Are Automatic Thoughts?, before moving into the exercises described below.

Once a client understands what an automatic thought is, introduce Handout 11, the Identifying Automatic Thoughts Worksheet, as a way for him to begin to identify his automatic thoughts. It may be helpful to let the client know that during the next session, he will learn how to challenge these automatic thoughts so they do not have such a powerful impact on his moods and behavior, and that challenging such thoughts requires identifying them first. You can explain to the client that although tracking the automatic thoughts may not make him feel better initially, it is a necessary precursor to challenging the thoughts effectively. In other words, this is the first step in a process.

Handout 11 consists of three columns that the client fills in: the situation, his mood, and the related automatic thoughts. Tracking these is the first step toward decreasing the frequency of distressing thoughts. As you review this handout with the client, explain that he may fill out the columns in any order (i.e., starting with a mood, a situation, or a thought, whichever is most apparent to him). We recommend that you practice filling out at least one copy of this handout with the client in preparation for asking him to complete it between sessions. Although it is preferable to choose a thought associated with the loss, any example will do.

Some clients will have difficulty naming moods or feelings. The "Recognizing Feelings" section of Handout 8, Feelings Skills, may be helpful to clients who have difficulty filling out the "Moods" column on the Identifying Automatic Thoughts Worksheet. Another potential difficulty is that clients may list a thought in the mood column, typically by prefacing it with "I feel . . ." For example, the client may list "I feel like I will always be alone" as a mood when it is actually an automatic thought. A simple guideline for distinguishing between thoughts and feelings on the worksheet is that feelings or moods can usually be described in one word. An example of a belief might be "I'm a terrible person," while the accompanying feeling could be "shame." Practicing together in session will help the client feel more confident when completing this exercise independently.

After you and the client have practiced completing an Identifying Automatic Thoughts Worksheet, you can then give examples of possible situations, thoughts, and feelings (based on previous conversations with the client) that the client can use to complete some additional copies of this handout on his own. Writing down the beginnings of an example together in session is an effective way of encouraging the client to continue this practice as an independent activity.

Challenging Automatic Thoughts

Once a client has some experience in recognizing automatic thoughts, you should introduce and practice techniques for challenging the distressing thoughts. To learn the technique of challenging automatic thoughts, she will use Handout 13, the Automatic Thought Record. This is essentially an expanded version of Handout 11. Clients use Handout 14, the Challenging Questions Worksheet, in tandem with Handout 13 to challenge distressing thoughts. The first three columns of the Automatic Thought Record are similar to those on the Identifying Automatic Thoughts Worksheet. The additional three columns are "Evidence That Supports the Automatic Thought," "Evidence Against the Automatic Thought," and "Alternative, Balanced Thoughts." During the session in which you introduce the technique of challenging automatic thoughts, you should complete an Automatic Thought Record together, which may require most of a session. It is often easiest for a client if you keep a blank copy of Handout 13 at hand and fill out the columns as the client generates the information. In other words, you can play the role of note taker during session to help the client practice completing an Automatic Thought Record before she tries it on her own.

When completing a practice Automatic Thought Record, you can copy the first three columns ("Situation," "Moods," and "Automatic Thoughts/Images") from the Identifying Automatic Thoughts Worksheet the client completed between sessions, or you can assist the client in generating new information for the first three columns of the Automatic Thought Record. If the client has generated more than one automatic thought, you might encourage her to choose the most distressing thought from her Identifying Automatic Thoughts Worksheet to work on in session. You can then use this worksheet in conjunction with the Challenging Questions Worksheet to explore and challenge the chosen thought. Handout 12 provides a Sample Automatic Thought Record. Many clients find it helpful to see a completed worksheet to gain a better understanding of the entire process of challenging automatic thoughts.

Choosing an automatic thought to question can itself be a challenge. The specific expression of the thought is important. Clinical judgment will play an important role as you assist the client in choosing the exact expression of the thought that you will challenge together. It is often useful to demonstrate the downward arrow technique to help the client arrive at an automatic thought she can challenge effectively.

Downward Arrow Technique

This technique is a method for questioning a client so that she arrives at the essence of the automatic thought. For example, the client might state that her deceased partner was perfect for her. This statement would be written at the top of the "Automatic Thoughts/Images" column of Handout 11 or 13. Employing the downward arrow technique, you would then ask what it means that her loved one was perfect for her. The client might reply, "He was my soul mate." You would draw an arrow pointing down from the initial thought, and write, "He was my soul mate" beneath it. If you then ask, "What does that mean for your future?", the client might say, "I'll never love anyone like that again." This could be the final thought under a downward arrow, or, if this is pursued further ("And what does *that* mean for your future?"), the final thought might be "I'll be alone forever." The downward arrow technique thus helps the two of you arrive at the essence of the thought—at what it ultimately means for the client.

The downward arrow technique often helps you and the client to discover the schema or core belief underlying the automatic thought. These schemas vary greatly from one client to another, but they often represent one of the five need areas listed in Table 2.2: safety, trust, esteem, intimacy, and control. These five areas can be referenced in order to help clients identify themes in their thinking. You should understand and use the need categories as a tool for identifying the schemas or core beliefs that drive automatic thoughts. Clients are often overwhelmed by the number of automatic thoughts they notice when they first start keeping track. Helping them to identify the underlying needs can be reassuring, especially when they are just beginning to learn how to identify and challenge automatic thoughts. Working on one automatic thought related to a particular need facilitates work on other thoughts related to that need.

Automatic thoughts are often severe or overstated and should match the emotions or moods the client has listed. Again, if there is more than one thought, circle the thought the client identifies as the most powerful or distressing. This is the thought she will address on the Automatic Thought Record.

The two of you then proceed to complete the next two columns of the Automatic Thought Record. Beginning with the "Evidence That Supports . . ." column, ask the client to tell you all the reasons she believes this thought to be true. Then record these reasons and ask questions to help the client to generate more reasons if applicable. When the client has listed all of the evidence she can for the automatic thought, direct her to Handout 14, the Challenging Questions Worksheet. This worksheet lists questions designed to help clients generate evidence against the automatic thought. This can be very difficult because people typically don't challenge their automatic thoughts. Automatic thoughts are habitual, are often long-standing, and may feel like the truth to the client. Ask the client to start by looking at the automatic thought she chose to circle on her Automatic Thought Record and questioning whether she has any general evidence against the thought. Once the client has generated as much evidence as possible, ask her to use the Challenging Questions Worksheet to try to generate more evidence against the automatic thought.

This is likely to be the aspect of the Automatic Thought Record with which clients will need the most assistance. People have often spent years believing their habitual automatic thoughts and actually generating evidence to support them, particularly when they are distressed. Although this may not appear rational, it is easier for them to continue to believe what they have always known and comfort themselves with evidence than to accommodate to new information that would alter habitual beliefs, even those that are negative. Although it may seem counterintuitive, people sometimes feel affirmed by "evidence" that they are correct, even in beliefs such as "I'm alone," because their worldview is confirmed.

The next step is to ask the client to go through each statement of evidence for the automatic thought and to ask herself whether it proves that the automatic thought is true. Together, you can use this process to generate more evidence against the automatic thought. In some cases, this can be as simple as rewording evidence that is overstated. For example, the "evidence" for "I'm a terrible person" might start as "I never do anything right" and evolve, upon examination, into "I sometimes do things correctly and sometimes make mistakes." As stated above, this process is often the most challenging part of completing the Automatic Thought Record. The accommodation of new information (i.e., evidence against an automatic thought) requires reexamining a network of interrelated assumptions about oneself, others, and the world (the assumptive world). This is a task most people do not take on unnecessarily, as it challenges their identities, their worldviews, and the foundation of their relationships. Because this aspect of the task can feel overwhelming or even terrifying, you may be tempted to offer contrary evidence yourself. However, it is especially important to strike the delicate balance between the roles of note taker and teacher in this part of the exercise. Whereas you can and should ask questions to help a client arrive at evidence for and against the automatic thought (*Socratic questioning*), you should try to avoid generating evidence yourself. Doing so usually invites the client to disagree, which is counterproductive.

The final step in completing the Automatic Thought Record is to create a balanced thought. The balanced thought is a statement that summarizes the information in the "Evidence That Supports . . ." and "Evidence Against . . ." columns. It is important for the client to understand that she doesn't have to convince herself of anything she doesn't believe. Challenging automatic thoughts is not the same as the "power of positive thinking." A client may still be convinced of her initial automatic thought by the end of the process. More often, however, the client is at least able to modify the thought so that it becomes slightly less harsh, if not to discount it. Even a slight modification in a habitual automatic thought can make a tremendous difference in mood. For example, when a traumatically bereaved client moves from believing that she is a bad person because she does not react to her sister's death the way her friends expect her to react, to believing that her way of reacting may not be typical but that it is not wrong, the "I'm bad" automatic thought may shift to "I'm different." Increased confidence and, eventually, increased self-worth may accompany this changed belief.

Clients may find that thoughts they have successfully challenged recur. Automatic thoughts are usually habitual, and clients will typically need to challenge them each time they surface. Over time, the distressing automatic thoughts will lose their power.

Clients may find it hard to challenge long-standing automatic thoughts or beliefs because they have difficulty dealing with the emotions the thoughts provoke. In this way, the cognitive processing technique overlaps with that of exposure. For example, a client may state that he should have checked his voice mail during his camping trip so he would have known that his father had died while he was out of town. When you prompt him to examine the thought more closely, the client may arrive at a simple and extremely distressing thought, such as "I never was a good enough son," and intense emotion may accompany this thought. The client may need some time habituating to this emotion alongside the need to process the thought cognitively.

Clients may also resist examining automatic thoughts because they relate to an important aspect of their lives, such as their upbringing or religion. For example, a Christian client may believe that if his faith were stronger, he would be able to accept the loss and would not be suffering. Challenging this thought may help the client to view all of his emotional reactions, including suffering after a loss, as part of a normal human response. Thus he might move from believing "I'm not a good Christian," to "God is with me in good times as well as when I'm struggling." Both skill and patience on your part will help clients to proceed with this process of challenging, even in the face of impediments.

You should try to complete at least one copy of the Automatic Thought Record with the client (and more as needed) in session to teach him the process. As noted above, you may find that you need to devote an entire session to this task. If you are short on time, the two of you may find it necessary to generate a few statements of evidence for the thought and then move on to the "Evidence against . . ." column rather than creating a comprehensive list for each column. The learning process typically continues for several sessions, as you both review in session the Automatic Thought Records the client generates at home.

It is important to repeat the rationale for cognitive work (Handout 9, A Model for Change) to your clients during the initial stages of teaching these skills. Completing the first few Automatic Thought Records is demanding and time-consuming. You can remind clients that they are trying to break a habit of thought they may have been engaging in regularly since childhood. It is important for them to practice this skill on paper until they are entirely comfortable with it. Ideally, they will begin to notice they are challenging their automatic thoughts when they have them during the course of their day. In this way, they will begin to replace old, damaging habits of thought with new, more balanced thinking habits.

Automatic thoughts tend to follow patterns. Identifying and challenging one thought will generalize to other, related thoughts. Understanding this may help clients feel less overwhelmed at the number of automatic thoughts they notice. For example, some clients tend to minimize the importance of anything positive that happens to them. Others engage in all-or-nothing thinking and tend to view things in extremes. Clients may benefit from having you help them identify such patterns in their negative thinking.

You can also use cognitive processing more broadly in this treatment approach. For example, you can use the techniques described above to challenge automatic thoughts concerning specific coping activities or social support. Some clients may find it helpful to work through their fears about exposure by using the Automatic Thought Record. You might ask a client, "What do you fear will happen if you allow yourself to feel your emotions?" If the client expresses fear, encourage her to give a vivid description of what would happen. Then explore the likelihood of the event, and/or the actual consequences of the event. Many clients say things like "I would never be able to stop crying," or "My family would have me put in an institution." Explore how likely the consequences are. For more realistic consequences ("I'd cry for several days and need help caring for my kids"), encourage the client to engage in problem solving and to weigh these potential costs against the long-term benefits. We invite you to think creatively about the use of the Automatic Thought Record and the Challenging Questions Worksheet.

Several handouts included in the Appendix or on the book's website supplement can technically be considered cognitive processing exercises, but have a definite emotional processing component as well. These include Handout 26, Account of Your Relationship with Your Significant Other; Handout 29, Letter to Your Significant Other; Handout 30, Exploring the Meaning of the Loss; and Handout S8, Continuing Your Relationship with Your Significant Other. These are often useful for a client who has progressed through most of the treatment. They offer opportunities to remember the deceased and the client's relationship with her, while both considering what she means to him and experiencing his emotions about the relationship and the loss. This can be especially helpful for clients who tend to avoid their emotions by intellectualizing the loss.

EMOTIONAL PROCESSING INTERVENTIONS

The emotional processing element of the integrated treatment approach is based on supported exposure to the thoughts, memories, and situations that trigger strong emotions. Put simply, supported exposure is a carefully paced, guided approach to facing fears that not only decreases avoidance and anxiety, but helps survivors to experience their full range of emotions. Its success depends on trust within the therapeutic alliance, and on a client having the resources with which she entered therapy or that were created or restored in the resource-building aspects of this treatment.

Cognitive-behavioral theory and available evidence suggest that guiding people to approach benign but feared stimuli slowly, beginning with the least feared and working toward the most, will help them learn to tolerate distress until it dissipates. This process also builds clients' confidence that they can handle these situations and emotions.

Such exposure activities are experiments in which a person tests his theories about what is actually dangerous in the world. The feared stimuli can be in the real world (e.g., airplanes) or in the client's memory or imagination (e.g., the memory of the phone call informing a man of his partner's death). In this treatment, you will employ different methods, depending on what the client is avoiding. There are two general categories of exposure activities: imaginal and *in vivo*.

Presenting the Exposure Rationale

Some clients have an intuitive understanding that facing their fears will be beneficial to them. These clients are often motivated to try imaginal and *in vivo* exposure. Other clients may be more fearful and hence more reluctant to engage in exposure activities, saying things like "I just want to put that behind me," or "I just need to move on." In these situations, it may be helpful to describe the importance of fully experiencing emotions in a safe environment without avoiding them. Earlier in this chapter, we have described the common fear that experiencing emotions about the loss will result in an inability to stop crying or to go on with life. Your reassurance, calm demeanor, and faith in the process are enormously helpful to clients at this stage of the therapy. The survivors' motivation to feel relief from intense suffering, combined with trust in you as the therapist, allows them to move forward into exposure. It is important to acknowledge that exposure can engender painful feelings. You should normalize clients' concerns about exposure, emphasize its effectiveness in decreasing long-term distress, reassure clients that they are capable of experiencing intense emotion without being disabled by it, and explain that the exposure element of this approach takes place within a broadly supportive treatment context. In other words, there are many strategies and supports in place that will allow clients to feel supported through this process.

You can explain that it is natural for people to want to avoid any person, place, activity, thought, feeling, or memory associated with negative emotions. Clients should understand that avoidance of feared thoughts and situations may help them feel better in the moment, but hurts them in the end. People avoid feelings and thoughts about loss because they are painful, but most clients will acknowledge that avoiding things that trigger emotions has not made the pain go away so far. In fact, it is likely that the clients have sought therapy because avoidance didn't work. Purposely facing their emotions allows mourners to regain control over them, and this control allows them to reinvest in life and to remember their lost loved ones in a fuller, healthier way. This is the exposure rationale.

In our sample treatment plan (provided on this book's website supplement), the rationale for exposure activities is presented in Session 6, about one-quarter of the way through the treatment. At this point, a client will have approached feared and avoided memories related to the loved one's death while completing activities such as the initial impact statement (Handout 5, Exploring the Impact of the Death) and looking at photographs of the deceased. The client must also overcome significant fear and anxiety to identify and challenge automatic thoughts about the loved one's death. Although these writing activities in previous sessions were not presented as exposures per se, they can be viewed as examples of situations in which the client was able to face fears. Even making the decision to seek therapy and come to the first session requires many clients to overcome their anxiety. You can remind the client of past success with these "exposures" to thoughts about the death, to put *in vivo* exposure into a more familiar context. In addition, many clients have already conducted informal *in vivo* exposures in their therapy work. Social activities and goals work often bring clients into contact with situations they have been avoiding, and typically prompt significant anxiety. Most clients will have conquered a number of these challenges by this point in therapy. Reminding clients of these successes may also reduce their fear about *in vivo* exposure.

Exposure is difficult work, but sticking with it alleviates pain. When clients create a safe environment and allow themselves to confront the painful thoughts, memories, and emotions, the pain will gradually lessen. If a traumatically bereaved client pushes himself to stay at a previously avoided restaurant for 45 minutes even though he may remain afraid, his anxiety will gradually fall (i.e., he will habituate to it), and he will experience less anxiety with each subsequent visit to the restaurant. Clients are often reassured by the idea of working their way gradually up the hierarchy with support, so that it doesn't feel overwhelming. The pain does not diminish as quickly as it does when they escape it by avoiding (e.g., leaving places that remind them of their significant other or working long hours to keep the focus off their grief), but the relief is more likely to be permanent through exposure activities. Escape and avoidance alleviate discomfort in the moment, but when clients escape by avoiding, the painful emotions come back full force the next time they confront those situations, memories, or thoughts. When clients purposely and repeatedly engage with what they have been avoiding, they will find that the painful emotions diminish, enabling them to move forward again.

Clients may avoid important aspects of life after a traumatic death because they serve as reminders of the loss. Behavioral exposure can help clients gradually approach an avoided person, place, or activity until they begin to feel comfortable again.

Imaginal Exposure

Much of the distress that traumatically bereaved clients report stems from thoughts and memories of the loss that they work hard to avoid. In imaginal exposure, the therapist asks the client to recount traumatic events in detail in the first person and the present tense, in either written or oral form. The client writes or tells this narrative repeatedly, with increasing sensory detail. This process evokes emotions that a survivor typically avoids. With repetition, the client experiences her emotions and learns that she can tolerate them. The more the client evokes the traumatic memory and finds that she is able to tolerate it, the less overwhelming the emotion becomes. At this point, the client can more easily process and begin to come to terms with the traumatic death. Imaginal exposure is used to help the client habituate to the anxiety caused by memories or other fear-provoking thoughts. Imaginal exposure is particularly useful in cases when *in vivo* exposure would be dangerous or impractical. The integrated treatment approach includes such exposure activities in the form of writing assignments.

Many of the writing assignments we recommend are imaginal exposure assignments. Those that are not specifically designed as imaginal exposure assignments contain elements of exposure, such as writing about the impact of the death (see Handout 5, Exploring the Impact of the Death). You may want to use the writing assignments in the order in which they appear in the Appendix, as this order represents the approach we used in pilot-testing the treatment. However, if you are comfortable with CBT or know your clients' needs, you may choose to use some or all of these activities in a different order.

The main written exposure assignments that ask the client to describe the "story" or account of the death or of finding out about it form the core of the emotional processing aspect of our therapy approach. Over the course of the 25-session sample treatment plan, a client is asked to write an account of the death three times (following Sessions 6, 7, and 8), and to read the account daily (see Handouts 16, First Account of the Death; 20, Second Account of the Death; and 22, Third Account of the Death). If you and the client are both able to do so, it can be helpful to schedule longer sessions (up to 90 minutes) for exposure work, and to try to schedule exposure sessions so that the client does not have to return to work, care for children or engage in other potentially demanding activities immediately after the session. A client who finds exposure work particularly challenging may want to schedule more frequent sessions during this process (e.g., twice weekly) for added support.

Choosing the Event to Describe

People experience the traumatic death of a loved one in individual ways, so a client should choose the event or the aspect of the event that caused the most distress. Some clients choose to recount receiving the phone call or hearing the knock on the door; others report finding their loved one's body; and some might classify identifying the loved one's body at the morgue as the most distressing event. Some clients were present when their loved one died, and may choose to recount that moment. Each client should also choose where to begin and end the "story," or the account of the death. Clients often feel that the events of the days prior to or after the loss are significant, and you should encourage them to include these. By attending carefully to the information each client chooses to include, you may identify obstacles to the client's mourning.

Guidelines for Writing Assignments

Encourage clients to write when they have ample time and no distractions. Advise them to begin at their own pace, giving only as many sensory and emotional details as they feel they can handle. Exposure should be challenging but not overwhelming, and most clients choose to report few details at first. The basic guideline for these writing assignments is that a client should write in such a way that she experiences her emotions as fully as possible without overwhelming herself. It is important for the client to feel a sense of control over this process, as an antidote to the loss of control that is the hallmark of a traumatic death.

Clients may use self-soothing skills such as breathing retraining before or after, *but not during*, a writing assignment because doing so would reinforce avoidance of the emotional experience. Exposure, particularly PE (see Chapter 7), is effective because it allows a client enough time to habituate to the emotion. If the client takes frequent breaks to calm down, she will not receive the full benefit of the activity.

Ask clients to write these assignments by hand. They should not type, edit, or rewrite the assignments. If clients are concerned that what they have written is not good enough, inaccurate, or in some other way "not right," it may help to assure them that they will be writing their accounts again in future sessions. You will also ask clients to write continuously. If they need to stop, they should draw a line indicating where they stopped and resume writing as soon as possible. These lines will help you to identify aspects of the account that may have been most distressing to each client. These assignments are repeated, and clients should be encouraged to include more and more sensory and emotional details in their accounts. The inclusion of such details tends to prompt the release and processing of emotions about the loss.

Focusing on a "Hot Spot"

If a client is having difficulty elaborating on or expressing feelings about a specific aspect of the account, it may help to use the "hot spot" technique. A "hot spot" is the specific aspect of the account that the client finds particularly distressing. This approach involves asking the client to write about only that segment of the account with as much detail as possible, and to read it repeatedly during the next session. The client can write the "hot spot" account at home, but she should read it multiple times in session because these accounts tend to be brief and it may require repetition before the client begins to feel less distress. If the client is unable to write the "hot spot" at home, you can ask the client to write it in session, and then read it repeatedly in session.

Reading the Account in the Next Session

When you have assigned a writing activity to be done between sessions, ask the client to read aloud what she wrote at the beginning of the next session. You can of course discuss and address any discomfort the client feels about reading the account. The goal is to collaborate with the client to help her feel comfortable enough to approach avoided memories and experience avoided emotions. If a client is particularly reluctant to read the account aloud, suggest reading just part of the account, reading while you look away, or having you read the account aloud. Ideally, however, the client will read the account aloud.

The confidence you display in the client's ability to write and read these accounts can make a tremendous difference in her feelings about the process. The purpose of exposure is to help clients overcome fear and anxiety by working through avoidance. You should support each client in doing exposures by working to make them achievable. Once the client has read the account to you successfully, ask her to read it multiple times on her own between sessions. Remind the client that she may use behaviors such as the breathing technique (Handout 7, Breathing Retraining), feelings skills (Handout 8, Feelings Skills), and other coping activities *after* completing the read-through at home.

You should help the client feel calm and fully aware of her surroundings by the time she leaves any session; this is particularly important during exposure sessions. Some clients report feeling "spacey" or "stuck in the story" and need more time to process their emotions, regulate their breathing, and feel grounded enough to leave. It is valuable to note the approaching ending of the session when you have about 10 minutes left. A statement like "I'm aware that we have about 10 minutes left" can help the client begin to orient herself to the ending and to leaving the office, and to engage in grounding or other coping skills if needed. The feelings skills that you have introduced early in the treatment are helpful in this regard, as is your caring presence.

In Vivo Exposure

In addition to avoiding memories of the traumatic death, survivors of traumatic bereavement also avoid people and situations that prompt distressing emotions related to the death. Clients may frame this type of avoidance as an inability to do certain things since the loss. Examples include avoiding paying bills because doing so is a reminder of the death of the loved one who used to pay the bills, avoiding seeking support from people who were associated with the loved one, and avoiding pleasant activities because the client feels that pleasure would be a betrayal of the loved one. Clients may report that they do not avoid these situations completely, but that they tolerate them with distress or they tend to escape from the situations early. *In vivo* exposure allows clients to habituate to such feared or anxiety-provoking stimuli. *In vivo* exposure is based on the same rationale as imaginal exposure: Facing anxiety-provoking situations allows clients to process and habituate to their emotions. Habituating to the emotions that these situations provoke decreases avoidance and reduces fear and anxiety. Research suggests that tolerating the fear for at least 45 minutes at a time, three times a week, allows clients to habituate to their fear (Foa et al., 2007).

Effective *in vivo* exposure exercises require careful planning with each client. The two of you will spend time discussing situations that the client avoids because they are distressing reminders of the traumatic loss. Together, you will then create a list of very specific feared or anxiety-provoking situations, which the client then rates in terms of how much distress they are likely to cause. You then instruct the client to approach the feared situations, beginning with the point in the hierarchy where the client feels mildly uncomfortable and working his way toward more difficult activities. We describe this process in more detail below.

Fear and Avoidance Hierarchy

It is important that the two of you collaborate in creating a list of feared situations. As mentioned above, the list should include very specific situations. After developing the list of avoided situations, the client ranks each situation on a 0–100 scale according to the level of distress it would provoke. The 0–100 scale is known as a Subjective Units of Distress Scale (SUDS). This scale gives you a common language or metric for describing the difficulty of many assignments; it will guide the two of you in choosing appropriate exposure situations to approach. More specifically, you will use the SUDS rankings to create a fear and avoidance hierarchy (using Handout 25, the Fear and Avoidance Hierarchy Form).

It is important to create a list that includes a wide range of distress ratings. This will provide the client with a sufficient range of exposure activities to help address his avoidance and gain confidence in his ability to do so through engaging in numerous activities. If a client has identified avoided situations that all fall within a particular range of the SUDS, encourage him to identify situations that seem easier or more difficult than those identified thus far. You may need to alter one avoided activity slightly to turn it into several. For example, if a client says she avoids going to the grocery store where she used to shop with her partner, you might ask her to rate driving to the parking lot and spending 45 minutes watching people go in and out. Alternatively, you could ask her to rate going shopping at the store with a trusted friend. For some people, altering the time of day or location of an activity (e.g., going at night or to a different store) changes the rating. It is important to spend adequate time exploring the list with the client, so that you will have a clear basis for the work.

Once the two of you have developed the hierarchy, you keep it, and you and the client choose situations as weekly assignments. This process provides a concrete plan for helping the client reengage in avoided activities: You guide the client in a "stepladder" approach to choosing *in vivo* exposure assignments. Clients with relatively good coping resources may choose to complete an exercise rated at around 40 or 50 on the 0–100 scale initially, and repeat the same exercise three or four times a week. Clients who are more vulnerable may start lower on the hierarchy. Clinical judgment will help guide where a particular client should begin. Regardless of where he begins, moving up the hierarchy by choosing increasingly distressing situations allows the client to get used to each level of distress before approaching the next level of difficulty.

In some instances, you may be able to accompany the client on one or more *in vivo* exposure activities during sessions. This support may help to lower the SUDS rating enough for the client to feel comfortable with the exercise. Use your judgment and consult colleagues, supervisors, and insurers (if necessary) before deciding whether or not to conduct exposure activities outside the office as part of a clinical session. The two of you can use the SUDS to keep track of the difficulty and helpfulness of exposure activities (whether these are conducted alone or with you).

Client Instructions for *In Vivo* Exposure Activities

The client should understand that the primary goal of exposure is to tolerate the distress of the situation for 45 minutes (although you may set a shorter goal if necessary to build the client's confidence). Clients often misconstrue the goals of exposure, so you should clarify that the goal is not for a client to feel calm, appear happy, or even complete the task well. As an example, a client may choose an exposure of having dinner at a restaurant that she used to frequent with her husband. The exposure would count as a success as long as she tried to remain at the restaurant and did not try to distract her attention from her emotions by reading a book or newspaper.

Ask the client to rate her anxiety three times on the 0–100 scale: just before the exposure, at its peak, and when she has completed the activity. This method will allow you to determine whether the client is habitually under- or overestimating the difficulty of exposure activities, and will allow the client to see the decline in difficulty of each exposure exercise over time.

You should ask the client to do the same *in vivo* exposure three times in a week. Some situations are very difficult to recreate in the same way three times. Very similar exposures can be substituted in this case. For example, a client may be uncomfortable initiating three different conversations with the same person. In this case, it is useful to identify three neighbors or new acquaintances with whom a conversation would provoke a similar level of anxiety. Clinical judgment is invaluable to this process. Consider what you notice as clients discuss activities and situations they avoid or tolerate with discomfort. You can use this information to modify exposures to provide the desired level of challenge.

Assessing client SUDS ratings during the exposures builds their confidence and eases them into the exposure work. As an example, a client may choose to pursue an exposure that is rated at a 20 (of 100) level of distress. He does the exposure activity three times in a week, 45 minutes each time. At the next session, he reports that by the last time, his distress level was a 2. He is now ready for the next exposure activity on the hierarchy, which he would initially have rated at 25 or 30. Clients gain confidence from each exposure, and since the activities are often related, conquering one makes the more difficult ones seem easier. Since the client (with your assistance) creates the hierarchy, modifies it as needed, and chooses where to begin, he regains a sense of control over his thoughts and memories.

It is fine to alter ratings or reassign the same exposure activities for a second week, based on information from the client. For example, if a client reports that an *in vivo* exposure prompted more anxiety than anticipated but she thinks she can conquer it, she might choose to attempt it again the following week. If a client believes that she rated the exposure activity inaccurately and it is too difficult to pursue at this point, she may decide to re-rate it with a higher distress rating and wait to try it until she has done the exposures that have lower distress ratings. The goal of each *in vivo* exposure is for the client to make it through the exposure without escaping the situation. You should congratulate the client enthusiastically for remaining in an uncomfortable situation for the agreed-upon time limit, even if she was anxious throughout the exercise. Your role will be to guide clients along their hierarchies. You want to ensure that they don't move up their hierarchies too quickly, but that they do move up as their anxiety in lower-ranked situations starts to diminish.

The nature of *in vivo* exposure requires that clients seek out real-life situations, which often include surprises. An exposure trip to a local restaurant rated at a 40 may suddenly jump to an 80 if the client unexpectedly encounters the best friend of his deceased wife. It is important to help the client realize that being unable to accomplish his goals in that situation does not constitute a failure, since it was no longer the exposure activity he had planned. When the client is able to go to the setting agreed upon in a session but is unable to remain in that situation, it is far more therapeutic to praise the client for his effort, explore the obstacles, and reassign the exposure than to frame it as a failure.

As with imaginal exposure, the client's *in vivo* exposure goal is to be able to experience her feelings and thoughts without trying to escape them. This can be difficult, especially for extremely anxious clients. The emotion-focused coping skills covered earlier in the book can be very helpful to clients in this process. Ideally, clients will use breathing retraining, Automatic Thought Records, or other emotion-focused coping skills to calm themselves when the exposure is over. However, it is sometimes difficult to gauge the level of *in vivo* exposures correctly. If a client finds herself in a situation that is too uncomfortable, practicing breathing retraining midway through the exposure in order to make it to the time limit is a far better alternative than escaping the situation. In general, however, the client should try to make it through the exposure without using self-soothing techniques, if such techniques inhibit the full experience of anxiety and the consequent learning that the anxiety will not destroy the individual and will pass on its own.

Suggestions for helping a client to engage in avoided activities include encouraging the client to use social support by calling upon a friend to be with him through the activity; advising the client to challenge automatic thoughts (e.g., "I will humiliate myself and lose a friend if I confide in her") that may be getting in the way; or reminding the client to utilize breathing retraining or another coping strategy in order to help decrease anxiety before beginning or after completing the activity. These coping strategies will set the stage for a successful exposure experience.

BEHAVIORAL INTERVENTIONS

If a client is finding that an automatic thought continues to cause distress even after several attempts at challenging the thought, the two of you can often design a "behavioral experiment" to test whether or not the automatic thought is true. For instance, if a client believes he cannot pay the household bills, you can work with the client to develop a plan to pay one or a few bills. This may require steps such as recruiting help from a friend or consulting his bank, which can be included in the plan. We have found it useful to agree with a client on a time by which he will have completed each step.

Behavioral experiments allow clients to test negative beliefs about themselves, the world, and their ability to operate in the world. In many situations, behavioral experiments are very similar to exposures, in that a client must overcome his anxiety in order to complete the experiment. As clients test their negative beliefs in the real world, they have opportunities both to gather new information. This process increases their awareness of the ways in which distorted or outdated automatic thoughts and associated schemas may be keeping them from moving forward.

Processing through Interaction: Activity Scheduling

Cognitive-behavioral theory suggests that individuals can learn new associations, even in the absence of overt cognitive processing, by interacting with the world. This concept is very useful with traumatically bereaved individuals who have come to view the world as inhospitable or to view themselves as unfit for the world. As described earlier, it is typical for these individuals to withdraw and avoid interaction with the world. The behavioral technique of *activity scheduling* is a form of behavioral experimentation in which a person forces himself to go out into the world in order to get feedback about its hospitability or his ability to cope with life.

Activity scheduling requires a client to compel herself to plan activities and pursue them, regardless of whether they are pleasurable at first. Continuing efforts at activity scheduling generally result in increased pleasure during the activities. It has been hypothesized that anxious and depressed clients tend to isolate themselves and engage in passive activities (e.g., watching television, sleeping) that give them no information about themselves or the world. Without the information gained by interacting with the world, people may have difficulty relinquishing their negative views. Activity scheduling has been shown to decrease depression and increase involvement with life (Jacobson & Gortner, 2000). The values and goals work described in Chapter 10 is a specific application of activity scheduling.

CLINICAL INTEGRATION

It was a clear December day, and the sun shone in through the window of Michele's office. She was meeting with Larry, a 44-year-old man whose teenage daughter had died in a hurricane 5 years earlier.

At some point about halfway through the therapy session, Michele noticed Larry lowering his eyes and picking at his fingernails. Having met with Larry for about 12 weeks now, she recognized these gestures as the ones often accompanying a particular automatic thought that continued to trouble her client.

"I noticed a shift just there as you were reading your written account of your daughter's death, Larry. Are you aware of any thoughts that you're having in this moment?"

"Um, yeah. Whenever I recount the horror of Lucy's death, I can't help but think that I should never have let her go to the Bahamas with Annie's family during hurricane season. I was her father, for God's sake! I should have known the weather in August was too unpredictable."

"OK," said Michele. "Let's pause here and explore this thought. You 'should have known about the weather in August in the Bahamas.' What does this mean for you—that you should have known?"

Michele and Larry had been identifying and challenging automatic thoughts for several weeks now, and so this manner of exploration was familiar to both.

Larry answered quickly, "It means that I should have protected my daughter. It means I failed as a father."

"You failed as a father?" repeated Michele.

"Yes. Parents are supposed to protect their children. I should have known. I should have protected her. I failed."

"And what does it mean for you now, if you failed?"

Larry's voice sounded more agitated as he spoke. "It means my father was right—that I'm a good-for-nothing jerk. He said I would never amount to anything, and it looks like he was right. I've amounted to a complete failure as a parent and as a man. I should have protected her; I should have kept her alive."

"Do you really believe you have that much power, Larry? To foresee the future and keep people alive?" Michele was surprised by her own voice as she asked the question. She usually encouraged her clients to ask their own challenging questions. The question startled Larry, too, and although he didn't answer, the slight blush of his face seemed to indicate that he was taking in her question.

Michele continued, "OK. We both know that this thought—that you failed as a father and as a man—is not new. And you've listed evidence in favor of and against this thought in the past. I want to focus on the related thought that your father was right—that you are good for nothing—and I want us to spend some time evaluating its legitimacy. This gets to the issue of self-worth that we have explored before. 'You are good for nothing.' Do you think you might be using all-or-nothing thinking here?"

"Well, maybe," replied Larry. "I know what you would say. And I know that on most days, I believe that being a construction manager and a volunteer fireman is good for something."

"And can you think of any other ways to challenge the thought that you are good for nothing? Feel free to use your Challenging Questions Worksheet to help you."

"I may be taking things out of context—you know, evaluating my whole life on the basis of Lucy's death. I do know that I loved Lucy. From the minute she was born, I used my anger toward my own father to fuel my desire to be the best father I could be. My wife tells me I was a good father to her."

"Is it possible that Nancy sees this issue more clearly than you do?"

"I suppose so."

"And what does it mean if, perhaps, you are good for something?" Emotion became visible on Larry's face as he slowly answered, "It means—it means my father was wrong." His voice quivered.

"Do you know what it is that you're feeling right now, Larry?"

"A lot of sadness."

"And what are you thinking about?"

"It's like my whole life is turned upside down. Maybe my father was wrong. Maybe the fear that I'd never amount to anything didn't have to be there all of these years. Maybe I would have been a better parent without the fear; or maybe it inspired me to be different from him. I'm not sure. It's all just a little confusing right now. I'm not sure what to believe."

Larry and Michele sat in silence for a moment. Michele wanted to provide the space needed for her client to take in this shift. Larry broke the silence: "I never thought Lucy's death would lead me here. It looks like I still have issues with my father and the way my father affected how I feel about myself."

CONCLUDING REMARKS

Losing a child unexpectedly is traumatic for surviving parents. This was certainly true for Larry; he was struggling with mourning his daughter's death as well as with the traumatic elements of her death, which gave rise to his belief that he should have prevented it. What is interesting within this example is the way in which this maladaptive belief quickly spiraled down to "I am good for nothing," and how *this* belief had its roots in Larry's upbringing. Often, this will be the case: The problematic beliefs that surface during times of stress or trauma have their foundations in clients' early years and interfere with their ability to process trauma or move through mourning. At other times, a belief may come into being as the direct result of the later traumatic event. For Larry, processing his daughter's death meant dealing with some childhood memories and familial dysfunction.

The fact that problematic beliefs surface during or are triggered by trauma is significant. Confronting the traumatic stress, in whatever form that might take, offers a person the opportunity to become aware of and then challenge these beliefs. In other words, exposure to the traumatic material and cognitive processing go hand in hand. Exposure also offers the opportunity to experience the emotions affiliated with the traumatic event and its aftermath. It is therefore a significant and foundational aspect of this treatment. In the example of Larry's therapy with Michele, we can see how the work of recalling the traumatic death as well as his traumatic childhood, and the work of challenging related problematic beliefs, enabled Larry to experience feelings such as helplessness, sadness, guilt, and confusion. Together, these elements are the work of our integrated therapeutic approach with traumatically bereaved clients, and they combined to help move Larry through the process of mourning for Lucy. In the next chapter, we provide a comprehensive framework for understanding this movement through mourning.

CHAPTER 12

Facilitating Mourning

"How did the date go?" asked Ross. He and Zac were eating dinner together at a local bar, as they did every Tuesday night. Best friends since childhood, they could talk about anything. They knew each other's histories, families, dreams, and insecurities. Ross had known Courtney and stood up for Zac as his best man when he married her. He had also been there for Zac when Courtney died unexpectedly 10 years ago. In fact, Ross had been there for his best friend every Tuesday night since Courtney's death. He had just recently convinced Zac to start dating again, using an online dating website. He was now asking about his best friend's recent first date.

"It was OK," said Zac. "We're just not a match, though."

"Well, tell me about the date anyway. I'm curious. I haven't been on many of my own recently, as you know." Ross had been going through a dry spell.

"We met for drinks. She's a vet. She talked about her work. She was nice. She laughed at some of my jokes. We had a good time. Something was just missing for me."

"Something or someone?" asked Ross, knowingly. "You're never going to find another Court, ya know. And that's not the point. Courtney's been dead for 10 years, Zac. It's time you started living your life again. Listen, man, I know how much you loved her. I also know that you idealized her when she was alive, and I think you've been idealizing her and your marriage since she's passed. I didn't lose my first wife; I divorced her. There's a big difference, and I don't pretend to understand everything you feel. But I know you, man, and although you spent a lot of time grieving in those first years after her death, I think you may still be stuck in some way." Ross paused, then added, "I'm saying all this because I care."

As discussed throughout this book, the elements of this treatment are designed to support the client's movement through the six "R" processes of mourning. As a reminder, the "R" processes are as follows: *Recognize the loss; React to the separation; Recollect and reexperience the deceased and the relationship; Relinquish the old attachments to the deceased and the old assumptive world; Readjust to move adaptively into the new world without forgetting the old;* and *Reinvest.*[1]

There are many reasons why traumatically bereaved clients may have more difficulty with the mourning process than those who lose loved ones through natural causes. For example, as

---

[1]There are two versions of the "R" processes. The first uses professional language, and is designed for treatment providers (see Rando, 1993, or Table 2.1 in this volume). The second uses less technical language, and is designed for clients (see Rando, 2014, or Handouts 3 and 6 in this volume).

discussed in Chapter 3, those who experience the sudden, traumatic death of a loved one have far more difficulty accepting the death, and its many ramifications, than those whose loved one died in other ways. Since the mourners had no opportunity to prepare for the loss, the initial weeks and months following the death can be more agonizing. In most cases, it is difficult for survivors of traumatic loss to call up memories of the deceased because these are often accompanied by disturbing images of the death. Moreover, survivors of sudden, traumatic losses are mourning the loss of the world as they knew it (e.g., they don't feel safe now), in addition to the death of their loved one. For all of these reasons, it is easy for traumatically bereaved clients to get stuck in the mourning process. As you assist a client in moving from acute grief through these processes (described below), you facilitate healthy accommodation of a loved one's death.

In this chapter, we provide a rationale for the importance of each "R" process and guidance for moving through them. Rando (1993, 2014) offers further details about this process. The "Rs" are broken down into subprocesses to clarify the most significant elements of each "R" process. We illustrate how specific types of resource-building elements can promote the mourning processes. In addition, we offer suggestions regarding how to draw from your knowledge of trauma processing to assist clients who appear to be stuck in the mourning processes.

In most cases, the "R" processes tend to unfold from one another, with earlier processes serving as prerequisites for later ones. For example, the main task of the fourth "R" process (*Relinquish . . .*) is a precursor to the fifth (*Readjust . . .*); change requires letting go. However, there are times when the "R" processes can overlap or occur simultaneously, such as the first (*Recognize . . .*) and second (*React . . .*). Because the course of mourning is nonlinear and fluctuates over time, some movement back and forth among the processes is common. For example, the mourner may vacillate between the second (*React . . .*) and third (*Recollect . . .*) "R" processes. The important issue is to track whether a client appears to be moving forward. That is, is the mourner working to accommodate the loss, or is he avoiding, resisting, or otherwise stuck within one or more of these processes?

FIRST "R" PROCESS: *RECOGNIZE THE LOSS*

In order to begin mourning, a survivor must acknowledge that the death has occurred, and come to an understanding of its cause (however incomplete and imperfect). In the first subprocess of this R, *Acknowledge the death*, the initial concession that the death has occurred is intellectual only. Emotional acceptance of the death typically takes much longer. If the death is not acknowledged, there is nothing to mourn. A lack of confirmation of the death (e.g., the body is not recovered, due to the loss of a boat at sea) makes it challenging to acknowledge the death. There is no proof to contradict the survivor's normal desire that this reality not be true. This is why treatment providers often encourage viewing the deceased's body after a sudden death. As discussed in Chapter 5, available evidence suggests that if a mourner wishes to view the body, doing so is usually beneficial, even if it has sustained significant damage (Bower, 2010; Chapple & Zieblanc, 2010). Unfortunately, relatives and friends often try to "protect" the mourner by strongly discouraging her from viewing the body.

If it is not possible to view the body, a survivor is more likely to deny the loss and avoid its implications. If the status of the loved one is unknown, such as when a loved one in the military is missing in action, it may be extremely difficult to commence with the mourning process. The mourner may be plagued by the following kinds of concerns: "Is my loved one dead or alive?",

"Maybe he is out there somewhere, but unable to come home," "Maybe he developed amnesia and cannot find his way back home," or "Should we be trying to find him?" (Rando, 1993). As we have discussed in Chapter 5, the distress of a person whose loved one is missing can be greater than the distress of someone whose loved one is confirmed to be dead.

The second subprocess, *Understand the death*, means developing an explanation of it that makes sense to the bereaved. Such accounts must explain the events that led up to the death and clarify how, why, and under what conditions the loved one died. Unfortunately, in many traumatic deaths, such information is lacking. For example, it may be unclear whether a death was a suicide, a homicide, or an accident. Not knowing why a significant other died or what led to the death is extremely upsetting for most survivors. Unanswered questions interfere with healthy mourning and can turn into unfinished business that adds to the client's distress. In addition, such questions can fuel feelings that the world lacks meaning, orderliness, or predictability. Others need not agree with the mourner's explanation, as long as it suffices for that mourner. For example, a mourner may insist that a loved one's death by gunshot was an accident, while others perceive the gunshot as deliberate and the death as a suicide. Although the explanation may not fit the facts of the death, it serves a psychological purpose at this point. The lack of fit can be addressed later.

Facilitating the First "R" Process

You can assist a client in recognizing the loss by facilitating those subprocesses that permit him to acknowledge and understand the loved one's death. A survivor typically requires repeated confrontations with the reality of the death in order to grasp what has happened. This process cannot begin until the mourner concedes that the death occurred. Your goal as the therapist is to help the mourner comprehend what has happened. It may take many months (and, in some cases, years) to recognize the reality of the loss on a consistent basis. In the interim, the mourner's ability to grasp the finality of the death and its implications fluctuates. This highlights the difficult, time-consuming nature of incorporating such a painful reality.

To assist a mourner with the first subprocess of recognizing the loss, *Acknowledge the death*, you must gently help the client to comprehend that the loss is permanent and irreversible. In almost all cases, this part of the mourning process is agonizing for clients. As Wolterstorff (1987) expressed it following the death of his son,

> It's the *neverness* that is so painful. *Never again* to be here with us, never to cry with us, never to embrace us as he leaves for school, never to see his brothers and sister marry. . . . Only our death can stop the pain of his death. A month, a year, five years—with that I could live. But not this forever. (p. 15; original emphasis)

It may be important to help the client build resources (see Chapter 10) as a foundation for acknowledging the death, so she can manage the feelings this acknowledgment is likely to evoke. Interventions to help the mourner accept the reality of the death may include discussing the absence of the significant other; the frustration and other feelings the client experiences now that her loved one is gone; and what it has been like for the client to go through her daily routine without the deceased. Rather than push the client to accept the fact of the loss, you can clarify what may be interfering with her ability to acknowledge it.

You can help the client recognize the loss through exposure activities, such as inviting her to bring in some photos of the deceased, or asking her to write a statement about the impact of this loss (see Handout 5, Exploring the Impact of the Death). Some mourners persistently avoid anything external (such as a person, place, object, or activity) or internal (such as a thought, feeling, or memory) that is associated with the loved one, in order to avoid acknowledging the death. Below, we describe some additional strategies you can employ to address such avoidance.

The inability to recognize feelings is often an obstacle to the client's acknowledgment of the death. It is therefore useful to introduce the concept of feelings skills or self capacities along with this "R" process—or in any case, early in the treatment (see Chapter 10 for a discussion of developing feelings skills, and Handout 8, Feelings Skills, for information on this topic designed for the client). Sometimes a mourner keeps refusing to acknowledge a death that you may believe she should have acknowledged by now (based on appropriate expectations for her, given her unique situation). If so, you could inquire what might be interfering with her ability to do so by asking her to complete, with as many responses as possible, the sentence "If I were to recognize my loved one as dead, that would mean . . .". For example, the mourner may respond by stating, "It would mean that I am all alone." Raising such questions can help both of you understand obstacles to be addressed. If the mourner has problems because an intact body is not available or there is no body, you can help her recognize that the death occurred by suggesting that she attempt to obtain and examine available data, such as newspaper articles, that could confirm or deny her loved one's death. If there is no body and hence no actual evidence of the death, you can encourage the client to consider circumstantial evidence, such as her loved one's continued absence, knowledge of the death of others, or the small chance of escape from the situation. This was the situation facing many families who lost loved ones in the 9/11 terrorist attacks.

As noted above, it will be important to the client to *Understand the death*—that is, to comprehend how it occurred. This subprocess involves the mourner's constructing a causal account of the death. You can assist with this subprocess by helping her identify what she does and does not know about the death, what she needs to know, and what will and won't be possible for her to know. If important gaps remain, you can work with her to strategize how to get additional information and/or how best to manage the feelings created by the lack of closure. It is important to be cognizant of the anguish many clients may experience if they do not have the information they desire. You can work with a mourner to assess the costs and benefits of pursuing particular kinds of information, such as police reports or traffic crash reports, as well as how she would deal with any distressing information she might receive. If the mourner is unable, despite considerable effort, to obtain information about how the death occurred, you can help with the feelings of anger and frustration that may emerge.

SECOND "R" PROCESS: *REACT TO THE SEPARATION*

Once a mourner has recognized the reality of the death, he must react to the separation it brings. This reaction involves three subprocesses. The first, *Experience the pain*, is one that mourners naturally want to resist. In the wake of a traumatic death, a mourner may be so overwhelmed or numb that it takes a while to feel the pain. This can further delay the process of reacting, since a person cannot process pain without experiencing it.

Traumatic death can bring excruciating pain. Here is where work on affect management (see Chapter 10) can be especially important. This is not to say that one must never avoid, delay, or minimize pain—only that one must use such actions as part of a plan to dose oneself and to learn to tolerate and process pain over time. The dual-process model, described in Chapter 7, provides guidance regarding how to work with the client so that intensely painful aspects of the work are alternated with activities that are restorative (such as going to see a film with an old friend).

Feeling the pain is also critical because, without it, the mourner will lack the experiences necessary to face the reality of the loved one's death. For example, a bereaved individual usually makes conscious or unconscious efforts to search for and recover the deceased. The failure to recover the loved one, and the pain associated with that failure, are what teach the mourner over time that the person is truly gone and that adjustments to this new reality are necessary. It typically takes many such "lessons" for the mourner to react to the death when it has come suddenly and unexpectedly.

The second subprocess is to *Feel, identify, accept, and give some form of expression to all the psychological reactions to the loss*. The mourner has to label, differentiate, and trace his feelings in all of their complexity and attempt to process each of them. The circumstances of traumatic death can bring many additional, often intense reactions beyond those commonly experienced in expected, natural deaths. You can assist the client in feeling and expressing his emotional reactions to the loss in ways that are appropriate and constructive for him in his unique situation. For many mourners, failure to do so can lead to adverse effects that come from unfinished business.

The third subprocess is to *Identify and mourn secondary losses*. For some, a secondary loss can be more difficult than the death. This was the case for the sister of a famous actress, who found it harder to lose the social status she had because of who her sister was than to lose her sister. She had envied her sister but had never been close to her.

As noted earlier, it can take months or even years for the survivor to become aware of the secondary losses associated with the loved one's death. For example, nearly 3 years after his wife died following an aneurysm, a man suffered a bad fall. His doctor told him that it was necessary to undergo hip replacement surgery. His recognition that his wife would not be there to care for him following this surgery, or any subsequent health problems, constituted a powerful secondary loss for him.

Facilitating the Second "R" Process

The first subprocess under *React to the separation*, *Experience the pain*, can be facilitated by broadening the client's perspective on her pain. You can do so by legitimizing and normalizing the client's pain. It is common for clients to infer from their pain that they are not moving forward. In addition, you can facilitate the mourning process by conveying that (1) the desire to avoid pain is natural and accompanies almost all major losses; (2) people vary in what is painful and in what strategies for dealing with the pain are most useful for them at any time; (3) successful mourning will help to alleviate the pain; (4) maintenance of pain as a testimonial or as a form of connection to the deceased is not healthy; and (5) there are strategies available to keep mourners from losing control or being overwhelmed with their pain, which tends to be the main impediment to this subprocess. You can convey to the mourner that she will be able to bear the pain, and help her develop the skills to do so.

It is useful to break the client's pain into its component parts and work on one at a time. For example, the mourner may feel angry that her partner has left her alone, frightened of her future as an aging single woman, and bereft of her partner's loving companionship. Each of these feelings can be addressed separately. In addition, you can tell your client that she can go as rapidly or as slowly as she wishes, and she can stop whenever she feels overwhelmed (Rando, 1993). You can also explain the rationale for alternating painful phases of the treatment with activities that are more restorative. Shifting between these types of activities, as the dual-process model would advocate, can energize the client so that she can deal with her pain more effectively.

It is important to recognize that some mourners do not view their pain as an aversive stimulus. They may regard it as the only way to maintain a connection to their loved one. If this is true for your client, the usual approaches to alleviating the pain will be ineffective because the mourner's suffering often comes from the thought of not having pain (Rando, 1993). In this case, you will need to work with the client to find healthier ways to maintain a connection with her loved one. (See the section on the fifth "R" process later for information about how to do this.)

There are several ways to assist a client with the second subprocess, which is to *Feel, identify, accept, and give some form of expression to all the psychological reactions to the loss*. Many factors may influence a mourner's style of expressing emotion following loss, including (1) beliefs based in the mourner's religion, culture, or ethnic identity; (2) coping skills; (3) habitual ways of expressing emotion; and (4) prior life events such as the early death of a parent, which can be triggered by the loss. It is essential to assess each client's particular ways of dealing with emotions. If the client feels uncomfortable with outward displays of emotion, such as crying, you could help her explore the obstacles and/or alternatives to expressing feelings in that way.

Conveying your desire to understand the full range of the mourner's feelings allows them to be addressed in treatment. In this "R" process, the emphasis may move from becoming aware of feelings to tolerating strong feelings, which is another dimension of affect management, a feelings skill. To support the client in reacting to the separation, it is essential to continue helping her build affect management and coping skills, as described in Chapter 10.

At any point when the focus is on the client's feelings, it may be useful to refer to Handout 8, Feelings Skills. (For further information on assessing self capacities, see Table 8.1.) Exposure activities, such as writing and reading an account of the death daily, can also help the client move through the "R" process of reacting to the separation. Both the process and the content of the activities strengthen clients' ability to manage strong feelings, opening doors to *Reacting*. (For more information on this work, see Chapter 11; Handout 16, First Account of the Death; and related handouts in the Appendix.)

Other approaches besides verbal techniques can help a mourner access unexpressed feelings. For example, you may wish to consider employing the *empty-chair technique*, also called *chair work*. Originally developed by Gestalt therapists, this technique is well suited for work with a survivor of a sudden, traumatic death. Ask the client to address an empty chair as if the deceased were sitting in it. You can ask the client to close her eyes if she is comfortable doing so and to initiate a conversation with the loved one, using first person and present tense. Explain that the client can tell the deceased anything she wishes—for example, conveying thoughts or feelings, or asking questions. Ask the client to imagine that the deceased can actually hear her. After the client has spoken, she then gets up and moves to the empty chair. Ask her to take the role of the deceased and continue the conversation. Of course, the client can become engaged in the dialogue without actually moving from chair to chair.

This technique plays a focal role in the treatment for complicated grief developed by Shear and her associates, who provide a detailed account of how to use it. Shear and Frank (2006) indicate that many bereaved individuals wish they could have one last conversation with the persons who died. Also, as noted earlier, some mourners are upset because they were not present when their loved ones died. Others are troubled because their last conversations with the bereaved were conflictual, and now there is no way to make things right. Shear and Frank provide a compelling example of how the empty-chair technique can assist a client in dealing with these painful feelings:

> For example, a client might say, "Did you feel that I abandoned you because I was not there when you died?" The response might be, "Of course not. I never doubted for a minute that you love me very much and that you would have been there if you could have." Although this may be the response the client wants to hear, it is also very convincing that the loved one would have, in fact, responded in this way. (pp. 300–301)

There are also several nonverbal techniques for becoming open to feelings. These include utilizing movement and physical activity; drawing or painting; creating a memorial garden with some of the deceased's favorite plants; or listening to music that reminds a mourner of the loved one. Nonverbal means of expression may be especially valuable for a client who has difficulty putting feelings into words. The goal is to help the client express his reactions to the loss in ways that are both acceptable to and therapeutic for him. Once the client has felt, identified, accepted, and expressed his thoughts, feelings, and memories, his emotions will become more manageable. He will be able to respond to them with greater ease. Although the client cannot choose his feelings, if he can identify them, he can decide how to respond to or hold them. Such choice begins to restore a sense of control to the survivor, which is crucial after traumatic bereavement.

If the mourner is having difficulty getting in touch with feelings related to his loss, you can help him review the relationship, the circumstances of the death, and the changes that have come about as a result of the death. Specifically, it can be useful to discuss the roles and functions the loved one fulfilled; all of the things the loved one did for and with the client; and the hopes, dreams, and plans for the future that involved the loved one's presence (Rando, 2014). As necessary, you will need to focus on any emotional numbing, avoidance, or other responses (such as guilt or fear of recognizing dependence upon the deceased) that could be interfering with this subprocess. These responses can be addressed by recommending tasks that the client regards as restorative, such as cooking dinner with a son or daughter. The tools described in Chapter 10 (developing self capacities and approaching avoided feelings) are also very useful.

The final subprocess, *Identify and mourn secondary losses*, involves working with the mourner to address the myriad secondary losses that accrue from this death. This concept helps clients to understand the pervasiveness of their losses. Specific examples of secondary losses include the psychosocial loss of a positive relationship with God and the physical loss of a house that one can no longer afford (see Chapter 2 and Handout 17, Secondary Losses, for more detailed discussions). Each one needs to be identified, labeled, and separated from the others. The mourner's reactions to each of them should be processed, just as they are for the death itself. As he reviews each of these secondary losses, a mourner may feel that he is experiencing a nonstop chain of losses. If the mourner is overloaded, it is important to help him manage the timing and dosing so he does not overwhelm himself by looking at secondary losses too soon, too rapidly, or too many at a time. This is also a valuable place to encourage the client to use the coping skills described in Chapter 10 as well as breathing retraining (Handout 7).

In addition to the work in session, the client can make a list of these losses between sessions for use throughout the treatment. Handout 1, Sudden, Traumatic Death and Traumatic Bereavement, as well as Handout 17, Secondary Losses, may be useful to this work. Exposure assignments, as described in Chapter 11, also fit well with work on secondary losses.

As this work progresses, you can reinforce the client for any steps he has taken to relinquish the previous attachments. For example, you might say, "It appears that you have learned to do many of the things your spouse used to do, such as paying the bills and managing the finances. How do you feel about taking on these responsibilities? How do you think your [spouse] would feel?" (Rando, 1993).

THIRD "R" PROCESS:
RECOLLECT AND REEXPERIENCE THE DECEASED AND THE RELATIONSHIP

The third "R" process paves the way for relinquishing inappropriate attachments so that the client can eventually establish new ones. It also enables the development of a realistic composite image, or internal representation, of the loved one. This process also helps you and the client discuss any unfinished business with the deceased. In the first subprocess, *Review and remember realistically*, the mourner reviews her relationship with the loved one. Ideally, this review will start at the beginning of their relationship. It should be both accurate and comprehensive, and include such things as how and when the mourner and the deceased met (if the deceased was a spouse or partner); how they grew important to each other; life milestones they shared; areas of serious conflict in their relationship; and their shared goals, values, and interests. A comprehensive recollection is important because any elements that are omitted can cause problems at later stages of the mourning process.

As noted above, a major problem for traumatized mourners is that thinking of their loved ones can trigger recollections (e.g., a gruesome death scene) that retraumatize them. This can seriously inhibit recollection, since survivors naturally try to avoid such memories. In addition, mourners may avoid this realistic review because of other negative emotions (such as guilt) that it may engender. Such avoidance interferes with subsequent readjustment.

In the second subprocess, *Revive and reexperience the feelings*, you can assist a mourner in experiencing the emotions associated with what he has remembered. The focus is on feelings because they constitute the "glue" underlying each attachment tie to a loved one. As the mourner experiences his feelings, he defuses the emotional strength of his former attachments to the deceased. Such reduction is necessary if the mourner is to be able to alter his former bonds with the loved one to take a new form that is more appropriate to the reality of the situation. Attachment ties that are affected include such elements as needs, feelings, thoughts, memories, assumptions, expectations, and interaction patterns. Although the memory of the tie remains, the power of underlying connective emotion is lessened so that it can be sufficiently modified or relinquished. Consequently, the mourner will have the emotional freedom to form new attachments in the future.

Facilitating the Third "R" Process

To help the client with the *Review and remember realistically* subprocess, you can encourage her to recall as many memories as possible of the deceased and the relationship. Ideally, the client will remember and review her full range of memories (e.g., good, bad, happy, sad, fulfilling, disappointing, etc.). It is helpful to think of this process as reviewing the client's life story with the loved one, looking at what he was and wasn't.

A complete and accurate picture of the loved one should emerge from this "R" process—one that captures the real relationship that existed. An inaccurate, idealized, or "sanctified" image signifies that some aspects remain unavailable to the mourner for processing, leaving her vulnerable to untruths that could emerge later (e.g., "He wasn't very considerate of my feelings").

Many mourners resist this process because it reminds them of things about their loved one, the relationship, or both that they would rather forget. In particular, they are likely to avoid material that could elicit such feelings as sadness, regret, embarrassment, anger, or remorse. For example, a woman who has lost her spouse may find it extremely distressing to discuss her husband's seductive behavior toward other women; instead, she may choose to remember his strengths. She may fear that addressing the former may invalidate the latter. Mourners who are angry at their loved ones may resist this subprocess (e.g., a mourner who is furious at a loved one for killing herself). Mourners may also wish to avoid discussing their dependency on their loved one. For example, a husband whose wife was killed might feel very uncomfortable describing all of the ways he relied on his wife, as this may engender feelings of helplessness, insecurity, or guilt.

Giving the mourner a rationale for moving through this process can help enormously. It may be useful to tell a traumatized mourner that although painful or traumatic memories can temporarily be disruptive and take precedence until integrated, these traumatic memories do not have the power to invalidate positive ones. You can also help the mourner appreciate that many memories are bittersweet because they include happiness (when recollecting events from the past), such as when a woman reminisces about the time when her husband took her on a cruise, and deep sadness, because such trips will never occur again.

The next subprocess, *Revive and reexperience the feelings*, allows a client to connect his feelings to his thoughts and other memories of the deceased and to experience them, which typically lessens their intensity. Both remembering the deceased fully and experiencing and integrating the feelings that such memories bring up will help the mourner to adapt and move forward.

In discussing the client's memories of the deceased, you may find it useful to ask her what she appreciated most about the deceased and what she did not appreciate; what she misses the most and what she does not; and what she wishes could have been different in the relationship. You can explore how realistic/complete the client's memory of the deceased is. You can also try to identify specific places where the client is stuck. For example, has the client under- or over-emphasized certain aspects of the deceased or of their relationship? If the client's memories of the deceased seem distorted or incomplete, what are possible places where she is blocked in this process? It can also be useful to acknowledge that all relationships include ambivalence, and then ask the client whether she is able to discuss both the positive and negative aspects of the relationship. If she can't do this, you can ask whether the client would be willing to talk about or question any fears she may have about discussing the omitted aspects of the relationship ("talking about talking about it"), which can give the client some emotional space and perspective. Handout 24, Positive and Negative Aspects of Your Relationship with Your Significant Other, may be useful in this process.

Of course, for a client who experienced a largely negative or ambivalent attachment to the deceased, recalling the negative aspects of the relationship may be the easier task. If this is the case, then it will be important to help the client to remember and articulate whatever positive aspects of the relationship existed.

Working with the client to identify and reexperience feelings constitutes one of the most challenging aspects of treating traumatic bereavement. Mourners often experience intense pain as they recount their feelings. As Rando (1993) has noted, this can be an excruciating time for both therapists and mourners because acute grief reactions fuel and are fueled by remembering and reexperiencing. The resources discussed in Chapter 10 will be particularly valuable in supporting clients in this process.

FOURTH "R" PROCESS: *RELINQUISH THE OLD ATTACHMENTS TO THE DECEASED AND THE OLD ASSUMPTIVE WORLD*

The first subprocess under the fourth "R" process is to *Let go of old attachments to the person who has died*. The material on continuing bonds, reviewed in Chapter 7, provides information that may be helpful in formulating this part of the treatment. The mourner must ultimately let go of old bonds to the deceased that are no longer appropriate, given that person's death. For example, a young man will have to give up his attachment to the expectation that his father would take care of him financially. Of course, mourners do not want to let go of former connections. Relinquishing these bonds is difficult and forces a mourner to contend with secondary losses and to cope with insecurity, anxiety, and the fear of losing his connection to the deceased. Nevertheless, when it becomes increasingly apparent that holding onto old ties, hopes, or expectations is useless and perhaps even harmful, a healthy mourner starts to give them up (Rando, 2014). He does not have to abandon all ties; for instance, he still can have feelings for the deceased. However, he must modify the old ties sufficiently to establish new ties that are more suitable. The new ties involve recognition that the person is dead and cannot return the mourner's emotional investment or meet his needs as before.

The other subprocess under this "R" process is *Letting go of one's old attachments to the assumptive world* that the death and its consequences have invalidated. In order to move forward, the mourner must give up specific assumptions predicated upon the loved one's physical presence in the mourner's life (e.g., "My mother will always be there for me," "We'll grow old together"), as well as any global assumptions that the loss has shattered (e.g., a child's death may shatter the assumption that "God protects the innocent"). Especially after a traumatic loss, a mourner has to surrender a number of assumptions pertaining to the self, others, life and the way it works, the world in general, and spiritual matters (Rando, 2014).

Facilitating the Fourth "R" Process

You can explore the disruptions in the client's assumptive world by highlighting violated or changed assumptions that have emerged in the work to date. Reviewing the client's initial impact statement (see Handout 16, First Account of the Death) is a useful way to identify assumptions that the death has affected. This can be followed by addressing automatic thoughts related to disrupted assumptions, as described in Handouts 9, A Model for Change; 10, What Are Automatic Thoughts?; and 11, Identifying Automatic Thoughts Worksheet.

Handout 23, Psychological Needs, can also be useful in identifying central assumptions about the world and related beliefs. You and the client can challenge automatic thoughts, helping her recognize her views of the world as they arise. This process will gradually decrease the power of these beliefs.

The client may experience intense pain while reviewing the ties that must be relinquished. You can help the client by normalizing the overwhelming desire to avoid letting go. As Rando (1993) has indicated, it is important to empathize with and legitimize the mourner's wish that things could be different. Nonetheless, you must, with compassion, maintain the position that they are not.

FIFTH "R" PROCESS: *READJUST TO MOVE ADAPTIVELY INTO THE NEW WORLD WITHOUT FORGETTING THE OLD*

This fifth "R" process is where much of the major action is in mourning. Letting go of the old, obsolete connections to the deceased and to the old assumptive world frees a mourner to accommodate the loss in his life. This occurs in four areas, each of which is a focus of a subprocess.

The first subprocess, *Revise the assumptive world*, involves modifying a mourner's assumptions to eliminate the painful discrepancy between what the mourner thought life would or should be like and what it actually is in the aftermath of the loved one's death. Ideally, the mourner will be able to let go of some of these assumptions and revise or combine some with others. The mourner may add new assumptions that reflect the way he perceives life now.

As with all trauma, basic global assumptions about such things as fairness in the world, the orderliness of the universe, personal invulnerability, and the trustworthiness of others are often shattered as a result of the death (Janoff-Bulman, 1992; McCann & Pearlman, 1990b; Rando, 2014). Still, one may be able to retain some assumptions. For example, while some of the mourner's global beliefs may have changed (e.g., "I can never feel completely safe again"), he can still retain some old beliefs (e.g., "It's worth doing whatever I can to take care of those I love"). He may add completely new assumptions (e.g., "I can't expect my partner to take care of me; I must learn to do it on my own"). One man who lost his partner had to revise his notions about fairness and predictability after the partner died suddenly in a boating accident, but he retained his belief in the goodness of others since so many people helped him afterward. A woman who lost her child melded some former assumptions with new ones (e.g., "I was naïve when I believed that God protects good people. I still believe in God, but I no longer believe that being good ensures protection from adversity"). Modifying such core assumptions can precipitate additional grief reactions, which you and the client will need to address.

Some changes to a mourner's assumptions happen quite quickly (as in the loss of feelings of safety after the murder of a loved one). Others may emerge over time or become more powerful as a result of events stemming from the tragedy. For example, a young man lost his fiancée in a motor vehicle crash perpetrated by a distracted truck driver, who was texting instead of looking at the road. He anticipated that the truck driver would be sentenced to some jail time and also lose his license. However, this did not occur. The truck driver received no penalty of any kind, and was back on the road within a week. This event confirmed the man's shattered assumptions about justice and fairness, which his fiancée's death initially violated. Her death provided a powerful lesson that "Life is not fair," and the man realized that this was something he would have to learn to live with.

In the second subprocess, *Develop a new relationship with the deceased*, there is a movement from a relationship of physical presence to one of physical absence. As discussed in Chapter 7, many professionals and mourners mistakenly assume that a mourner has to let go of all connections to the deceased. Rather, if the mourner desires continued connections, they must be transformed. A healthy new relationship with the deceased must meet two criteria (Rando, 1993). First, the mourner must truly comprehend the death and its implications, which should be reflected in his expectations of, symbolic interactions with, and connections to, the deceased person. Second, he must continue to move forward adaptively into his new life in the absence of his loved one. For example, he might take active steps to spend more time with his grandson. If the mourner is not able to do these things, it may be too early for him to develop such a new relationship, or he may be maintaining an unhealthy connection with the deceased. For example, he may be so focused on the deceased that he cannot engage constructively in day-to-day activities. (We refer readers to Rando [1993, 2014] for more detailed discussions of this issue.) It should be noted that in some cases, a continued connection with the deceased may be unhelpful or even detrimental to the bereaved. This may be the case, for example, if a survivor was neglected or abused by the person who died. If the bereaved is left with such a negative legacy, discussing this in treatment can be invaluable. This can help the bereaved to attain valuable self-knowledge (e.g., "I deserved to be with someone who treated me better").

The third subprocess, *Adopt new ways of being in the world*, involves adding, relinquishing, or modifying aspects of the mourner's life to accommodate the losses and unmet needs the death has created. The number, extent, and types of changes depend on the particular relationship that existed between the mourner and the deceased, and the specifics of that person's involvement in the mourner's life. The mourner will have to find ways to meet the needs that the deceased previously met for her, or to learn to do without having these needs met. In almost all cases, the mourner will have to adopt new roles, skills, behaviors, and relationships to compensate for what was lost with the loved one's death. For example, a parent who loses a spouse now must assume the roles and responsibilities of parenting that the partner previously fulfilled.

The final subprocess, *Form a new identity*, involves integrating the new and old selves so that the mourner's new self-image reflects all the changes he has undergone. For example, after a spouse dies, the mourner may develop a new identity, viewing himself as more independent. A further transition that the mourner must undertake at this time is to change from a "we" orientation (comprising the mourner and the loved one) to an "I" orientation. This will involve relinquishing, modifying, or taking on new ways of thinking, feeling, and being that reflect the reality of the loved one's death. Over time, the mourner will usually benefit from developing some perspective on what he has lost and gained. He must recognize and mourn what has changed, affirm what continues, and incorporate what is new.

Facilitating the Fifth "R" Process

The previous process of relinquishing defunct connections to the deceased and the old assumptive world (the fourth "R") frees the mourner to create new connections to the deceased (and ultimately to new people) and to develop new assumptions about the world. The first subprocess, *Revise the assumptive world*, is challenging for clients because in addition to global assumptions they may have held all their lives, they must relinquish or modify any assumptions that were predicated on their loved ones' presence. It can be helpful to encourage a mourner to identify what has remained the same for her, despite all that has changed. Seeing that some things are unchanged, even with all that has happened, can provide some measure of reassurance and promote a sense of security. At proper times, the mourner can be encouraged to test out her revised or new assumptions to determine their validity. For example, someone who has lost a spouse may feel that she will never again be able to take a vacation because traveling alone would intensify her feelings of loss. After working on this belief, the client may develop a new one, such as "Traveling by myself will be difficult, but I can do it." Planning and taking a short vacation, even a weekend away, can be a test of this new assumption.

This is also a natural place to work with automatic thoughts, since such thoughts are indicators of assumptions or beliefs about the world. Because automatic thoughts often become habitual, clients may benefit from challenging them to determine whether they still hold true (see Chapter 11). Mourners can have difficulty with this subprocess if they fail to change assumptions in order to avoid the reality of their loved ones' deaths. If so, you can confront this issue gently at the proper time.

The second subprocess is *Develop a new relationship with the deceased*. As long as they meet the two criteria above (i.e., a mourner must comprehend the death and move forward adaptively) for a healthy new relationship, there are many ways that a mourner can maintain meaningful connections to a loved one (Rando, 2014):

1. Appropriate identification with a loved one occurs when a mourner adopts the attributes or views of the deceased. For example, a son may attempt to be as patient with his own children as his father was with him.

2. Mourners can benefit from both personal and collective bereavement rituals. A ritual can take the form, for example, of planting a tree in honor of the deceased each year on her birthday.

3. Possession of tangible objects—including, for example, photographs, mementos, gifts, or the loved one's creations (e.g., artwork)—can be comforting because they provide the basis for a connection that does not rely on the loved one's physical presence.

4. The surviving family members and/or social group can benefit from such activities as telling stories or sharing information about their loved one. Active reminiscing allows survivors to keep their loved one's memory alive by reminding themselves of what kind of person he was. This can be particularly beneficial to mourners who are concerned that they may forget what their loved one was like, and thus lose contact with him forever.

5. Some individuals are comforted by maintaining certain routines that were part of the relationship, such as doing things that they used to do with their loved ones. For example, having coffee in the morning while gazing out into the garden, a formerly shared activity, can be a valuable connecting behavior.

6. Purposeful use of triggers can stimulate a connection with the deceased. For example, a client may listen to a loved one's favorite songs, which will remind her of the life they shared together.

7. Daydreaming and fantasizing allow survivors to interact symbolically with the deceased. As long as a mourner recognizes a fantasy for what it is, and does not use it as a substitute for engagement in life, this process can be beneficial.

8. Communication with the deceased loved one, which includes "talking" with the loved one or expressing one's thoughts, feelings, or requests for guidance, allows for continuing connection.

9. Reflecting the loved one's values in the mourner's day-to-day life can continue the loved one's legacy. By acting on his values and concerns, and considering his perspective on subsequent decisions, the mourner can retain a healthy connection.

In recent years, there has been interest in connections in which a deceased loved one serves as a moral compass or guide (see, e.g., Klass & Walter, 2001; Marwit & Klass, 1996). Glick, Weiss, and Parkes (1974) found that at 1 year following the loss, 69% of those who lost a spouse expressed agreement with the statement that they try to behave as the deceased would want them to. Similarly, Stroebe and Stroebe (1991) found that at 2 years following the death of their spouses, approximately half of the respondents indicated that they consulted the deceased when they had to make a decision. Many similar kinds of attachment behavior have been described in the literature, including relying on the deceased as a role model, incorporating virtues of the deceased into one's character (Marwit & Klass, 1996; Normand, Silverman, & Nickman, 1996), and reflecting on the deceased person's life and/or death to clarify current values or value conflicts.

Some mourners believe that concrete reminders of the deceased will help them live a life that honors that person's memory. For example, John got a tattoo following the death of his older brother, George, who was killed in an industrial explosion. The design of the tattoo incorporated the letters of his brother's name. "George was the adventurous one," John said. "I have always been reluctant to try new things. Now I push myself a bit. The tattoo helps me to imagine that he is encouraging me. This happened last month when I went whitewater rafting."

Those working within the continuing-bonds tradition (e.g., Klass et al., 1996) have frequently discussed legacy work as a way of maintaining an appropriate bond with the deceased. For example, it is common for people to honor their loved one's memory by becoming involved in social action. As one mother indicated, "I felt compelled to do everything I could to reduce the chances that what happened to my child would happen to others." Legacies of this type are often referred to as living memorials. Karla Frye-McGill established such a memorial for her 10-year-old son Bradley, who was fatally shot in the back. A 14-year-old had been playing with a gun, firing it out of the second-story bedroom window in his apartment, when Bradley was killed. As Mehren (1997) has explained,

> As a teacher, his mother, Karla Frye-McGill, channeled her grief into developing a gun safety program for children. Using her family's tragedy as the focus, she began her own curriculum in her school in New Mexico. In the first year alone, she visited more than seven hundred New Mexico schoolchildren. Soon Frye-McGill joined a task force to address child safety issues. She persuaded colleagues to fund a firearm injury prevention curriculum, using the facts from real firearm deaths of children as its foundation. Inspired by and dedicated to Bradley, the program is now in place in elementary and middle schools across New Mexico and, Frye-McGill notes, "the concept of the curriculum could be used anywhere in the world." (pp. 78–79)

As Lewis and Hoy (2011) suggest, creating a legacy to honor a loved one's memory can play a vital role in facilitating the healing process. These authors discuss how therapists can assist their clients in creating meaningful legacies. They recommend starting with "the deceased's unique features—of personality and character, accomplishment, human passion" (p. 318) and developing a legacy that embodies these qualities. According to Lewis and Hoy, the creation of such legacies can help survivors draw strength from the evidence that their loved ones are still having an influence in this world. This can help the mourners to go forward without the living presence of the loved ones.

As we have discussed in Chapter 10, many people use Facebook Memorial Groups and other memorial websites to create a lasting testament to their loved ones' lives. In most cases, these websites also provide a continuing connection to the deceased and the people who were important to him.

You can work with a client to develop healthy ways of using these resources to relate to and stay connected with a lost loved one. Handout S8, Continuing Your Relationship with Your Significant Other (available on the book's website supplement), may be useful in working on this process.

Others in a mourner's life may mistakenly conclude that continued connection with the deceased is pathological. In fact, it is not uncommon for therapists to view such behaviors as "talking" to the deceased as pathological and inappropriate. Available evidence suggests, however, that such "interactions" are normative (see, e.g., Klass et al., 1996; Klugman, 2006; Sanger, 2008–2009). In a telephone survey, Klugman (2006) found that 69% of the respondents reported having conversations with their deceased loved one. Additional ways in which a mourner may feel connected with the deceased include an overwhelming sense of the loved one's presence; the physical sensation of being touched, held, or kissed by the loved one; dreams in which the mourner believes that the deceased was actually present; feeling watched over and protected by the deceased; or the movement of objects believed to be a sign from the deceased. Evidence suggests that these ways of maintaining a connection are very common. In the survey by Klugman, 55% of respondents felt the presence of the deceased, and 37% reported seeing a vision of the deceased.

In our experience, these ways of maintaining ties to the deceased are comforting to some mourners. Some benefit from the belief that although their loved ones are dead and will never come back to life, they may still exist in some form. As one husband indicated, "When my wife died, I found it unbearable that her spirit was gone forever. One night I had the actual physical sensation of my wife next to me in bed, and we embraced. It was incredibly comforting to learn that at some level, she still exists." In addition, these experiences allow survivors to believe that the deceased are content and in a good place. This belief can be particularly important to bereaved parents.

It is surprisingly common for survivors to contact psychics in order to maintain contact with their loves ones. This phenomenon occurs with many kinds of losses, but appears to be most prevalent following the death of a child. Although systematic studies are rare, Feigelman, Jordan, McIntosh, and Feigelman (2012) assessed the frequency of consultation with a medium among parents who had lost children to suicide, drug overdose, or other causes. They found that across several types of child loss, 30% of parents reported seeking out psychics. However, this figure was dramatically affected by type of death. Among parents whose children died of natural causes, just 13% turned to psychics. Approximately 30% of parents whose children committed suicide or whose deaths resulted from an accident consulted with psychics. Among parents whose children died of drug overdoses, 54% contacted psychics. We address this issue in some detail because consultation with a medium is prevalent among the bereaved, but rarely discussed. Moreover, if it is not handled carefully, it can drive a wedge between clients and therapists and jeopardize their relationship.

In our experience, most bereaved parents are almost desperate to know where their child is. They want to know whether their child is safe and comfortable. They are often concerned about whether the child is calling out for them, and whether he is upset that they have not responded to his cries. The anguish associated with these unanswered questions sometimes leads parents to contact a psychic. In many cases, they receive the answers that they were hoping for—that their child is comfortable and happy. This gives them some peace of mind, and allows them to focus on other important things, such as their relationships with their surviving children. Seeking out a psychic is also common among those who had a troubled relationship with the deceased. In such cases, the person who died typically expresses regret and asks for forgiveness. (For more information about the role of psychics in facilitating grief resolution, see Sormanti & August, 1997; Walliss, 2001.)

Do those who seek out the services of a psychic find them helpful? Although more data are needed, available evidence suggests that much of the time, people view psychics as beneficial. In their book on the death of a child from suicide and drug overdose, Feigelman and colleagues (2012) asked survivors to identify sources of help that they found to be very helpful. They also asked respondents to identify sources that they viewed as providing little or no help.

Those who sought the services of psychics reported the second highest rating for helpfulness of all sources studied, with 34.6% of survivors indicating that this was very helpful. Only support groups for survivors of suicide were rated higher (43.8%). Since participants for this study were recruited through such support groups, this latter finding may be artificially inflated. The percentage of people rating psychics as very helpful was slightly higher than the corresponding percentage for general bereavement support groups (31.6%), and was also higher than the rating for bereavement counselors (27%) or psychologists/psychiatrists/social workers (25.7%; these categories were grouped together for this study). Participants rated psychics considerably higher than members of the clergy, who received the lowest rating of all the sources of help that were studied (21.5%).

For bereaved parents who consulted psychics, the percentage viewing that source as "of little or no help" was quite low (24%)—lower than the percentage of any other source of help except support groups for survivors of suicide (22.2%). Of particular note, the percentage rating psychics as "of little or no help" was lower than the percentage for the psychologist/psychiatrist/social worker category, where 33.3% of respondents felt that they had received "little or no help." As Feigelman and colleagues (2012) have expressed it, "The help bereaved experience from psychics is likely to remain an enduring feature in the bereavement resource landscape" (p. 145). Of course, it will be important to replicate these findings with larger and more representative samples; nonetheless, these data suggest that many of us may need to reevaluate our beliefs about the benefits of consulting a psychic. It seems possible that psychics can engage with survivors in a sensitive and intuitive way, and at a very personal level. It is especially interesting to note that individuals with solid academic credentials have begun to move into this area. Allan Botkin, a clinical psychologist, has developed a treatment approach based on EMDR that purportedly facilitates communication between survivors and their deceased loved ones (Botkin, Hogan, & Moody, 2005).

It is important not to pathologize clients who turn to psychics. In fact, many bereaved persons choose not to disclose consultations with psychics for fear they will be considered crazy (Rando, 2014). As Rando states:

If a bereaved person wants to consult with a psychic, it's my obligation to help them secure referrals for individuals reputed to be "legitimate" in their field. It's not my place to dissuade them or scoff at their need. It *is* my place, and my duty, to talk with them about what they hope to gain from the consultation and how they'll cope with what they might hear. It's my responsibility to psychologically process it with them afterwards.

Again, we maintain that as long as it meets the two criteria described above for a healthy relationship with someone who has died (comprehending the death and moving forward into one's new life), there is no problem with maintaining connection to the loved one in the ways we have described above. It will take some time before a mourner can reach the point where she can simultaneously meet both of these criteria. If it is too early in her mourning process and she has not yet had the time and experiences to recognize the reality and implications of her loved one's death, she won't be able to make the transition to a symbiotic relationship with the deceased. In that case, many of these ideas, such as the purposeful use of triggers, could elicit distress. This is another opportunity to work with automatic thoughts. For example, a mourner may state that she cannot look at old photos because she will not be able to survive the pain. The underlying automatic thought could be "I'll die if I feel my grief." If she needs to protest the death continually, or is unwilling to accept the need for a new relationship because she insists on living in the past where the loved one was physically present, it may be premature for the mourner to develop or benefit from a new relationship with the deceased.

Revising the assumptive world and developing a new relationship with the deceased require new behavior patterns on the mourner's part. Changes in behavior are reflected in the next subprocess, *Adopt new ways of being in the world.* You can work with the mourner to identify unmet needs as described earlier. The two of you can then determine the best option among (1) meeting the need herself; (2) finding someone else to meet the need for her; (3) determining other ways to get the need met; or (4) learning to do without getting the need met (Rando, 2014). Should the mourner lack the necessary information or skills to move forward, you can assist her in identifying such gaps and strategize how to fill them (e.g., securing vocational training if she needs a new job). The social support network is an excellent resource in this process, and Handout 18, The Importance of Enhancing Social Support, can be helpful here. We also recommend encouraging clients to set personal goals (see Chapter 10 as well as Handout S1, Personal Goal Setting, available on the book's website supplement). Supporting them to achieve these goals can help clients adopt new interests, activities, and relationships. *In vivo* exposure activities (described in Chapter 11) can also be helpful in allowing them gradually to test new ways of being in the world.

There are many reasons why problems may occur in this subprocess. For instance, a mourner may refrain from making changes in order to deny that his loved one is gone or because he does not want to go on in the loved one's absence. Certain personality traits (such as insecurity, dependency, or poor self-image) or the results of personal traumatization from the death (such as feeling that another catastrophe can happen at any time) can interfere with moving forward into the new world. The mourner may also lack the skills needed to adopt new behaviors or to meet his needs. He may restrict his world by not going out or talking with people he doesn't know well in an attempt to ensure control and protection. Beliefs that he cannot function without the loved one, a desire to punish himself, feelings (often guilt or anger), thoughts (often negative), or omissions or commissions involving the loved one can also be complicating factors. If any of these interferes with this subprocess, you can help the mourner identify and process such obstacles. It may be necessary to remind the client compassionately that nothing can change the reality of the loved one's death.

The "R" subprocess *Form a new identity* focuses on helping the mourner adjust her self-image to reflect the changes she has undergone. Although many aspects of the mourner's former identity may remain, a new identity is now required that integrates the old and new aspects of the self. It often helps the client to understand that most people define themselves in the frame-work of their relationships with others; when an important relationship changes, so too does a person's sense of who she is. As the mourner alters her assumptive world, her relationship with her departed loved one, and her ways of being in the world, these changes—whether losses, gains, or modifications of what existed before—alter her sense of self. You can acknowledge that parts of herself that were developed within her relationship with the deceased (e.g., her co-parent self) have died too. If this is the case, it is important to mourn such losses along with the primary loss of the deceased. You can invite the client to remember and honor those parts of herself, both in memory and in her new relationship with the deceased. For instance, she can commemorate the anniversary of her marriage to her husband, wherein she honors that special piece of her history as his wife. The key is to do this in ways that reflect a healthy relationship with the deceased and that don't prevent her from moving forward when the time is right.

You can further assist the client by facilitating the crucial process of narrative reconstruction (Neimeyer, 2001, 2012; Neimeyer et al., 2010). It will be helpful to acknowledge and address any anxiety the mourner has about the changes in her self-image. These include such issues as the mourner's fear of the unknown, insecurity over possible consequences of the new identity, or desire to minimize additional secondary losses. The mourner may also have trouble forming a new identity if she relied too much upon her loved one, finds she has little else to define her besides the old relationship, copes poorly with emotions or relationship changes, or feels the relationship was the best thing in a less-than-satisfactory life (Rando, 2014). Your work with the client will help her develop an identity that does not perpetuate her acute grief, inhibit her from moving forward, or limit her (such as the survivor of a public tragedy who is expected to remain focused on that event forever). *In vivo* exposure activities can be designed to allow gradual testing of the new roles and relationships that involve the new identity.

SIXTH "R" PROCESS: *REINVEST*

The mourner must eventually reinvest the emotional energy that was once endowed in the relationship with the deceased in ways that are life-affirming and gratifying. New attachments can provide the mourner with some of the emotional fulfillment that was lost with the death. The reinvestment, however, need not be in a person who has the same role as the one who died, or even in a person at all. A mourner can reinvest in new causes, roles, relationships, activities, projects, and passions—anything that can bring enjoyment and satisfaction. The material in Chapter 10 on values and goals should assist clients in identifying new pursuits and carrying them out.

Facilitating the Sixth "R" Process

You can convey that reinvesting does not mean that the deceased disappears from the client's life. The client may find it helpful to hear that the deceased will always be a part of himself and that nothing will erase this. The task is to figure out how to integrate new aspects of his life and new investments with the old.

It is useful to acknowledge to the client that he may not be ready to reinvest in life. The client may benefit from hearing that reinvestment is often a long process that will probably take place gradually, and that he may be able to reinvest his energies in some things or relationships sooner than in others. Clients may find it valuable to explore what reinvesting in a new interest or new relationship means to them, or to pursue ways in which they have already reinvested or would like to reinvest someday. The process of investment can often be facilitated by working with a client to identify and pursue his most important goals, as noted previously.

Many mourners believe that it is an insult to the memory of the loved one to enjoy life again. It may be necessary to explore a client's beliefs to be sure he knows that the length and amount of his suffering do not constitute a testimony to his love for the deceased or proof that he is not "betraying" the loved one. Furthermore, it is important to address any fears the client may have that he may be hurt in the future if he invests in someone else whom he could lose, or that others could perceive him as not having mourned his loss enough. Mourners will need additional intervention if they are extremely dependent or anxious, lack social or communication skills, have excessive fears of the unknown, or worry that reinvestment signals the end of their involvement with their loved ones. These interventions can take the form of building resources and exploring automatic thoughts.

The reinvestment process can also be affected by the type of death. If the death occurred as a result of suicide or murder, for example, the mourner may find it awkward to reinvest in social endeavors. He may believe that his presence makes others uncomfortable, and this may in fact be the case. Gentle guidance can help such clients attain the courage to invest in the skills to manage interpersonal situations.

CLINICAL INTEGRATION

Zac and Courtney had been together for 20 years when Courtney died in a bicycle accident on an unseasonably warm day in December. Zac was lost after Courtney passed away. In the years since her death, he had slowly picked up the pieces of his life—returning to work, forcing himself to go out with friends, working out at the gym. His zest for life was gone, though. And his friends kept telling him he was living in the past. His best friend, Ross, had recently made the observation that he idealized his marriage to Courtney, remembering it in a unrealistic way. This was what Zac reported to Susie, the grief counselor, when he first met her. Several sessions later, Susie would challenge him about his idealization.

"Zac, we've been talking about the importance of remembering Courtney in a realistic and complete way. So far, she sounds like an angel. She sounds really, really great, and your love for her is obvious. Your marriage sounds as though it was marked by mutual respect and genuine caring. It's inspiring. I'm also remembering that you told me that Ross thought you idealized the marriage. Could this be true? Does it seem to you that there are things about Courtney or your relationship with her that you're leaving out?"

"No. She was special. We were a great couple. Everyone we knew envied us."

"What was one thing you wished could have been different? One thing that could have been better in your relationship?" Susie wanted to explore how realistic Zac's picture of his relationship was. She knew it was important for him to remember Courtney in a complete way, and she wondered whether holding on to an ideal image somehow protected Zac from relinquishing an attachment that was no longer possible.

Zac seemed to be thinking. "Well, when Court was alive, I wished we had more sex. It seems so stupid and unimportant now. But I think 15 years ago, that's how I felt."

Susie tried not to show her surprise. From Zac's earlier description, their relationship had sounded so perfect. "Sex is a big deal, Zac. Although it's more important to some couples than to others, sex is an element of every relationship, whether present or absent. It sounds as though you would have liked it to be more present, and it sounds as though you haven't allowed yourself to really think about or feel that."

Zac suddenly felt confused. He wanted to take back everything he'd just said. He felt as though Susie were seeing something within him that he didn't want to see himself.

"It's really OK to have some mixed feelings about your relationship, Zac. No relationship is perfect, and no one person can satisfy all of our needs. All relationships contain some disappointment. I'm wondering how it feels for you to acknowledge a disappointment in your relationship with Courtney."

"I feel really guilty."

"What do you imagine would happen if you just allowed yourself to acknowledge the disappointments? If you allowed yourself to accept this as part of the story?"

A tear rolled down Zac's cheek. He reached over for the box of tissues on the nearby table. "I'm afraid I'd be moving away from Courtney. I'm not sure if I can explain it any other way. It just feels like I'd be putting distance between us, and if I did that, she might leave me. How crazy is that? I'm afraid my dead wife might abandon me!" Zac's sense of humor softened his self-criticism.

Susie laughed along with him. "Remind me to have you challenge that thought—that it's crazy to feel that way. A little work may help you to see that it's not crazy at all. For now, I want to stick with a very significant insight you just shared. There is a fear that putting distance between you and Courtney might lead to her abandoning you. You're afraid of losing the connection you have with her, even in her death, if you were to move on in some way. Does this sound right?"

Zac nodded.

"And can you see how this could keep you stuck?"

Zac nodded again.

"I'm going to suggest that we work on helping you to remember Courtney and your relationship as realistically as possible. You and she both deserve this: that the reality of your relationship be preserved. As we do this, it's important that you know that I know how much you loved her, and still do. I know that this was, in fact, a special relationship—a relationship that really worked. And I know that alongside of all that, there may have been disappointments, too." With that, Susie began to wind down the session and asked Zac to write a realistic description of Courtney for their next session. Zac thanked Susie and rushed out of their session, late for dinner with Ross.

CONCLUDING REMARKS

This chapter has presented a comprehensive framework for understanding and facilitating the process and evolution of mourning as described by Rando (1993, 2014). Our task as therapists is to facilitate this process for clients: to help them to move through their mourning, as Susie was doing with Zac in the example above. Zac was struggling with the third "R" process, *Recollect and reexperience the deceased and the relationship*. Susie correctly ascertained that his capacity to relinquish unviable attachments to Courtney would increase if he was able to remember her in a more realistic way; she asked him to write a realistic and comprehensive description of Courtney in order to facilitate this process. Susie also alluded to challenging one of Zac's beliefs that was associated with this process of realistic remembering (cognitive processing); and she assessed Zac's associated thoughts and emotions, inviting these inner experiences into the therapy room (emotional processing). She might also emphasize drawing on extra social support in the weeks to come, or engaging in breathing retraining or self-care activities in an effort to utilize resources that would assist him in moving through a potentially painful time within the therapy (resource building).

In more general terms, Susie's work demonstrates awareness of the various treatment elements and how they can fit together for a particular client. The "R" processes provide a framework for the evolution of mourning. As well, they suggest interventions for facilitating this process. Depending on the reasons why a client might be stuck, and depending on what kinds of support might be most useful to him, other interventions can be utilized along the way. As we have emphasized throughout this book, the context of a traumatic death brings about some unique obstacles to moving through mourning. As you read through the case examples, you may want to consider where in the mourning process our characters might be, as well as what (if anything) keeps them stuck in their mourning and what interventions you might use to address these obstacles.

PART V

CHALLENGES IN IMPLEMENTING THE TREATMENT APPROACH

CHAPTER 13

Treatment Challenges

Joan was shot at close range with a semiautomatic handgun while at work. On what was until then a normal April day, a former employee entered the corporate offices where Joan worked, got off the elevator on the sixth floor, and began randomly shooting people before he was tackled from behind by a security guard who happened to be close by. Joan died en route to the hospital from multiple gunshot wounds, despite emergency personnel's efforts to control the bleeding. Her two young adult sons were in shock upon hearing that their mother was one of the fatalities in this local tragedy. "My mom wasn't supposed to die at the age of 48," said Joan's older son, Seth, when he began therapy with Dr. Lecia Taylor almost 2 years after his mother's death. Seth's younger brother, Danny, was also struggling with acceptance of his mother's death—and, as Seth was beginning to suspect, Danny seemed to be managing his struggle in problematic ways.

Several weeks into his therapy, Seth, looking exhausted, reported to Dr. Taylor his belief that his 21-year-old brother had begun using illicit drugs. He further reported having had several sleepless nights since the last session. Seth then told Dr. Taylor that he needed to talk about this issue, rather than focusing on the death of his mom.

In this chapter, we discuss challenges in working with traumatically bereaved clients. The first section focuses on aspects of the treatment that you may find challenging and provides guidelines for identifying them. The second section provides a model for addressing clinical hurdles. The chapter ends with a discussion of your possible responses to working as a therapist in a paradigm that may be unfamiliar to you.

POTENTIALLY CHALLENGING ASPECTS OF THE TREATMENT

The elements of this integrated treatment approach form into a whole that is greater than the sum of its parts. By focusing on specific components of this approach, we hope to identify why some of these elements may seem challenging to implement. The descriptions of potential difficulties associated with each treatment component serve, in and of themselves, as a sort of intervention or aid for all of us who do this work. Recognizing ourselves in these descriptions gives us labels for our experiences as well as potential relief, knowing that our responses are expectable. The goal for all of us who wish to use this treatment approach effectively is to maintain awareness of our responses and to make decisions from that awareness.

Within each component of our treatment, there are various approaches to addressing the challenges presented. We describe some of these below, in the section entitled "Challenges Arising from Working in a Different Paradigm." In general, the best approaches to these aspects of the treatment are (1) to increase your knowledge and understanding through study of the relevant material in this book and other sources; (2) to practice the treatment elements and note both the clients' responses and your own; and (3) to obtain consultation from clinicians who are familiar with the treatment approach or components that you find challenging.

Development of Self Capacities

Therapists accustomed to working with people who had adequate childhood attachment experiences may not have familiarity with adult clients with interpersonal trauma histories. Often these latter individuals may be reasonably capable and effective in the world (or have strong ego resources, to use CSDT terminology as described in Chapter 2). In contrast, they have great difficulties regulating their internal states by tolerating strong feelings, maintaining a sense of self-worth, and gathering support from an internal psychological experience of positive others (i.e., they may have underdeveloped self capacities). These clients have often been termed "resistant." One way of understanding so-called "resistance" is that it signals something a therapist doesn't yet understand about the client, and may require modification of the treatment to meet a client's needs.

It's understandable that therapists may feel confused or impatient with clients who strongly resist emotions, avoid relationships, or react strongly to seemingly small slights. Yet these behaviors are common in clients with complex trauma (Courtois & Ford, 2009; Pearlman & Courtois, 2005). Therapists with their own complex trauma histories may have difficulty tolerating rapidly shifting or intense emotional states, whether these are their own or their clients' (Pearlman & Saakvitne, 1995). If this is the case for you, seeking additional consultation and support can be helpful, as can using the resource-building strategies discussed in Chapter 10 for yourself. Using breathing retraining (see Handout 7) to regulate your own physiological arousal, for example, can be helpful for therapists with or without trauma histories after sessions in which clients express strong feelings or report gruesome details of a violent death.

This treatment emphasizes the importance of resource-building activities within the context of a supportive therapeutic relationship as a path to developing three self capacities: affect management, self-worth, and inner connection with benign others (Pearlman, 1998). Unless you assess—and, where indicated, build—traumatically bereaved clients' resources, therapy may not produce the desired success with the exposure work. This is particularly likely when clients have complex trauma or are otherwise particularly strongly affected by the death of their loved ones.

One factor that makes an important difference between effective trauma processing via exposure and retraumatization is the adequacy of a client's self capacities. Understanding this is part of the preparation that is an essential element of providing a healing as opposed to a retraumatizing experience. Therefore, building or strengthening a client's self capacities, in addition to assessing them along the way, is a key part of this treatment approach. This process takes time and requires patience from you as the therapist. This patience will be enhanced by understanding that clients' early experiences may not have allowed them to develop the internal capacities needed to tolerate the strong affective responses that sudden, traumatic deaths can trigger. Individuals who have had early experiences of abuse or neglect often suffer physiological effects that correspond with their sometimes exquisite emotional sensitivity or emotional reactivity (Schore, 2001). Knowing this can move you and your clients alike toward a greater and more compassionate understanding of these affective responses. We discussed the development of self capacities in Chapter 10 and in Handout 8, Feelings Skills. This process is beautifully articulated in Jon Allen's (2013) book *Restoring Mentalizing in Attachment Relationships*. (See Pearlman & Courtois, 2005, and Saakvitne et al., 2000, for more on developing and maintaining a therapeutic relationship with a client suffering from complex trauma.)

Trauma Processing

Cognitive Processing

As discussed in Chapter 7, cognitive therapies for PTSD have strong research support (Foa, Keane, & Friedman, 2000; Resick & Schnicke, 1993). Cognitive restructuring work with automatic thoughts and the beliefs that underlie them is a significant aspect of this treatment. This approach addresses problematic beliefs or automatic thoughts actively and directly. Therapists who are accustomed to discussing negative cognitions only as clients bring them up may not feel comfortable actively encouraging clients to look for them. Those who view affect as the core aspect of problematic responses to life circumstances may not feel comfortable highlighting thoughts (although highlighting cognitions certainly does not imply ignoring affect, as we elaborate below).

Even those therapists who would describe their approaches as cognitive may find this element to be challenging because of the structured format we recommend for the exploration of cognitions (by using worksheet-style handouts—e.g., Handout 11, the Identifying Automatic Thoughts Worksheet). The structured format is important for two reasons. First, it gives clients a sense of active participation in their treatment and provides them with concrete tools to use outside of treatment sessions. Second, this approach ensures that each problematic belief receives detailed attention.

If you are not a cognitively oriented therapist, you may find that the skills involved in identifying and challenging beliefs take practice. We have included information in Chapter 11 to help you learn these skills, and we invite you to give this approach a try. Some of us who had not used worksheets such as Handout 11 in the past were surprised and pleased to see how well clients responded to them. Novice users have also commented on the depth of this work. They have noted, for example, that this approach allows problematic beliefs to come to the surface much sooner than do traditional methods. Otherwise, such beliefs may remain unexpressed and pose obstacles to accommodating the loss.

Emotional Processing

Similarly, exposure treatment can feel uncomfortable if you are not familiar with it. You may feel that talking about potentially painful topics will be harmful to a client. In U.S. mainstream culture, we learn not to talk about dying, death, and bereavement, which is one reason why it is so difficult for many Americans to process the loss of a loved one. Those social norms can easily carry over into the therapy room. Alternatively, you may simply be accustomed to allowing a client to determine when she is ready to address a particularly sensitive topic. For these reasons, you will want to be alert to the danger of collaborative avoidance. As described in Chapter 7, research has consistently shown exposure treatment to be an effective means of helping clients with PTSD. If you understand the critical importance of exposure to recovery, you can help clients to approach rather than avoid painful material. Of course, one still must be sensitive to clients' feelings and respectful of their right to choose whether, when, and how to engage in a particular exposure activity. Each client is the best judge of her own capacities, and you must respect the client's instincts and preferences. That said, it is also your responsibility to encourage each client to participate to the best of her ability. It is possible to deliver an exposure treatment gently, supportively, and compassionately. This is the art of psychotherapy, and it is what we have worked to create and support within this integrated treatment approach.

Focus on Loss and Mourning

As discussed throughout this book (see especially Chapter 12), we use Rando's six "Rs" to guide clients through the mourning processes (Rando, 1993, 2014). Focusing on the active tasks of mourning may be challenging for some therapists. Trauma-trained therapists may not be familiar with treatments for grief. Moreover, therapists with more general practices may be unfamiliar with the subtleties of grief-related issues. Therapists may also find that the work activates their own losses; they may then tend toward shutting down or avoiding aspects of processing their clients' losses that they find most challenging personally. In the next chapter, we address both the effects this work can have on therapists and the needs of therapists related to these effects, with suggestions about how you can meet such needs in your own practice.

Structured Treatment

The active and directive approach needed to implement a structured treatment may not be the norm for many therapists. Although it will be challenging at times, if you choose to use it, you should find that the structure offers many advantages. It can provide a level of confidence for both you and the client. It helps the two of you manage potential avoidance. It provides the foundation for an introduction to and overview of the treatment elements, so that the client knows what to expect. (You may want to give the client Handouts 2, Orientation to the Treatment, and 3, Treatment Goals and Tools, to provide additional information about the treatment approach.) In addition, a structured approach may be particularly appealing to traumatic bereavement survivors. These individuals may be uncomfortable with open-ended or unstructured therapy for fear it would open up painful feelings or last forever.

One of us (Christine H. Farber) who pilot-tested the treatment generally works from a client-centered and intuitive approach to therapy, which is open-ended. She found that the structured nature of the treatment acted as a container, which allowed for deep, intensive work in a safe, effective, and relatively quick way. Interestingly, the narrow focus of the treatment approach (i.e., one particular death) allowed themes that were more pervasive in a client's life to emerge in high relief; they became easily identifiable and thus more readily available for exploration. Both clients and therapist experienced a sense of empowerment within the treatment and a deep sense of satisfaction with its completion.

Relational Focus within a Structured Treatment Approach

The unique nature of this treatment is nowhere more evident than in its focus on the relational aspects of structured therapy. Therapists who do not use structured approaches sometimes characterize these as "impersonal." The clinical literature presents many structured approaches in outline or list formats, which may lead therapists to believe that these approaches lack relational components. The true nature of CBT and structured therapy then gets "lost in translation" because most authors, for good reason, tend to focus on the details of how to do it and the theory behind it, while the relational aspects of implementing the therapy remain implicit.

Throughout this book, we address the many issues this survivor population faces, while making the relational aspects of the therapy explicit. We recognize the individuality of each client and therapist; the importance of empowering the client; the sensitive nature of the issues the treatment approach addresses; the need for explicitly addressing the client–therapist dynamics as appropriate; and the power of a planned therapy ending for someone who has lost a loved one without saying goodbye. All of these elements call for a collaborative relational approach that includes the client as a partner.

Relational therapy, as the term is used by the writers based at the Stone Center at Wellesley College, means that what happens between a therapist and client—their interactions with and experience of each other—is part of the "conversation" between the two parties (Jordan, Kaplan, Miller, Stiver, & Surrey, 1991). Our use of the term also includes adjustment of the treatment to each individual client, collaboration on goals, respect for the client's sensitivities, and awareness of the client's authority about his own needs. The most skillful application of this approach will include balancing all of these matters with the tasks outlined in the treatment description, including the resource-building, trauma-processing, and mourning work.

Psychoeducation and Independent Activities

Both psychoeducation and independent activities between sessions are essential to the success of this treatment approach. These processes require a level of activity that may not be familiar to some therapists. Furthermore, both processes lead a therapist into the role of educator and coach in a way that may be uncomfortable to those who practice from a more receptive, intuitive, relational, or psychodynamic stance. Certainly, at the outset of the treatment, you will have a lot of information to share, and you may feel ill at ease with how much of the time you are talking. The independent activities require you to check *in* with a client, which may feel like checking *up* on him. Some clients will not be surprised that you are doing a lot of the talking, and some may experience relief that they are not expected to know what to do or say on their own. Whatever a client's reaction may be, it is important to respond to it in ways that build the therapeutic relationship and further the treatment goals.

Focus on Termination

For therapists who have not worked on their own issues related to loss, abandonment, and endings, the focus on termination in this treatment approach, as well as the process of ending itself, may be challenging. As a therapist, you can become attached to clients, and even without a personal loss history or with a planned ending, you may feel a sense of absence when clients leave. Rynearson, Johnson, and Correa (2006) have observed, "Therapists may have difficulty accepting that their role as rescuer or advocate is no longer needed" (p. 151).

Termination can be particularly disruptive for you if a client ends the treatment prematurely. You may feel surprised, frustrated, angry, or abandoned if the ending is not adequately planned and accomplished. (See Chapter 9 for more on termination in this treatment.) If you have your own traumatic loss history, an unplanned or premature ending can renew feelings of loss.

Although these feelings are natural, it is essential that they not color treatment decisions. A client in time-limited therapy often expresses a wish to continue treatment as the ending approaches. You and the client must consider this wish as a feeling, not as a mandate. There may be good reason to continue the treatment (such as the client's unresolved trauma or loss issues that further treatment might address successfully). However, we strongly recommend that you work with clients to process their feelings before making any decisions. In addition, we recommend seeking consultation to process your own feelings about ending, so that these responses do not unduly influence your behavior with clients.

Rynearson and colleagues (2006) have noted that therapists working with this population may distance themselves as treatment draws close to the end. Traumatically bereaved clients are likely to feel such a withdrawal and experience it as another loss. Rynearson and colleagues stress that it is important for therapists to "control their own anxiety [and] sustain empathy" (p. 151).

GUIDELINES FOR IDENTIFYING TREATMENT CHALLENGES

The guidelines provided in the box on the next page are a tool to help you identify challenges such as those outlined above, which may not be immediately clear to you while in the midst of the treatment. It may be helpful to revisit these guidelines once you are engaged in the treatment.

RESPONDING TO CLINICAL HURDLES

Human beings bring some element of unpredictability and surprise to all of our experiences, and therapy is no exception. Responding to the unexpected requires sound clinical judgment based in theory, science, and experience. When you use your clinical judgment creatively, it contributes to the effectiveness of the treatment and to the personal and professional rewards of the work for you. In this section, we anticipate some of the issues and challenges you may encounter while implementing this therapy approach. We underscore the importance of using your clinical judgment. We also offer a framework for thinking through additional challenges and dilemmas you may encounter. This framework supports the best use of your clinical experience, judgment, and creativity.

The Four "E" Strategies

The key to managing challenging client responses is the following four "E" strategies: *Explore, Empathize, Educate,* and *Encourage* (reinforce). The effective use of these strategies will be based on your knowledge of the treatment approach and its underlying philosophy, on your clinical experience, and on your clinical judgment based on your work with each client. We describe and illustrate these strategies below, offering guidelines that will help you to address three specific challenges—staying on task, lack of treatment progress, and worsening symptoms—as well as providing a process to use with other issues as they arise.

Identifying Treatment Challenges

- What are the indicators that something challenging is happening?
  - Unexpected or unusual emotions (yours or client's)
  - Unexpected or unusual thoughts (yours or client's)
  - Unexpected or unusual behaviors (yours or client's)
  - Treatment not progressing as expected
- If something unexpected is happening, what might be some of the reasons?
  - First (or an early) time you've done this type of treatment (or some aspect of it)
  - First time working with this client population
  - External events or processes in your personal or professional life
  - External events or processes in the client's life
  - Unexpected turn of events in the therapy (e.g., client reveals important material that shifts the focus from the target death)
    - Could the client be introducing this issue in order to avoid working on the target loss?
  - Avoidance on your and/or the client's part
  - Lack of adequate self capacities on the client's part
- What might help you work with this challenge?
  - Review relevant portions of this book.
  - Find additional relevant readings (see the References list for possibilities).
  - Seek clinical consultation with someone who has experience with this population or with those elements of the treatment with which you're currently working.
  - Gather more personal support for you or the client. (For the client, this could take the form of resource building; for you, this could mean, e.g., clinical consultation, personal support, journaling, or resource building.)
  - Discuss with the client what's happening in the treatment (e.g., "We seem to be stuck. I think that this is because of X Y Z [observations]. Do you have any thoughts about it?").
  - If the client seems stuck, review the elements of the treatment with her that best address the obstacle she is facing.
- If all else fails, what would be the advantages of seriously modifying or even ending the treatment at this point?
  - What types of changes might allow the client to benefit from the treatment?
  - Would another approach to treatment be likely to benefit this client more at this time?
  - If the right decision is to end this treatment, how can that be done most constructively? (See the "Focus on Termination" section of this chapter. See also Chapter 9, as well as Handout S2, Ending Therapy [available on this book's website supplement], for ways of thinking about ending treatment.)

Staying on Task

Part of your role as the therapist is to keep the treatment on track and to motivate and gently guide each client through the process. Common issues that can arise in all treatments—missed sessions or incomplete independent activity assignments, for example—may be more significant in this treatment because staying on task and completing the independent activities are essential to the effectiveness of the work. Furthermore, such issues may be signs that a client is avoiding the difficult emotions associated with the loss.

A main premise of this treatment approach is that many traumatically bereaved clients are stuck because they have been avoiding painful memories, feelings, and thoughts. As emphasized throughout this book, this treatment approach invites clients to experience the pain of their loss consciously and intentionally, while calling on a variety of supports in doing so. Consciously experiencing pain with adequate support allows the clients to process or work through the elements of their responses to the loss. This in turn helps clients to continue their movement through the six "R" processes (Rando, 1993). In attending to the need to stay on task, you will experience a heightened attention to the issue of avoidance. Whereas in a nondirective therapy you would go with the flow, in this treatment approach you will be asking yourself, "How do I keep us on task?" This question will lead to potentially productive musing about avoidance.

Let's consider the following example: Melinda comes into session and introduces material that falls outside the purview of the treatment. Initially she sought treatment in order to address the deep feelings of grief she still holds after losing her mother in a boating accident 3 years earlier. On this particular day, she comes in distraught and tells you that she and her boyfriend have been fighting again. In some treatment approaches, it is possible and even preferable to follow the client's lead. Because this therapy is focused on a particular loss, however, you will need a strategy for addressing Melinda's concern within the frame of the treatment approach. This entails evaluating the needs and motivations that underlie the specific concern or behavior. You might ask yourself, "Is Melinda avoiding the loss work? Does she need to attend to this other issue before she can focus on the work at hand? Or is this somehow related to her loss work?"

When the dilemma of staying on task presents itself, more often than not the issue you will need to evaluate is whether going "off task" is motivated by or will support avoidance in some way. This attention to avoidance will keep the treatment moving and promote its effectiveness. Still, remaining focused on the target death can be challenging. The processes listed below will help you to sort out avoidance-related concerns.

Explore. Based on your knowledge of the treatment approach and its philosophy, your clinical judgment, and your experience with this client, what might help the two of you to stay on task? The first step is to understand why the client is behaving as she is. A conversation with the client about a missed session or forgotten independent activities can illuminate her understanding of the reasons for the behavior. Of course, it is possible that the client is unaware of or unable to articulate her fears about facing potentially painful feelings. If you believe these fears are part of the problem, you can suggest this to the client, respectfully and compassionately. In many cases, naming the dilemma in which you find yourselves opens up collaborative exploration. In the example of Melinda above, you might simply observe, "I know your relationship with Thomas is difficult for you right now, and I'm also aware that going down this path today will take us off track. I know that your goal in coming here has been to feel better about the loss of your mother. I'm wondering whether there is a connection between what's happening now between you and Thomas and your feelings about your mother's death."

Empathize. This treatment approach, like all change-supporting activities, is tough. It will be helpful to remember that your main task is to keep the treatment moving by embodying the openness to try new things, take risks, express emotions, and change. *Compassion and empathy are the foundations of support that will allow the client to progress through the treatment.* This last statement probably strikes you as self-evident. Even so, you may find compassion and empathy particularly difficult to maintain if you are feeling frustrated or under pressure to keep the treatment on track. At these moments, it helps to go back to basics: Try to identify with the client, and imagine (or recall) what it's like to lose a loved one unexpectedly and traumatically.

Expressions of empathy are often helpful in moving clients through avoidance: "This is really hard, isn't it? I know at least part of you wants to do it, and I believe you can."

Educate. Reminding the client of the rationale for this treatment approach and the particular elements of it can help her to renew her commitment. Tailoring this rationale to each client's situation is valuable. You might say something like this: "We both know how hard it has been for you to experience the feelings of grief about your mom's death. We also know that this has kept you feeling stuck for a long time. This approach is the best way we know of to help you to get unstuck."

Encourage (or Reinforce). In this treatment approach, you play many roles as the therapist, including teacher, companion, and coach. Encouraging, or reinforcing, largely falls within the role of coach. Taking the time to acknowledge, highlight, and praise a client's success at facing a painful feeling, completing a treatment task, and being fully present in sessions can provide essential support to clients. It's easier for clients to do something daunting if they know that you are in their corner, noticing their struggles and acknowledging their successes, however small they may seem. You might say, for example, "Good job. I know that was a hard independent assignment, and you did it!" or "I want to make sure we both acknowledge the victory of your visiting the gravesite. It took a lot of courage, and you worked hard to get yourself ready to face this challenge." Remembering to wear the hat of coach will go a long way in this treatment.

As you use these strategies, you will gain a fuller picture of what will help you and a particular client to stay on track. When in doubt, remember that you always have several choices in session. These include (1) naming the dilemma (e.g., "We had planned to move to a new task today, and yet it seems like the activities from our last session might need more attention"); (2) consulting with the client (as in the example of Melinda above); (3) suggesting that you spend part of the session talking about the current situation (in the example of Melinda, the boyfriend) and part of it doing what was planned for that session; (4) suggesting that you continue as planned if the client feels able to do so; and if not, (5) spending this session on the current situation and returning to the treatment plan next time. A sixth option often arises as you *Explore, Empathize, Educate*, and/or *Encourage*: (6) understanding how the client going off track can be brought into the frame of the treatment. In the Melinda example, you might come to appreciate how much Melinda misses being able to talk with her mother about her relationship issues. This might lead to a discussion of secondary losses that is in line with the session tasks for the day or another important treatment element. The path to take depends on the nature of the challenge; the relationship between you and the client; and, ultimately, your clinical judgment and the client's priorities.

Lack of Treatment Progress

Another challenge comes about when a client's symptoms seem not to be improving or he is remaining entrenched in the difficulties with which he came into treatment. With this particular challenge, evaluation entails assessing where the client is stuck. You can use the six "Rs" and Handout 11, the Identifying Automatic Thoughts Worksheet, as tools to run through possible ways of understanding where the client is stuck. In addition, your clinical judgment may help you understand the lack of movement and determine how to address this challenge. What does your clinical judgment tell you about the client's difficulties? Are you aware of a particular memory, emotion, belief, or activity that the client seems to avoid, skirt around, or gloss over? Can you identify any patterns that would help you understand the lack of progress at a deeper level? For example, does the client consistently not complete independent activities that relate to one of the "R" tasks, to social support, or to exposure tasks? Each of these patterns will invite a different solution (see Chapter 12 for information about moving through the "R" processes, Chapter 10 for more on social support, and Chapter 11 for exposure tasks). The "E" strategies will also help you to evaluate and respond to this category of challenges.

Explore. If a client continues to seem stalled in the same ways that brought him into treatment in the first place, it might be helpful to explore this together. Are you and he on the same page? Does he in fact feel as though nothing has shifted? If so, what is his understanding of why and how he remains entrenched? If not, what are some changes that he has noticed? Have you noticed any changes in the client, and if so, can you share these observations with him? You may also want to explore which aspects of the treatment have been particularly difficult for the client and whether any have been either tolerable or helpful from the client's perspective.

In exploring the client's understanding of his lack of movement, do you notice any resistance to "getting better"? Do you notice avoidance of aspects of the treatment, or avoidance of aspects of his experience? Referring to self-care activities, one client told a therapist, "I don't go for that fluffy stuff you want me to do between sessions." Upon exploration, the therapist learned that the client's feelings came to the surface when he engaged in self-care activities. The therapist concluded that an emphasis on feelings skills (Chapter 10) would be useful to this client. This discovery led to an increased emphasis on managing emotions, which helped the client to move through the rest of the treatment.

Empathize. Empathize with the difficult feelings a client may be experiencing, as well as with the strategies he may be using to avoid such feelings. For example, you might say, "I understand that your daughter's piano lesson conflicted with our meeting, and I'm also wondering whether you had some misgivings about coming to see me last week. Our work together is challenging, and sometimes it's hard to keep going." This will help both of you to remember that you are in this together, that motives are sometimes complex, and that you will continue to work toward the client's treatment goals.

Educate. After exploring where the client is stuck and empathizing with him, educate him about what you have observed and what strategies you might use to address the challenges. In doing so, you provide a collaborative foundation for moving forward. Education about the rationale of the treatment as a whole (Handout 2, Orientation to the Treatment) and about its individual elements (Handout 3, Treatment Goals and Tools) will help map out the territory ahead in a way that holds hope for healthy accommodation of the loss. You might say, for example, "I know you are feeling stuck right now. I believe that if we continue to explore your belief that getting better is a betrayal of your son, you will eventually break through this stuck place. Remember that what we tell ourselves and what we believe may be distorted. Challenging such beliefs is part of the process of recovering from trauma and adapting to loss."

It can help to remind the client of the exposure rationale—that avoidance prolongs pain in the long run (see Chapter 9)—while empathizing with the fact that avoidance can seem like a better approach in the moment because the client does not want to experience painful feelings, and because he may have difficulty believing that doing so will help him move forward.

Encourage. Finally, it will help to encourage or reinforce what the client has been doing that will help him to move through the mourning process. Clients may not recognize the value of, or give themselves credit for, small steps toward their goals. You can support them by noticing and naming these steps.

Worsening of Symptoms

It is not unusual for individuals in this treatment, as in other treatments, to experience a worsening of symptoms before feeling better. Engaging with painful memories, thoughts, and emotions definitely hurts at first, which is why people avoid them. However, this engagement will allow people eventually to move through the pain and bring it to tolerable levels. Again, you can use the four "E" strategies as a framework to help you evaluate what a client needs when she is getting worse, as well as why she may be getting worse. As you evaluate such challenges, you will want to look for whether the worsening symptoms are a result of increased engagement with painful thoughts, memories, and feelings. Alternatively, are the worsening symptoms a result of a client's increased resistance to confronting the pain? This is also an expectable response in this treatment approach. Are symptoms worsening due to the normal fluctuations found over the course of traumatic bereavement? Are these symptoms caused by reactions to external events (such as legal trials or major life changes that the survivor must face without the deceased)? Finally, you will want to evaluate whether the client needs more support to tolerate and eventually move through her symptoms, and if so, what kind of support would be most helpful.

The client's sense of daily well-being is very important. Can the client manage her day-to-day life and current symptoms? If she is having greater difficulty managing, what additional supports might she need? If she becomes symptomatic in ways that interfere with her daily life, she probably needs more support. This will be true whether the pain results from rigid avoidance or from distressing thoughts and feelings. Such symptoms may include dissociation, substance overuse, self-harm, aggression, increasing depression, social withdrawal, self-sabotage, suicidality, and psychosis, among many possible others. None of these responses is in itself a reason to discontinue the treatment. You and the client must decide together whether and how the treatment can continue. There is little doubt that more support (e.g., independent activities, more frequent sessions, more social support, or a medication consultation) is indicated at a time like this.

In addition, the hierarchical approach to avoided thoughts, memories, or situations is fluid. A client may initially assume that recounting a specific memory or visiting a place she used to visit with the loved one is low on her fear and avoidance hierarchy, but later may realize that she underestimated the distress caused by the memory or the situation. In this case, you should normalize the experience of "guessing wrong" about the hierarchy and help the client choose a different, less distressing memory to recount or exposure to pursue. Clinical consultation with therapists who do similar work can be an invaluable resource as you make such decisions.

Explore. Exploration of this challenge involves formally or informally taking an inventory of the client's symptoms and their intensity. You might begin with a conversation about the client's understanding of her symptoms and level of well-being. Do you both agree about whether the symptoms are getting worse or better? Are some getting worse and others better? How does she understand why this might be so? Assessment strategies, such as those we recommend in Chapter 8, can provide crucial information about treatment gains that may accompany increased symptoms in other realms. How are the worsening symptoms interfering with the client's day-to-day activities? Might symptoms be worsening because the client is not moving through the mourning processes? In addition, it can be useful to explore what activities have helped the client to feel supported in the work. To what extent is the client engaging in the independent activities? (This means not only whether she is doing the work, but how she is doing it. Is she actively engaging or just going through the motions? Is she attempting tasks that are too challenging or not challenging enough?)

The next step might involve using structured interviews and/or pencil-and-paper measures, which can provide invaluable information under such circumstances. For example, portions of Rando's (1993) GAMSII instrument (described in Chapter 8)—such as Topic Area H, "Mourner's self-assessment of healthy accommodation of the loss now and in the future" (pp. 679–680)— can offer information about the client's perspective on her progress and coping. The Inner Experience Questionnaire (Brock et al., 2006), a paper-and-pencil measure of self capacities, may also be useful. (For additional information on assessment, see Chapter 8.) Gathering this information will help you with your evaluation of (1) what is causing the worsening of symptoms; and (2) what supports, changes, and/or skills the client might need in order to tolerate and move through the pain.

Empathize. Use your clinical judgment and knowledge of how the client has been moving through the treatment to help you decide how and when to express empathy. If it seems as if the client is getting worse because she is defending against some aspect of the process, you might say, "I know this is particularly frustrating for you right now, especially because you've been working so hard. I have a hunch that if we keep at it and focus on the beliefs you hold about [for example] getting better, you will begin to feel better. I do realize how difficult this is." If it seems as though the symptoms are getting worse because the client is engaging with painful memories, then it will be helpful to empathize with and normalize this.

Educate. If the client notices increased intrusive symptoms, anxiety, or depression because she is beginning to open up to the pain of her loss, then it is important to hold onto the knowledge that this is an expectable part of this treatment and to share this understanding with the client. It can be very useful to explain that the pain often gets worse before it gets better, and to remind the client that it does get better. Part of the purpose of exposure is to elicit feelings that mourners have often suppressed. As clients decrease their use of certain defenses (such as dissociation, denial, and avoidance), they may become more symptomatic. Harvey (1996) found that traumatized clients often exhibited either no improvement or a worsening of trauma symptoms in the early part of therapy, while simultaneously showing positive changes in authenticity and meaning. Such information provides a framework for clients to understand their distress, which usually motivates them to continue the work. If a client is holding onto protective strategies more tightly, and therefore avoiding more intensely, then it will be necessary to go back to the rationale for the treatment as described in Handout 3, Treatment Tools and Goals, and Handout 9, A Model for Change. You may need to review the rationale repeatedly, pointing to examples in the client's life of how engaging with the pain of the loss opens things up, and avoiding shuts things down. When asked what they fear will happen if they allow themselves to experience fully the emotions related to the loss, clients often describe fears of crying without ever stopping or being so distressed that they cannot function again. Gradually allowing themselves to experience their feelings decreases these fears. Clients come to see that they can allow themselves to acknowledge and experience their pain without being overwhelmed by it. Handout 13, the Automatic Thought Record (described in Chapter 11), may be useful in challenging catastrophic thoughts about what might happen if they experience the emotions they have avoided until now.

Encourage. As described above, reinforcing a client's progress (however substantial or limited it may be), and holding hope for the future, are significant aspects of working collaboratively with the client and supporting him within a strong alliance.

Attend to safety. Addressing a worsening of symptoms entails careful attention to a client's safety. If you believe that the client may be unsafe to himself or a danger to others, safety must become the primary focus. *Safety is always the top priority.* If you have questions about the client's safety, we urge you to rely on your foundational clinical skills and professional resources to assess safety and respond in an ethical, supportive, and respectful manner. This is one of those moments when we recommend veering from the structure of the treatment approach. Many of the tools we provide will be helpful to establishing and maintaining safety (e.g., feelings skills, social support, self-care activities). If safety is in question, then these tools should be used solely in the service of establishing it. Putting on hold exposure work or exploratory work that opens up feelings or memories may be the best course of action. Once safety is established and maintained consistently for some time, you can talk with your client about whether resuming other aspects of the treatment will be helpful. Clinical consultation with peers, your supervisor, or a more experienced therapist is also an important element of helping a client to stay safe and deciding whether to continue with any aspect of the treatment approach.

CHALLENGES ARISING FROM WORKING IN A DIFFERENT PARADIGM: STRONGER AND WEAKER SUITS

Our approach is unique in its combination of elements to treat traumatic bereavement. As previously described, the core treatment components include developing resources (self capacities, coping skills, social support, bereavement-specific strategies, values, and meaning); cognitive and emotional processing of trauma; and moving through the six "Rs" of mourning. All of this takes place within the context of a strong therapeutic relationship. The treatment approach encourages use of psychoeducation and independent activities. With all of these components, it is likely that you will find areas of greater and lesser familiarity. In addition, you may have positive or negative reactions to certain treatment techniques or philosophies of treatment, based on your experience or on other, more subjective factors.

Identifying Stronger and Weaker Suits

It is natural that we all have, and usually prefer to work within, our "stronger suits." We may have discovered our stronger suits in our initial professional training, from workshops or self-guided study, from mentors or clinical supervisors, and from our own experiences as therapy clients. Most of us will recognize these strengths. These are the conceptualizations and techniques that we use naturally and intuitively with most clients. They are often well represented on our bookshelves and in the list of conferences we've attended. When we're working from our

244 CHALLENGES IN IMPLEMENTING TREATMENT

strong suits, we feel energized and perhaps even passionate about our work, as if we're in our comfort zones.

Strong suits can include content areas of knowledge or information, process areas of techniques or information, clinical populations, and skill areas like assessment or treatment. For example, one of us (Laurie Anne Pearlman) works most comfortably doing relational psychotherapy with adult clients with complex psychological trauma adaptations. Another (Catherine A. Feuer) works most comfortably with children and adults in a CBT framework. A third (Christine H. Farber) considers her strong suit to be individual psychotherapy with adult clients who are experiencing various life transitions. She prefers to work within a humanistic framework that acknowledges spiritual dimensions of life experiences.

"Weaker suits" are those areas to which we have not been exposed as therapists, in which we have not had a lot of interest, which we have not had a chance to practice and use, or in which we simply lack skill. They may also be weaker suits because we do not feel open to learning about or developing them. These are the areas with which we are less comfortable—the areas that require us to stretch ourselves professionally and possibly personally as well. Working outside our strong suits most likely entails doing things that are less familiar, and we all have tendencies to drift toward the habitual. Of course, the hazard of this drift away from the elements and techniques that are less comfortable is that we will inadvertently shortchange our clients.

The box below is a tool for identifying your own stronger and weaker suits. You can use this awareness both while sitting with clients and when planning for professional development.

Identifying Your Stronger and Weaker Suits

- You know you're working from one of your strong suits when . . .
  - Your physiological indicators are on "go": You feel calm and relaxed, maybe even slightly aroused physiologically.
    - Your energy level is good.
    - Your stamina and endurance are strong.
  - You feel confident and optimistic.
  - You feel creative.
  - Time seems to fly by.
  - You have a sense of flow.
  - Your mind seems to be working very well.
  - You and your client seem to be "in synch," moving forward together throughout the session.

- You can recognize your weaker suits when . . .
  - Your physiological indicators are on "interference": You feel physical discomfort, as if you're coming down with something—aches and pains (e.g., stomach, neck, back, head), fatigue, drowsiness.
  - Your energy is low; you lack interest.
  - You find it difficult to concentrate or stay on task; your mind may wander.
  - You find yourself looking at the clock more often than usual.
  - You exhibit negativity and/or feel self-doubt.
  - You feel as if you and your client are at odds with each other or simply not connected.

Building Your Weaker Suits

Successful application of this treatment approach requires identifying and strengthening the areas that may be less familiar to you. This book provides the background necessary to develop those less familiar areas. Building a weaker suit requires self-awareness and openness to learning. *The best approach to building a weaker suit is study, coupled with practice and consultation.* We strongly encourage you to read the relevant material in Parts I–III and then to employ the approach, using the material in Part IV for guidance. Specific consultation on particularly challenging elements is a good way to work out rough spots. For example, if you are new to exposure treatment, you might want to arrange some consultation sessions with someone experienced in that approach. Someone who is less familiar with resource-building work may want to consult with a colleague who has done more of it with traumatized clients.

Practicing this treatment approach provides an opportunity for you to expand your therapeutic tool box, while also learning about yourself and the process of transformation through grief. As a step toward growth, we encourage you first to identify your stronger and weaker suits; then to identify what you might need in relation to each area for growth (e.g., information, skills, knowledge, support, self-awareness, experience); and finally to develop a plan that suits you. Your plan might include one or more elements from the following list:

- Continuing education: Books, journals, websites and other online resources, workshops, conferences
- Consultation: Peer or expert, individual or group, time-limited or ongoing
- Training: Online or live
- Study group: Peer or facilitated
- Your own psychotherapy

It is also worth remembering that sometimes all of us struggle with a lack of confidence rather than a lack of competence. Clinical consultation can also be a place to explore this issue.

CLINICAL INTEGRATION

Dr. Taylor could feel a lump forming in her throat at the beginning of her session with Seth when he asked to talk about his brother's possible drug use, thereby veering off their treatment plan. She believed that maintaining their focus on Joan's death was the right thing to do. She had witnessed a lot of clients understandably avoiding the issues they came into therapy to address by presenting other concerns in sessions. Dr. Taylor worried that she would enable Seth's avoidance by following his lead on this day. At the same time, it was clear to her that he was having difficulty focusing on anything other than his worries about his brother's alleged drug use. As she sat across from Seth, Dr. Taylor felt confused and concerned. She was unsure how she would respond to his request.

"Dr. Taylor?" Seth was worried that he had lost his psychologist to her own thoughts. She suddenly seemed distant.

"Yes, sorry, Seth. I'm here. I was just thinking about which direction we should head today. Listening to you, I found myself feeling concerned. I can see how upset you are today, and we can certainly take some time to talk about your brother. My concern is that this would take us off track." Dr. Taylor had made the decision to address this issue directly. Seth was listening. "Before we explore the situation with your brother, I'd like to ask you a few things. Does that sound OK?"

"Yes, sure. I just don't know what to do about Danny."

"I can only imagine how challenging this must be for you—to be worried about Danny during this time that has been so difficult for both of you." Seth seemed to relax a bit upon hearing Dr. Taylor express some empathy. "Let me ask you this: How were you feeling after we discussed doing *in vivo* exposure last week? And how were you feeling as you anticipated coming to therapy this week?"

"I felt pretty anxious, actually, the day after our last session. The thought of being at my mom's place and beginning to sort through her belongings, as we had discussed, felt overwhelming to me. I just haven't wanted to get rid of any of her stuff." Seth began to tear up. "I don't want to let go."

"I understand something about how difficult this must have been for you. Facing these kinds of things can be really hard. You said the thought of being in your mom's house was overwhelming. Did you actually go into your mom's place?"

"Yeah, I did. I lasted for about 25 minutes, but then I felt too panicky. When I started to think about getting rid of some of her things, I not only felt anxious, but also angry. I just don't want to feel all of the grief."

"Twenty-five minutes is a good start, Seth. In terms of our work together, it's an accomplishment. I know it didn't feel good, but you got through it. It must have been difficult to come in here today, knowing we were going to talk about the exposure activity, and that I would likely encourage you to do more of this."

"It was."

"Maybe you were also feeling anger toward me? Not wanting to experience those feelings, and here I am giving you activities to do between sessions that ask you to do just that?"

"I'm not sure. I know I was feeling irritable all week. But the thing with Danny is real. He looked high one day last week, and there was another day when he wasn't at class as he said he would be. I'm worried about him." Seth's body language suggested increasing agitation.

"Let's explore that," suggested Dr. Taylor. After asking Seth more directly about his experience with *in vivo* exposure, she felt more comfortable moving into an exploration of his feelings and concerns regarding Danny. She also had a hunch that the situation with his brother was related to his feelings of grief and anger about his mother's death. "Tell me more about Danny."

"I'm furious with him. He's destroying himself rather than coping with our mom's death. At least that's how it feels. He's so angry that she's gone. I'm so angry that she's gone. And my mom was the only one who could ever get through to him. I don't know how to help him, and I'm mad at her for being killed—for putting me, and him, in this situation." Seth's voice grew stronger, even as tears were welling up behind his words. "And I feel guilty for being angry at her," he added in a softer voice. "You can't be mad at someone for having been murdered!"

"Actually, you can be. And of course you're angry. In addition to missing Joan as your mother, you miss her as Danny's mom. This is one of those secondary losses we've talked about. Also, it sounds to me as though you really empathize with your brother's pain. And I imagine that facing his potential drug use is not unlike going to your mom's house. Both have required you to come face to face with the anger and pain and loss that are within you. Both confront you with the reality that your mom is gone."

Seth was now crying quietly. No longer agitated, he seemed instead to sink into his grief as he sat back in his chair and covered his face in his hands. Dr. Taylor sat with him, quietly. She knew that they could continue to explore exposure activities and the emotional processing that these activities served. For the time being, her client was in the midst of this processing, and she allowed him space for just this.

CONCLUDING REMARKS

Throughout this chapter, we have explored some common challenges that you may encounter while implementing this treatment approach, as well as guidelines for how to manage them. The example of Seth and Dr. Taylor illustrates how these challenges might manifest themselves in a particular therapy. It might not surprise you to learn that Dr. Taylor struggled with the structured nature of this approach, as well as with the implementation of exposure activities. She was aware that these were her weaker suits, and she had a tendency to compensate for her limitations by "following the rules" more closely with these aspects of the treatment. When Seth asked to address a situation that seemingly fell beyond the scope of their therapy and might have been related to avoidance, Dr. Taylor experienced some of her own anxiety, as it touched on vulnerabilities of which she was aware.

Dr. Taylor offers us an example of how to manage challenges effectively. In various places throughout the session, she chose to address her dilemma directly: She let Seth know of her concern that the topic of Danny's drug use could lead them off track, and she directly *Explored* his reactions to doing exposure work. She also collaboratively explored how Seth's responses to exposure work might have been related to his concern about his brother, and in doing so she expressed *Empathy* both directly and indirectly. By addressing her concerns directly with Seth, Dr. Taylor also provided *Education* with regard to the difficulty of exposure and the importance of the structured nature of the treatment, and she reinforced (*Encouraged*) both how Seth was feeling and the good work he was doing.

As readers and clinicians, we can imagine the challenges that Dr. Taylor, or any of us, might need to address in order to work with this approach effectively. Our final chapter addresses the potential effects on us as therapists of working therapeutically with the traumatically bereaved.

CHAPTER 14

Effects of the Treatment on Therapists

It was a brisk, bright October morning, but Mala was having difficulty getting out of bed. She had gotten enough sleep, the sun was up, and she could smell her coffee brewing. Her trouble with waking up on this particular morning confused but didn't surprise her. She had been feeling this way on and off for several weeks now. Her difficulty in getting going was accompanied by a sense of dread about being at work, and on some level, she was aware of this connection. With a sigh, she got going.

Mala had begun working at the Health Clinic 17 years earlier. She started out as an intake specialist before pursuing her master's degree in social work and then becoming a licensed independent clinical social worker. Mala was now the clinic's director, and for the most part she enjoyed her work. She took pleasure in the challenges of her career and especially liked the supervisory work she did with the counseling staff. Over the last few months, however, she'd started feeling tired, unenthusiastic, and even a bit defeated. Whereas Mala had initially dismissed this experience as a phase, telling herself, "This too shall pass," she was beginning to disbelieve her own pep talks.

On this particular day, as the work day drew to a close and she realized she was anticipating the next day of work with anxiety and dismay, Mala decided to call Nathan—a fellow social worker, mentor, and confidant with whom she had consulted in the past whenever she felt stuck in some way. Mala felt tears in her eyes as she picked up her phone and dialed his number.

This chapter addresses the effects that this work can have on you, the therapist. We discuss those responses that relate to work with a particular client under the heading "Countertransference." We discuss under the heading "Vicarious Traumatization" those responses that result from therapies with multiple trauma clients over time. We then move to a discussion of training and consultation as ways to support yourself in the work. The chapter also highlights the rewards of working with traumatically bereaved survivors.

Many factors contribute to our own responses to the work, and it may not surprise you to read that in certain ways, our responses parallel those of traumatically bereaved individuals. Put simply, these individuals struggle with the difficulty of accepting and accommodating a reality that they wish were not true. Likewise, we therapists may have difficulty remaining open to clients' symptoms and adaptations, struggle to accept particular elements of this treatment approach, or experience resistance to our own responses to it. The guiding principle of this chapter is that self-awareness is the key to ethical, effective, and fulfilling therapeutic work. We address each of these effects, as well as how to create support for yourself in order to provide the best possible treatment while honoring your own needs and feelings.

COUNTERTRANSFERENCE

The work of mourning can raise strong feelings in you as a therapist, as well as in clients. A variety of factors will influence your *countertransference* responses (all of your responses *to a particular client*). These include your personality, coping style, and strategies; experience with your own losses; family history; and current life stressors. Your comfort with and confidence in this treatment model can also affect countertransference responses. So too can the specifics of each client's presentation, as well as the client's ways of coping with and managing the loss. The details and specific nature of the death may influence countertransference responses as well. Although there are many possible sources of countertransference responses in trauma work (Dalenberg, 2000; Danieli, 1994; Pearlman & Saakvitne, 1995; Wilson & Lindy, 1994; Wilson & Thomas, 2004), several responses to the combination of trauma and loss are particular to this work. We delineate some common responses in Table 14.1.

Sources of Countertransference in Traumatic Bereavement Treatment

Whatever the source of countertransference may be, awareness is essential to using these responses constructively to help a client (for more on using countertransference constructively with trauma clients, see Dalenberg, 2000; Pearlman & Caringi, 2009; Pearlman & Saakvitne, 1995; Saakvitne et al., 2000). Here we discuss some of the common responses you may experience when using this approach to working with traumatically bereaved clients.

TABLE 14.1. Common Countertransference Responses to Sudden, Traumatic Death and Traumatic Bereavement

- Related to a client and her adaptations
  - Compassion for a client who suffers so terribly
  - Assumption of a client's attitude that life is not worth living without the significant other or that all meaning has vanished
  - Grief consonant with a survivor's grief
  - Frustration with a client who is unable to take in the many positive elements in his life
- Related to the death
  - Shock, horror, or disgust at the sometimes violent or otherwise horrific details of the death
  - Anger at those who may have created, allowed, or contributed to the death or its aftermath
- Related to the therapy
  - Annoyance with a client who is not fully engaged with the treatment
  - Yearning or resentment that a client is receiving treatment that wasn't available to the therapist in her own losses
  - Worry that the therapy isn't "enough"
  - Satisfaction at being able to help someone who has suffered deeply
  - Love for a client who struggles to thrive and move on, against various challenges
- Related to the therapist
  - Guilt about having a comfortable life that hasn't included losses such as the client's
  - Fear that the therapist will lose a loved one or will die suddenly, leaving his significant others to mourn his death

Responses Related to Client Adaptations

Many survivors of sudden, traumatic deaths have spent years struggling with their reactions to their losses. For some survivors, the grief is very visible. One type of client with visible grief is a person who, years after the death, cries readily, has not dealt with the loved one's belongings, and has not developed or maintained an intimate or meaningful relationship with anyone new. In other cases, particular manifestations of grief may not be obvious to the survivor or those around her. For example, a client may present with psychosomatic difficulties but no reported emotional problems (or perhaps no evident or reported emotions). With other survivors, substance abuse or social or sexual withdrawal may be the main clue to unresolved trauma and grief. As a therapist, you will have a variety of responses to each presentation, finding some more challenging than others.

As an example, a client who has overt, intense signs of grief or trauma may elicit feelings of sympathy, compassion, concern, aversion, dismay, and/or anxiety. You may feel an intense need to do something to relieve the client's suffering. You may feel helpless and hopeless, perhaps echoing the client's feelings. If you feel inadequate to conduct the treatment, you may then feel ashamed, annoyed, or angry with the client, and/or resentful of the client's needs and demands. As another example, a resigned or resistant client may evoke feelings of powerlessness, helplessness, or annoyance. Further countertransference responses may come about as you react to these inner experiences—for example, moving toward overactivity, overinvolvement with, or withdrawal from the client.

Responses Related to the Death

Many of the events that lead to sudden, traumatic death include aspects that are senseless, shocking, violent, or untimely. Therapists often feel revulsion; fear that such things could happen to themselves or their loved ones; or anger, despair, or cynicism about people who cause such tragedies or about human vulnerability. As a therapist, you may find yourself moving away from gruesome details during sessions when it would be therapeutic for a client to give voice to them. If you fear a similar fate for your loved ones, you may experience the impulse to blame the client, in an effort to ensure that the same thing won't happen to you.

You may also identify with individuals who were involved in the death. This could include those who contributed to the death or whom others perceive as responsible. For example, you might think, "How awful for that doctor to have misdiagnosed and then lost her patient," or "I can imagine what the driver of the vehicle is feeling now." All of these responses are understandable; being aware of them will give you the choice not to act on them in ways that would be countertherapeutic.

Responses Related to the Therapy

In Chapter 13, we discuss aspects of this particular treatment approach that may be challenging for you. Such issues can evoke countertransference responses in a particular therapy. For example, one therapist struggled with teaching feelings skills. When she worked with a client who was much older than she was, her struggle became more pronounced: She experienced herself as condescending and thus tended to minimize these aspects of the treatment. After exploring her responses with a colleague, she came to understand that her client often did not get the support he needed because others saw him as unusually self-sufficient. The therapist also had not seen his vulnerability.

Alternatively, you may feel annoyed with a client or disappointed in yourself (or both) if a client continues to exhibit distress while not engaging adequately with the treatment. These responses may lead you to exhibit impatience, which may arouse guilt or resentment in the client. As with any lapse in empathy, the client may feel alienated or abandoned, which in turn can affect her motivation.

In the presence of a highly distressed traumatically bereaved client, you may worry that the therapy is too complex, particularly if you are new to this treatment approach. This response can lead to a lack of confidence in the treatment and/or impatience with its pace. In turn, you may convey that lack of confidence to the client, undermining his hope and motivation. Alternatively, you may skip the resource-building elements and move prematurely to the exposure elements, or skip essential "R" processes that the client has not yet completed, unwittingly robbing him of important dimensions of adaptation to the loss.

Responses Related to the Therapist

Your particular responses may depend on such factors as your theoretical orientation, personal style, history, and current life circumstances; similarities between you and the client; and consultation resources available. Most of us have experienced losses of loved ones, whether through death or other types of separations. Many of us also have personal histories of traumatic loss. Identification with a client along any dimension (e.g., age, gender, life situation, and particularly the nature of the traumatic loss) can raise significant challenges. The client and his situation may reawaken your own loss and grief experiences. One danger for the treatment is that, based on your own experiences, you may make assumptions about who this individual client is and what he needs. It is easy in this case to lose sight of the particulars of the client's situation and needs, and then to veer from empathic engagement.

Batson, Fultz, and Schoenrade (1987) described an important and relevant distinction between *empathy* and *personal distress*. They depicted empathy as a process in which one imagines the experience as happening to the other person (the client, in this case). They explained personal distress as arising when one (you as the therapist, in this case) imagines the experience as happening to oneself. They reviewed evidence suggesting that whereas personal distress ("What if this happened to me?") seems to motivate people to reduce their own aversive arousal, empathy ("How terrible that this happened to her") seems to motivate people to address the other's needs. This observation has important implications for the ability to respond constructively to clients in distress. If you are experiencing personal distress as a result of your interactions with a client, you may unconsciously attempt to find ways to reduce your own distress. For example, you may collude in avoidance with a client (e.g., by redirecting her when she talks about her deceased loved one); forget important information the client has shared; feel sleepy or distracted in sessions; or fail to return client phone calls or prepare adequately for sessions.

Personal traumatic experience can come into play when therapists and clients have endured the same traumatic events at the same time, such as natural disasters or community violence. Tosone (2006) has termed such experiences *shared trauma*. Hurricanes, earthquakes, wildfires, floods, terrorist attacks, and group violence can affect the lives of everyone in a community. When therapists lose loved ones in such events, it is imperative to engage in clinical consultation with an experienced consultant as they find their way through their work with traumatic loss survivors. We also strongly recommend that survivor therapists take time to process their losses in their own psychotherapies before and during their work with survivors.

In addition to losing loved ones, therapists may experience other losses in natural disasters or community violence. These may be tangible (e.g., loss of home or other property) or intangible (e.g., loss of security, predictability, or connection to the community). These losses, too, will affect countertransference responses to survivor clients. Therapists must understand them in order to provide the best possible care.

If you have lost a loved one and mourned the loss without the kind of expert assistance you are now providing to a client, you may yearn for the same kind of help, or regret that it was not available to you. If you are unaware of these feelings, you may unwittingly withhold (or "forget") essential elements of the treatment, such as the compassionate support, resource-building elements, careful work with automatic thoughts, or exposure elements that would be vital to the client's recovery. Alternatively, if you have never lost an important loved one, you may feel guilt in your relief that you have not experienced such a loss.

Perhaps too infrequently discussed are the "positive" countertransference responses therapists may have for their clients. As a therapist, you may feel deep respect, admiration, or parental love for a client who struggles to thrive and move on against various challenges. As with all countertransference responses, and as discussed in more detail below, bringing such inner experiences into awareness and using them in therapeutic ways is the ultimate goal. We encourage all therapists to express feelings of respect and admiration (*love* is generally too strong a word for appropriate use in psychotherapy), although this must be done with sensitivity (Dalenberg, 2000; Kahn, 2006). It is essential to observe a client's response to such expressions, to discover whether they are motivating, embarrassing, or alienating to the client. Of course, when treatment goes well, you will feel rewarded and satisfied with the work, as well as happy for the client who has reclaimed his life. It is often appropriate to let the client know how pleased you are with her progress.

It is common for these various responses to exist in combination with one another. For example, you may feel constrained by the structured nature of the treatment approach or impatient with a client who you feel isn't progressing, while remaining unaware of the activation of your own traumatic loss history. Clinical consultation can be useful in sorting out the various contributing factors to countertransference responses; such differentiation is essential to using them constructively to move the treatment forward.

Managing Countertransference Responses

Paulo sat down with Marta, a new client who came in because she had felt emotionally frozen ever since the death of her infant daughter a few years earlier. Paulo had started to see some traumatically bereaved clients since losing his father in an automobile accident a year before. He had been engaged in his own psychotherapy, and felt he might have something special to offer to other mourners.

As Marta began to tell the story of her loss, Paulo increasingly thought about his own grief and mourning. How could he make sense of the depth of the pain he had experienced, when measured against that of losing a young child? His father had been elderly, not in excellent health, and probably not too many years away from a natural death. In contrast to Marta's infant daughter, his father had led a long and satisfying life.

Paulo's guilt began to get in the way of hearing Marta's story. He began to reassure her that her frozen response was normal. He also stated that her husband, who insisted she come in to therapy, sounded insensitive. He thought that he would not use the exposure elements of the treatment because he thought it would be too much for Marta; instead, he would focus on offering warmth and support.

It seems clear that in this example, Paulo was carried away by his countertransference responses to Marta and her story; these responses interacted with his own feelings. Paulo's recent loss made it difficult for him to stay focused on Marta and to consider her needs without comparing his situation to hers. His assessment concerning the appropriateness of exposure was probably colored by his wish to avoid his own deep feelings of loss. One hopes that he sought consultation before abandoning a treatment approach—exposure—that might provide Marta with some relief from traumatic bereavement.

Our guidelines for managing countertransference come from the *Risking Connection* trauma training curriculum (Saakvitne et al., 2000). *Risking Connection* advises clinicians to (1) notice countertransference, (2) name it (for themselves and possibly with the client), and (3) use it to move the treatment forward. Although these steps sound simple, it may not be easy to implement them. We opened this section with a clinical illustration to bring life to the simple, yet challenging, process of working with countertransference. Paulo first needed to notice that this therapy was eliciting a particular set of inner experiences that could cloud his judgment and interfere with his ability to offer therapeutic intervention. Consultation with colleagues, personal therapy, and clinical experience all contribute to the skill of noticing even subtle shifts of inner experience. Even experienced therapists with well-developed self-awareness can miss countertransference clues, especially without tools to help. We cannot easily will ourselves to be cognizant of thoughts, feelings, and beliefs that exist outside of our conscious awareness. For this reason, tools and activities that require reflection on and expression of inner experience are invaluable to effective and ethical work. Journaling, peer consultation, our own therapy, and self-awareness checklists (e.g., Saakvitne et al., 1996) are examples of useful tools for noticing, naming, and constructively working with countertransference.

Some of the guidelines suggested in Chapter 13 (see the "Guidelines for Identifying Treatment Challenges" section and the accompanying box) may be beneficial. In addition, worksheets such as those in the appendices of *Risking Connection* or in the workbook *Transforming the Pain* (Saakvitne et al., 1996) may be useful, as they were developed specifically to support trauma workers in identifying their countertransference. As mentioned, professional consultation, whether with peers or more experienced clinicians, can also provide a forum for noticing various thoughts, feelings, and behaviors. These might suggest a need for more attention to a particular treatment relationship; for deciding whether and how to name these responses with the client; and for using them constructively to help the client.

Another clinical example can illustrate how managing countertransference effectively can contribute to moving a therapy forward. Ms. Black, a 45-year-old woman whose son had been shot and killed in a hunting accident the previous autumn, came to treatment. She presented the story of the death without much emotion, avoiding eye contact with the therapist, Dr. Owens. She repeatedly stated that she didn't think therapy could help her, that it couldn't bring back her son, and that she was only here because her trusted primary care doctor had asked her to see this therapist. At the end of the first session, she told Dr. Owens that she didn't think she would come back, but agreed to an appointment "just in case." The therapist felt concerned about Ms. Black's situation. She had described considerable social isolation, evidence of depression (loss of interest in everything she had once enjoyed, including difficulty eating, sleeping, and concentrating), and recurring intrusive thoughts about the shooting. Dr. Owens, who was opposed to hunting, felt angry about the death, which seemed completely avoidable ("Why did the son go hunting by himself? Was he wearing one of those orange vests?"). In addition, he wanted to engage this client, both for her sake and because this was his first referral from her doctor's busy practice.

Ms. Black returned the next week for a second session. She started out by saying, "Now don't think just because I'm here that I'm coming back again." Dr. Owens embarked on a discussion of the treatment, moving into both psychoeducation and assessment issues. In the middle of the session, the client said that she didn't think this treatment approach would work for her.

The therapist decided to bring his countertransference into the room. After noticing what he was feeling (eagerness, frustration, anxiety, worry, compassion, annoyance), he named it: "I'm aware that I have a lot of feelings right now about your situation. You have had a horrible loss, and you may have lots of confusing feelings about it yourself." To his surprise, Ms. Black said quietly, "Really, Doc, the worst of it is that I can't help blaming my son for his own death." Tuning into his own countertransference responses, Dr. Owens responded, "That really feels terrible, doesn't it? I think some of the information and activities that are part of this therapy can help with that." The client seemed to relax for the first time and tentatively decided to continue with the treatment. The therapist felt relieved to have a way of understanding his countertransference and how it resulted in his tendency to blame the victim, perhaps in identification with the client. Furthermore, the client's ability to respond to his statement gave him hope for their future collaborations.

What did Dr. Owens do in the example above that seemed to help his client? First, he noticed his own feelings and made them explicit to himself. If he had not wondered about his own reactions, he might have agreed that the client should not come back; he might have had difficulty expressing warmth toward her; or he might have found himself becoming disengaged. Instead, Dr. Owens reflected on his feelings in a way that allowed him to move into the client's experience. Then, with this awareness as his foundation, he made a decision to share some of his feelings with his client. He named them for her in a general enough way to give the client space for any responses she wanted to share: "I'm aware that I have a lot of feelings right now about your situation. . . ." Finally, he was able to use this process to move the treatment forward: "You have had a horrible loss, and you may have lots of confusing feelings about it yourself." In this example, a therapist's awareness of his countertransference issues became a primary tool in the therapy.

VICARIOUS TRAUMATIZATION

In this section, we describe the specific ways in which working with survivors of sudden, traumatic death *over time and across clients* can negatively affect therapists. Although our focus here is on these negative effects, or *vicarious traumatization* (VT), we follow this section with a discussion of ways that working with traumatic bereavement clients can enrich therapists.

We define VT as the negative transformation that takes place in a therapist through empathic engagement with traumatized clients and a commitment or sense of responsibility to help (McCann & Pearlman, 1990c; Pearlman & Saakvitne, 1995). Its hallmark is disrupted spirituality (Pearlman & Caringi, 2009)—a concept that is both difficult to define and yet recognizable to many. Nonetheless, most of us have a sense of what *spirituality* means. We use the term here in its broad sense to refer to those aspects of life that are intangible and that reflect a connection with something beyond our material selves. In the context of VT, we draw on Neumann and Pearlman's (1992) work to describe spirituality as an awareness of intangible aspects of life, including a sense of life's meaning and hope for the future. Whereas countertransference refers to our responses as therapists to individual clients, VT describes our responses across clients, over time. Both countertransference and VT are inevitable aspects of psychotherapy with trauma survivors. Both can be harmful to clients. If we are not attuned to these responses, they can lead us to engage in countertherapeutic, unethical, or harmful behaviors with clients. In addition, unaddressed VT can harm us by shattering our worldviews, damaging our spirituality, and interfering with our personal relationships, as elaborated below.

As described in detail elsewhere (McCann & Pearlman, 1990c; Pearlman & Caringi, 2009; Pearlman & Saakvitne, 1995), VT arises from an interaction between aspects of the client and aspects of the therapist, all in a particular social and cultural context. In this chapter, we focus on special issues in VT that relate to work with traumatically bereaved clients. For an excellent review of the effects of trauma work on therapists more generally, see Elwood, Mott, Lohr, and Galovski (2011).

Sources of VT

The Clients

Although VT responses and adaptations will be unique for each therapist, some responses to traumatically bereaved clients are more common than others. These include responses to typical adaptations of this survivor population, as well as to traumatic death itself. (See Chapters 3 and 4 for more about these adaptations.) Many mourners come into treatment because they are stuck in their lives. They are carrying deep traumatic grief and many other personal and interpersonal problems. Over time, as a therapist working with this population, you may develop your own deep grief in response to the grief—both expressed and unexpressed—of your clients. Working with clients' grief may lead you to become numb to your own feelings as a way of managing your grief. Alternatively, you may develop a chronic sense of outrage or become cynical in response to the senseless loss of vitality and potential. Your own fear of losing a loved one suddenly, as it accumulates across clients, can lead to emotional reactivity, preoccupation or obsessions about death and loss, overprotection of loved ones, or hypersensitivity to potential danger. You may also feel compelled by your clients' pain to do more than you should to assist them. Examples of this would be making yourself available without limits, consistently allowing sessions to run over in time, neglecting to ask for payment, and other behaviors that ultimately can lead to burnout.

Loss of meaning is at the core of psychological trauma—a fact that is evident with this population. As described in Chapter 3, survivors of sudden, traumatic death often struggle with the "why" questions: "Why me? Why him, not me? Why now?" As they attempt to make sense of their losses, they also face the task of rebuilding their lives, which have often been shattered by both primary and secondary losses. The disruptions in meaning and hope that characterize traumatic death are also signature symptoms of VT. As a therapist doing this work, you may enter into your own search for meaning, or you may find that the way you once understood life no longer seems to work for you. Like your survivor clients, you may face the task of rebuilding a worldview that can accommodate the fact that such profound losses happen all around us and can happen to you.

The Therapist

Adams and Riggs (2008) assessed defensive styles in 129 graduate students in clinical and counseling psychology. They found that "a self-sacrificing defense style characterized by reaction formation and pseudo altruism" (p. 31), which the authors describe as a "need to maintain an image of the self as kind, helpful, and never angry" (p. 29), was associated with greater vulnerability to VT. Conversely, "the student therapist's use of adaptive coping mechanisms such as suppression, sublimation, and humor decreases the likelihood of experiencing vicarious traumatization" (p. 31).

In his 2004 review, Bride found that although the evidence was not entirely consistent, the preponderance of the research supported a relation between therapists' personal trauma histories and VT. The research on this link has not yet explored specific aspects of trauma history that may be associated with greater VT vulnerability. However, Adams and Riggs (2008) found that defensive style moderated the effects of personal history on VT. It seems possible that therapists with unacknowledged or unaddressed trauma histories may experience more VT than do those who are aware of their histories and have worked to understand the effects of traumatic events on their lives (Pearlman & Saakvitne, in press). Of course, a specific personal history of concern in working with traumatically bereaved clients is a history of traumatic death in a therapist's circle of intimate others.

Various authors have suggested that empathy may be the mechanism through which VT comes about (Pearlman & Caringi, 2009; Pearlman & Saakvitne, 1995; Rothschild, 2006; Wilson & Thomas, 2004). A therapist with a personal loss that has not been adequately addressed may be more likely to identify with his clients by recalling his own experience or imagining the clients' losses happening to himself, which can elicit personal distress (associated with feelings of alarm and upset; Batson et al., 1987). This could reawaken unresolved memories or feelings related to trauma and loss. "Wounded healers" (to use Carl Jung's term) may have greater empathy for clients with trauma histories similar to theirs; such empathy could be an asset, helping clients feel understood. On the other hand, wounded healers who have not fully explored the effects of their own histories on their work may violate boundaries with clients in ways that are at best not helpful and can cause serious harm (through, e.g., revealing their own loss histories to clients without clinical reasons to do so or suggesting that what will help the client is the same as what helped the therapist).

When these responses emerge across a professional's therapies, they can create clinical difficulties in the treatments, as well as personal problems for the therapist. The therapist may find her own grief (and trauma, if she experienced a traumatic death) reactivated and then avoidanything that intensifies it, including whatever aspects of the treatment she finds most difficult.

The challenge for all therapists is to identify, address, and ideally transform VT when we experience it. As in our approach with clients, we advocate an integrated approach to painful feelings, thoughts, and imagery, as a way to transform VT. We describe this approach below.

Identifying VT

Risking Connection (Saakvitne et al., 2000) and *Transforming the Pain* (Saakvitne et al., 1996) provide self-assessment tools for identifying VT. Stamm (2005) has developed the Professional Quality of Life Scale (ProQoL), which allows therapists to assess their *compassion fatigue* (Figley, 1995), compassion satisfaction, and burnout. Although the compassion fatigue construct differs from VT in its focus on symptoms rather than on changes in the self of the helper (Hug-gard, Stamm, & Pearlman, 2013), Stamm's measure provides potentially useful information about the impact of the work on therapists who assist trauma survivor clients.

The important question is not "Do I have VT?", but rather "How is this work affecting me in ways that resemble trauma, if in a milder form?" You can ask yourself (and your loved ones) how you have changed during the time you have worked with traumatically bereaved clients, and whether and how these changes might relate to the work. Changes in relationships, affect management, and spirituality, as well as the presence of such trauma symptoms as intrusive imagery and dissociation, suggest the possibility of VT and the need to attend to the effects of the work. In the following sections, we discuss both coping with and transforming VT.

Addressing VT

If you become aware that you are experiencing psychological, behavioral, or spiritual changes as a result of trauma work, or foresee that you may, you can and must take action. Such action is an ethical imperative, as addressing VT is essential to providing good clinical services. Activities that focus on rest and play can help you *cope* with VT. These activities include hobbies, travel, creative endeavors, time with friends and family, and so forth. You can use the checklist on pages 261–262 to assess how you are doing in your efforts to address VT. *Transforming* VT requires attending to meaning and hope, as discussed below.

Coping with VT

Researchers have found support for the value of strategies such as educating oneself and others about the effects of traumatic events; obtaining assistance and support from others; using humor, active coping, and planning; countering isolation (in professional, personal, and spiritual realms); developing mindful self-awareness; expanding perspective to embrace complexity; engaging in active optimism and holistic self-care; maintaining clear boundaries; creating meaning; processing with peers or supervisors; and exercising (Follette, Polusny, & Milbeck, 1994; Harrison & Westwood, 2009; Killian, 2008; Pearlman & Mac Ian, 1995; Schauben & Frazier, 1995). In contrast to the work of these researchers, Bober and Regehr (2006) found no association between indicators of VT and coping strategies employed. They maintain that a focus on individual coping unduly individualizes the problem; instead, they recommend interventions at the organizational level, perhaps because the strategies they studied were generic (e.g., leisure and recreation) rather than specific to VT (Pearlman & Saakvitne, in press). Others have argued for the importance of organizational changes for those working in agencies (Bell, Kulkarni, & Dalton, 2003; Fawcett, 2003; Jordan, 2010; Munroe et al., 1995; Pryce, Shackelford, & Pryce, 2007; Rosenbloom, Pratt, & Pearlman, 1995), although not in place of individual interventions. We focus on a few of these strategies below.

Building good personal support networks within your community is an important aspect of coping with VT. Communities allow us all to exercise other aspects of our identities, so that in addition to "therapist," we engage with the world as "partner," "pianist," "jokester," "gardener," and a host of other identities. Our communities hold our values, joys, and sorrows with us and remind us that we are part of an interconnected web, which can counter the isolation of trauma.

Another aspect of addressing VT is the use of self-care. Just as we do for clients, we strongly recommend that all therapists—and particularly those working with traumatically bereaved clients—develop solid self-care plans and revisit/revise these plans as their needs change over time. Norcross (2000) has described self-care strategies that have received empirical support in the literature. On the basis of his research, Norcross has emphasized the importance of recognizing and addressing the hazards of clinical practice rather than denying them. He suggests thinking in terms of strategies (such as exercise in general, or building community) rather than specific techniques or methods (such as running or swimming, or going out with friends twice a week). In addition, the research supports using multiple strategies (e.g., exercise, relaxation, and social support). Norcross further recommends attending to stress levels and making choices wherever possible in establishing routines. One therapist found that daily morning exercise helped her feel centered, although it meant not arriving at the office until 9:30 A.M. (a choice she was able to make). Another scheduled his most challenging clients first thing in the morning, when he was freshest.

Norcross (2000) further recommends making the work environment soothing and supportive rather than depressing. One trauma therapist bought fresh flowers for her office weekly—an expense she found worthwhile in elevating her mood, especially as it reminded her of life in the midst of working with death. Norcross also suggests using relationships—personal psychotherapy, peer consultation groups, and loving personal relationships—for support in this work. In addition, focusing on what can be changed rather than on what cannot is valuable in avoiding paralysis. A counselor working in a community mental health clinic consistently reminds herself that accepting the work hours and arranging her schedule as well as possible within that frame is a healthier way of working than railing against the 8:00 A.M.–5:00 P.M. schedule. Finally, focusing on the rewards of the work—both small and great—is a very important way to sustain oneself in this challenging work, as we discuss below.

The way we do our jobs as therapists can increase or mitigate our VT. Pearlman and Caringi (2009) have presented recommendations about ways of working that can help to prevent or ameliorate VT. Some of these strategies are ways of thinking about the work (such as working from a theoretical base, staying connected to our own experience while sitting with clients, and focusing on process rather than outcomes). A second group of strategies includes practice recommendations, such as managing boundaries thoughtfully, writing progress notes after sessions (as a way of containing affect), using countertransference responses to promote each client's growth, and doing something between sessions that engages the body (e.g., stretching), the spirit (e.g., meditating), or creativity (e.g., sketching).

Rothschild (2006) has recommended attending to bodily experiences while working with traumatized individuals—for example, adjusting one's body posture as a way of managing neurobiological mirroring responses. She describes this process as unconsciously mimicking the client's facial expression or body posture. Additional ways of working protectively include diversifying one's work (another empirically supported process; Norcross, 2000) to include clients who have not experienced trauma or loss, or work other than psychotherapy, such as teaching and writing; expressing feelings about the work through creative activities, such as drawing or making music; establishing professional networks for vital interpersonal support; taking breaks within each day, across the week, and across months; creating an attractive and comfortable work environment; and finding capable clinical supervision or consultation. Some of these suggestions have been noted above as well.

Finally, Pearlman and Saakvitne (in press) have described some trauma-specific strategies for use in coping with VT. We describe and elaborate some of these in the box on the next page as they apply to traumatic-bereavement-related VT.

Strategies to Reduce Traumatic-Bereavement-Related VT

- *Manage exposure to trauma material*. In addition to limiting the number of weekly sessions or percentage of your caseload represented by traumatically bereaved clients, the following strategies for managing exposure may be helpful:
  - *Choose your listening distance*. Pearlman and Saakvitne (in press) note that you can choose to listen to potentially shocking stories from a distance, remaining connected to the client's experience while retaining an awareness of the present moment. You can imagine watching the terrible scene on a video screen and controlling the speed and volume as a way of feeling some control and regulating your responses (an Ericksonian technique), just as you might invite your clients to do.
  - *Choose whether to visualize*. Visualizing the story as the client tells it brings you into closer contact with potentially traumatizing material. Staying with the client and her feelings while she is recounting the story, rather than immersing yourself in the material, is a more therapeutic stance; as one therapist commented, "I have to keep one foot on the shore, or we'll both drown." If you choose to visualize, or find yourself doing so, try not to imagine the events happening to yourself, but stay grounded in the client's experience as she is reporting it to you.
  - *Stay connected to your inner resources*. Thinking about things you find comforting or soothing can help you regulate your internal states while sitting with a highly distraught client or listening to a gruesome account.
  - *Stay in the present*. Keeping in mind that the events the client is recounting took place in the past and that the client survived can be helpful. The loved one is deceased, but there is life in this room now, where your attention belongs.
- *Respond to signs and symptoms of VT*. Outside of sessions, monitor and manage intrusive imagery, avoidance, hyperarousal, dissociation, and loss of meaning.
  - *Use protective imagery*. You can change the intrusive imagery in your mind or add protective elements such as guard dogs or bodyguards to the scene.
  - *Regulate your nervous system*. Like your clients, you can use breathing, relaxation, and cognitive appraisal (or reframing) to calm your body and soothe your emotions.
  - *Notice changes in core beliefs*. In parallel with your clients, you can experience alterations in your beliefs related to your own and others' safety, trust, esteem, intimacy, and control. One way to notice such changes is to identify a theme in the aspects of the client's story that affect you most deeply. It's likely that troubling images or thoughts have tapped into your core beliefs. Understanding this will allow you to process and integrate the new information into your existing central beliefs. They usually become less intrusive and manageable this way. This work can lead to "vicarious posttraumatic growth" (Arnold, Calhoun, Tedeschi, & Cann, 2005).
  - *Stay connected*. A common experience among trauma survivors is a sense of disconnection. This can also be part of your experience of VT. Reconnecting with your inner experience and with supportive others is an important antidote to VT.

Based on Pearlman and Saakvitne (in press).

Transforming VT

In addition to coping with VT, we may be able to transform it. The hallmark of VT is disrupted spirituality. Hence the key to transforming VT is (re)connecting with and (re)discovering the intangible aspects of life and our participation in these nonmaterial aspects of life. This includes finding or creating meaning and reestablishing hope. To be clear, our assumption is that being human entails more than a material and tangible existence, and therefore that spirituality is an inherent quality of each of our lives. Neumann and Pearlman (1992) have defined *spirituality* as "an awareness of ephemeral aspects of life." Here we use the word *intangible* in place of *ephemeral*, as these spiritual issues may be enduring rather than transient. According to Neumann and Pearlman's research, spirituality includes meaning and hope, awareness of positive and negative aspects of life, valuing of nonmaterial aspects of life, and an open focus (i.e., a willingness to encounter all of life's offerings). If VT is the process of negative change within the self of a therapist, then transforming VT requires attention to the self, including inner experience (feelings, thoughts, beliefs, worldview, etc.) and transcendent experience (sense of meaning, hope, connection with something greater than oneself, etc.). In other words, it requires attention to spirituality, broadly understood.

Paths to developing this spirituality include activities and practices that cultivate an awareness of our connection with and participation in the intangible aspects of life: practicing meditation, reflection, or prayer; engaging in significant social or political movements (such as working to address some of the causes of sudden, traumatic death); participating in community; creating art; and being fully present in each moment.

Allowing the work to transform us through engaging with the pain and sorrow is another path to growth. Rather than trying not to feel the pain, opening ourselves to it and growing as human beings through the deeper comprehension of all dimensions of life and the interconnected web of human existence is a way of benefiting from the work. This engagement also allows us to offer those benefits to our clients. When we integrate our clients' pain into our own life experiences, we deepen our understanding of human strength and resilience. Through this process, we expand what we have to offer others who share their tragedies with us. We have referred to this effect as *vicarious transformation* (Pearlman & Caringi, 2009; Pearlman & Saakvitne, in press). You can use the checklist on pages 261–262 to assess how you are doing in your efforts to address VT.

TRAINING AND CONSULTATION: SUPPORTING YOURSELF IN THE WORK

Training and Continuing Education

When any of us takes on a new clinical population or wants to learn a new approach, we need more training. As we have described in Chapter 13, it can be useful to "build our weaker suits"—that is, to try to pick up training in less familiar areas. For this treatment approach, training in CBT; the treatment of complex trauma, grief, and bereavement; or relational psychotherapy can all be useful additions to a personal knowledge base.

Clinical Consultation

Self-awareness and good clinical consultation are essential for all therapists, especially those of us working with traumatically bereaved clients. You may find that at times, self-awareness may prompt you to refer a client elsewhere for services because the client's concerns are too close to your own unprocessed issues. In such situations, the most ethical and beneficial thing you can do for a client is to find someone else to help her. Of course, you must convey this plan with sensitivity to the possibility that the client will experience it as yet another loss over which she has no control. You might choose to say something like this: "The nature of your loss evokes something from my own experience that would make it difficult for me to give you the help you deserve. I'd like to refer to you to a colleague who I think can be more helpful to you."

A Checklist for Addressing Vicarious Traumatization (VT)

We invite you to photocopy this checklist and use it on a regular basis to increase your awareness of how you are addressing your VT. The activities below relate to working protectively, resting and playing, or transforming your VT.

In the space before each item, write the number of times you engaged in each activity in the past week. (Use your best estimate if you are uncertain.) At the end, add up your numbers to give yourself a total score. See how your scores compare across weeks and across months. Do you think you are making progress in addressing your VT?

During the past week, how many times have you . . .

_____   1. Engaged in a hobby, such as collecting or researching something not related to your work?

_____   2. Planned a trip or traveled to an interesting place?

_____   3. Engaged in a creative endeavor, such as writing, drawing, or quilting?

_____   4. Spent time with friends?

_____   5. Spent time with family?

_____   6. Consulted with colleagues?

_____   7. Asked for support from others?

_____   8. Used humor/laughed aloud?

_____   9. Discussed your reactions to your work with a colleague?

_____   10. Acknowledged how challenging this work is?

_____   11. Engaged in a new strategy for self-care (such as physical exercise, using social support, or getting away from your work regularly and frequently)?

_____   12. Engaged in new techniques for self-care (such as taking swimming lessons or going dancing) within an existing strategy (such as physical exercise)?

_____   13. Loafed around doing nothing?

_____   14. Written in a journal or participated in another form of self-exploration (such as seeking therapy or counseling)?

_____   15. Reflected on the rewards of working with traumatically bereaved clients?

_____   16. Thought about your work with traumatically bereaved clients within a theoretical framework?

_____   17. Attended to your own physical and emotional experience while sitting with clients?

_____   18. Focused on process (what you are doing with your clients) rather than outcomes (whether they are feeling better)?

(continued)

A Checklist for Addressing Vicarious Traumatization (VT) *(continued)*

_____ 19. Thought about and managed boundaries carefully?

_____ 20. Written progress notes after sessions with traumatically bereaved clients?

_____ 21. Used countertransference responses to promote a client's growth?

_____ 22. Done something between sessions that engages the body (e.g., stretching, moving) or the spirit (e.g., meditating)?

_____ 23. Intentionally changed your body posture or facial expression while sitting with a traumatically bereaved client, in order to manage mirroring (i.e., unconsciously mimicking the client's posture or expression)?

_____ 24. Engaged in professional work other than treating traumatically bereaved clients?

_____ 25. Taken breaks within each day? Across the week?

_____ 26. Increased the attractiveness or comfort of your work environment?

_____ 27. Engaged in clinical supervision or consultation for your work?

_____ 28. Engaged in meditation, reflection, or prayer?

_____ 29. Engaged in a significant social or political movement (such as addressing one of the causes of sudden, traumatic death)?

_____ 30. Engaged with one of your personal or professional communities, such as your faith community or professional society?

_____ 31. Noticed yourself being present in each moment?

_____ 32. Used more than one strategy to address VT?

A decision to refer is best made as early in the treatment as possible (when you become aware of the conflict), and after consultation with a colleague who can help you sort out your responses and develop a referral plan that is in the client's best interest.

Clinical consultation can also be useful when you are assessing your ability to stay present with a traumatically bereaved client. Rather than a one-time analysis, you must continually review your ability to engage effectively with the client. As described in the case of Paulo and Marta above, similarities or differences between a therapist's story and a client's can make it particularly difficult to stay present. Even experienced therapists who feel prepared to work with survivors of sudden, traumatic death can benefit from ongoing expert consultation when working with survivor clients (Pearlman & Saakvitne, 1995).

For example, Chris had been meeting with José for 5 weeks when she decided to seek consultation with a colleague. Conducting the integrated approach for traumatic bereavement was not new to her, and she had seen many clients who, like José, had lost a spouse. Chris was therefore surprised to find herself feeling remarkably sad during and after their sessions, as well as increasingly anxious more generally. She was relieved as soon as she made the call to Suni, a colleague with whom she had consulted many times before.

"So," said Suni, in the midst of their consultation session, "do you find yourself identifying with José in some way?" And just then, it hit her: Chris realized she was identifying with his dead wife! In other words, she was relating to her client, having empathy for him, as she would for her own husband if he were to experience her death. "Talk about close to home," thought Chris, and tears welled up in her eyes. Internally, Chris connected with her experience of cancer 2 years earlier, with her husband's fear and sadness, and with her own guilt about being sick. The sessions with José were triggering this whole experience, though it had been outside of her awareness until now. Meanwhile, Suni watched Chris's facial expressions and tears, and somehow felt that this sadness was connected with her experience of cancer. She was then able to offer her friend and colleague the support she needed to sort out her feelings and to channel her empathy to work effectively with José throughout the remainder of their treatment.

This example illustrates how a consultant can help identify a therapist's blind spots. A consultant can also suggest alternative clinical intervention approaches, self-care strategies, and other resources, as well as ways of working self-reflectively (Pearlman & Caringi, 2009). Good clinical consultation can also help to ameliorate VT.

Of course, the potentially powerful meanings and affects related to sudden, traumatic death can touch all of us, including those of us who have not experienced such a loss. In our view, informed ongoing clinical consultation is essential for all of us—therapists with and without sudden death histories, at all levels of experience and expertise—in order to support ethical and effective trauma treatment and to help us to thrive in our professional lives.

What constitutes good trauma therapy consultation? Here are some qualities that apply to therapist consultation related to the treatment of traumatic bereavement. (Pearlman & Saakvitne, 1995, also address this issue.)

- *Respectful.* Perhaps the most important element of a useful therapy consultation is that the consultant respect the therapist's knowledge, experience, positive intentions, and courage in opening his work to a consultant.
- *Collaborative.* In a relational therapy or therapy consultation, the parties share power. Each person understands where her own and the other's expertise lies, and seeks collaboration with the other.
- *Experienced.* Of course, the best consultant to a traumatic bereavement therapist is a professional psychotherapist who has experience with this population. A psychotherapist with experience in both loss and trauma and the combination of the two is likely to have a lot to offer. If such a person is not available, a consultant with trauma experience who is open to learning about traumatic loss, or one with bereavement experience who is open to learning about psychological trauma, will be the next best resource. Consultants with special expertise in CBT may also be extremely helpful.
- *Generous.* A useful consultant offers her expertise generously. That doesn't mean telling the therapist how to practice, but rather sharing information as well as her own clinical experience, including mistakes.

Another type of consulting arrangement that can be supportive is a peer support group. A group of clinicians who talk about their therapies (with their clients' consent) in a confidential professional forum can provide information, support, and opportunities for reflection on the work. This can also be a place to process countertransference responses. The group need not be one that works solely with traumatically bereaved clients or that works solely with this treatment approach. The essential element is that the participants develop mutual trust and respect, allowing them to give and receive constructive feedback.

REWARDS OF THE WORK

Working with traumatically bereaved clients has tremendous potential benefits for us as therapists. The most obvious benefit is the satisfaction that comes from being able to facilitate positive change in a client. It is a tremendous honor when clients entrust us with their pain, fear, grief, and vulnerability. When our clients achieve personal growth, we who have been their partners on that journey are also rewarded. Some of the clients who benefit from this treatment have been struggling, suffering, deadening themselves, living circumscribed lives for years. It's a wonderful experience to be part of positive change for such individuals.

In addition, mastering a complex treatment approach like this one is gratifying. Some of the elements of the approach are likely to be new to each of us. Learning stimulates us and keeps us engaged in our professional lives. We can integrate the information and skills gained from working this way into our work with other clients, expanding the benefits to others.

Finally, as we accompany our clients in their struggle for meaning, we will face questions of meaning in our own lives. Our clients' ability to endure their terrible losses can inspire a kind of *vicarious resilience* (Hernandez, Gangsei, & Engstrom, 2007). What makes life worth living? Why do we do the work we do, and how does it fit into the bigger picture? How can awareness of the finitude of life inform how we live the time we have left? Grappling with these issues deepens our humanity. What a gift to have a job that can do that!

CLINICAL INTEGRATION

Nathan saw a vaguely familiar number when he looked down at his buzzing phone. "Hello, this is Nathan," he said, unsure of who the caller might be.

"Hi, Nathan. It's Mala. Do you have a few minutes to talk?"

"Mala! Of course I have a few minutes for you. How are you?"

Mala described her recent fatigue and the related anxiety, which seemed to have something to do with her work. She described being confused by these feelings and asked whether Nathan had time to meet with her for some clinical consultation. They set up three appointments over the next month, and Mala felt her worry begin to lift.

Over the next few weeks, Mala and Nathan explored two specific clinical situations as the focus of their consultation. The first was Mala's supervision of a young woman who was finishing her social work internship at the clinic. Mala liked and identified with Keisha in many ways. She was confused, therefore, also to discover some resentment toward her, related to Keisha's struggles as a working mother. Keisha was trying to sort out whether she could continue this work and still be the kind of parent she wished to be to her three small children. She was spending some of her supervision with Mala trying to clarify this issue.

The second situation was a 5-month long therapy in which Mala was working with a traumatically bereaved client—a woman, Patty, whose son had died 3 days after birth. Whereas Mala usually found her work with bereaved clients to be especially fulfilling, she was having a difficult time with this therapy.

During one of their consultation sessions, Nathan asked Mala what she felt when sitting with Patty in her grief and mourning.

"I feel mostly numb," said Mala.

"OK. Stay with that numbness," coached Nathan. "Let the numbness—the lack of feeling—fill up space, and just allow yourself to be with it." Nathan paused to allow space for Mala's inner experience. "Now ask that space, 'What would be there if the numbness weren't?'"

Mala's closed eyes began to water. "There is so much sadness. And grief. It all feels so heavy." Nathan repeated back her words, allowing her to take in the feelings and connect with her new experience. He was aware that Mala had miscarried a pregnancy 2 years ago—a loss that was devastating for her at the time. Nathan found himself thinking about this, wondering whether Mala, too, was in touch with this loss.

"I'm thinking about my miscarriage," Mala said, and opened her eyes to meet Nathan's. Over the course of that hour, it became clear that she was experiencing a countertransference response in her work with Patty. She identified with Patty's grief and felt it as though it were her own. However, because Mala had worked with her grief at the time of her loss, her grief had been outside her awareness, so she hadn't been able to process much of what she had been experiencing in her work with Patty.

Clarity also began to emerge about a different yet related countertransference response within her supervisory work with Keisha. Mala felt jealousy toward Keisha because she was a mother. In part because she liked Keisha so much, and in part because she did not want to identify as a person who could feel jealous of someone for having children of her own, Mala had managed to push these feelings aside. Nathan's nonjudgmental attitude allowed her to accept these feelings more easily. Mala again felt relief upon naming the experiences she was having.

These first consultation sessions proved helpful to Mala. After continuing to consult with Nathan for an additional month, Mala noticed several shifts in her experience. First, her therapy with Patty deepened. Acknowledging her own grief to herself allowed her to process her losses. Once she began to do so, the need to repress the awareness of her miscarriage and her associated feelings dissipated, and she was free to use her emotional awareness to work more effectively with Patty. Second, she noticed that her resentment of Keisha also lifted. Rather than feeling jealousy toward Keisha, she focused on the truth of her disappointment about not having children of her own. Mala then felt more compassion for Keisha; she understood Keisha's concern that her work might negatively affect her availability to her children. The joy of supervisory work returned for Mala, and she started to conceptualize her work as a clinical supervisor as a way of engaging her own maternal instincts and energy.

A third important shift that occurred for Mala involved Nathan's observation that she was experiencing VT. Mala became more aware of how easily she identified with both clients and supervisees and how much she wished to help each group. She began to glimpse the ways in which her countertransference responses interacted with an overall sense of VT and compassion fatigue. She understood how these processes, when unrecognized, had contributed to a sense of futility and dread in her work, and how this had then precluded the productive use of countertransference reactions as well as her own self-care away from the office.

These insights inspired Mala to address VT and compassion fatigue more directly as she consults with other therapists. She came to appreciate how her own supervisory work contributed to the professional development and personal well-being of her colleagues—a realization that energized her ongoing work.

CONCLUDING REMARKS

Working with a traumatically bereaved population presents us with rewards and challenges. As we've discussed throughout this chapter, these challenges include effectively managing counter-transference responses and ideally transforming VT. These therapeutic phenomena can touch us at our core. As therapists, our own inner experiences, life challenges, and encounters with psychological transformation become part of our tool boxes. In other words, we use our *selves* to do our jobs. Doing this job ethically and effectively requires awareness of our own limitations and vulnerabilities, as well as sensitivity to the vicissitudes of our inner experience, behaviors, and habits. In this chapter, we have outlined some of the factors that contribute to countertrans-ference and some sources of VT with this particular population. We have also offered strategies for addressing both.

The example of Mala demonstrates how countertransference and VT can manifest them-selves, how they can interact with one another, and how helpful clinical consultation can be in addressing these phenomena. Like our clients, we can become stuck in our own processes of moving through a situation, a therapy, or a challenging time in life. It is the very nature of our professional role to overlap with personal experience, and it is up to us to bring awareness and sensitivity to this. We owe it to ourselves and to our clients.

In concluding this chapter and this book, we'd like to emphasize a point that we have alluded to within this chapter. We hope that both clients and therapists who work with this treatment approach will encounter *spirituality*, as defined by Neumann and Pearlman (1992) to include meaning and hope, awareness of positive and negative aspects of life, valuing of nonma-terial aspects of life, and openness to all of life's offerings. In many cases, a traumatic death will evoke these issues and related questions for survivors, regardless of what they do with the vari-ous elements named above. Likewise, as therapists who work with survivors of loss, trauma, or traumatic death, we are likely to experience such spiritual elements within our work. Working actively with these issues and related questions and exploring paths to developing spirituality (e.g., meditation or creating community) can contribute to satisfaction and self-care within the challenging work we do. It is our sincere hope that the information provided throughout this text also contributes to your confidence, satisfaction, and self-care in your traumatic bereave-ment work and beyond.

Handouts

This Appendix contains handouts referred to in the text, which are also available on the website (*www.guilford.com/pearlman-materials*). You can photocopy these handouts or download them. There is also a list of supplement handouts that are available only on the website. Permission to photocopy the handouts is granted to purchasers of this book for personal use only.

Some of these are psychoeducational in nature; others are rich in detailed exercises for independent activities that will help the client move through the treatment. Although the handouts are written for the client, many provide useful information for you, the therapist, as well. You may use them in any order or combination. We present them here in this order to provide an overview of the treatment's flow, rather than to prescribe an exact sequence for their use. Permission to photocopy the handouts is granted to purchasers of this book for personal use only; additional copies can be downloaded from the website supplement.

LIST OF APPENDIX HANDOUTS

Nine additional handouts are available for downloading at this same website supplement *only* (*www.guilford.com/pearlman-materials*). These handouts have numbers beginning with S (Handout S1, etc.) and do not appear in this Appendix.

Sudden, Traumatic Death and Traumatic Bereavement

Human life continually involves loss. All change—whether positive or negative, wanted or unwanted—involves loss. Few losses in life are as painful as the sudden, traumatic death of a significant other. (We use the terms "significant other," "deceased," and "loved one" interchangeably throughout these handouts.) We hope that in reading this handout, you'll recognize at least some of the difficulties you have been experiencing, and will see that others have had similar problems. We also want you to know that you have every reason to expect things to get better—that you can get a handle on these problems, diminish their effect on you, and regain a footing for proceeding with your life.

TYPICAL, ON-TIME DEATHS VERSUS SUDDEN, TRAUMATIC DEATHS

In addressing how the death of a loved one affects people, psychologists often distinguish between *typical, on-time* and *sudden, traumatic* deaths. Typical, on-time deaths include those that we expect to occur during the course of our lives, such as the death of an elderly parent from natural causes. Following such a death, it is common to experience grief and mental anguish. Feelings associated with grief typically include an overwhelming sense of loss, as well as strong yearning or longing for the person who has died. It is common for survivors to feel a profound sense of emptiness, as though a part of them had died. They often lose interest in the world around them. In many cases, they speak of generalized pain or heaviness in the chest. In addition, they may cry easily, find it difficult to eat, and experience physical symptoms such as headaches or stomachaches. Although these symptoms can be painful and debilitating, they typically subside within several months to a year or so after the death.

Evidence suggests that the psychological repercussions following a sudden, traumatic death are very different from those of a typical, on-time death. The survivors of a sudden, traumatic death usually experience all of the sadness and emptiness associated with grief, as well as a host of trauma symptoms. Many survivors develop symptoms of *posttraumatic stress disorder* (PTSD). They may have intrusive thoughts, flashbacks (feeling as if the terrible experience is happening all over again), or nightmares about the events surrounding the death. They may do things to avoid confronting the pain associated with the loss, such as staying away from activities or places related to the significant other's death, or numbing themselves emotionally. In the wake of a sudden loss, people may have difficulty sleeping or concentrating, find they're more irritable and more easily startled, worry that something bad may happen to another loved one, and catch themselves repeatedly scanning the environment for danger.

The combination of grief and trauma symptoms can overwhelm a person's capacity to cope. Because sudden, traumatic deaths occur without warning, they provide a shock to the system that can have lasting psychological, physical, and spiritual effects. Unlike most typical, on-time losses, traumatic deaths often cause intense distress that continues over an extended period of time.

(continued)

TRAUMATIC BEREAVEMENT: TRAUMA AND GRIEF SYMPTOMS

Following a sudden, traumatic death, survivors' lives are often shattered as they attempt to cope with the tragedy and its aftermath. Feelings of safety, security, and trust can be deeply undermined. Survivors usually experience powerful feelings of confusion and anxiety, as well as the depression and mental anguish typically associated with grief. Trauma symptoms may include feelings of horror and anxiety on the one hand, and a sense of disconnection and feelings of unreality, on the other. Some people cannot remember significant parts of what happened; others are plagued by memories or feel as if they are reexperiencing or reliving the event through painful flashbacks.

In general, survivors of a traumatic death may find it extremely difficult to move on with life—for example, by pursuing new interests. They may start to behave in ways that are not in their best interest, such as increasing their use of alcohol or other drugs. In many cases, these symptoms, along with the grief symptoms described above, interfere with the survivor's ability to function in many domains of life. The loss may place great stress on the survivor's relationship with her spouse and surviving children. Such symptoms can also have an adverse impact on the survivor's performance at work. Relationships with other family members and friends are also likely to suffer. This occurs in part because those in their social environment do not know what to say or do. As a result, survivors of traumatic loss often find themselves withdrawing from others and spending more time alone.

Survivors of traumatic death must contend with a number of additional issues that are difficult and painful:

1. It is much harder to accept the death of a loved one if it occurred suddenly and without warning. When a death comes about as a result of natural causes, the surviving family members have the opportunity to prepare for what lies ahead, and to say goodbye. This is not the case with a sudden, traumatic death. In most cases, family members learn of the death after it has occurred. There is no chance to prepare for the death or to convey feelings of love. Survivors are shocked and overwhelmed by what has happened. Consequently, it is hard for them to accept the death. They may know intellectually that their significant other is dead, but find themselves expecting that person to walk through the door or call on the telephone. This makes it difficult for the mourning process to begin. Difficulty accepting the death is one reason why it can be so hard to part with the significant other's possessions.

2. Survivors have to contend not only with the death of their loved one, but with the shattering of their most basic assumptions about the world. These include beliefs that the world is predictable and controllable, that the world is meaningful and operates according to principles of fairness and justice, and that they and the people they love are safe. The shattering of these core assumptions can have a profound impact on subsequent life. Many people question the value of working toward long-term goals because they know that they can lose everything important to them in an instant. Survivors of a traumatic death that was caused by another person are also likely to have difficulty trusting others, since they may believe that the person who caused the death could not be trusted.

3. Following a traumatic death, survivors typically report that they are unable to make any sense of, or find any meaning in, what has happened. This adds to the distress they experience as a result of their loved one's death.

4. In many cases, the sudden, traumatic death of a loved one can undermine faith in a loving, caring God. Many survivors cannot understand why God failed to protect their loved one. This can result in anger, disillusionment, and feelings of betrayal.

(continued)

5. People who lose a loved one under traumatic circumstances are typically preoccupied with issues of causality, responsibility, and blame. They may feel that someone should be held accountable for the death, and they may become angry if nothing is done. If there is evidence that the death resulted from the actions of a specific person, survivors may feel angry if that person fails to acknowledge what he did. They may also experience anger toward the perpetrator if he fails to show remorse. In addition, it is common for them to experience self-blame and guilt. People may ruminate about ways they could or should have prevented the death or how they could have rescued the person. They may also experience guilt about events that occurred prior to the death, such as having an argument with the deceased.

6. Depending on how the death occurred, survivors may believe that it resulted from the negligence of others. Survivors usually judge such deaths as preventable, which results in intense feelings of anger. They typically conclude that if the person who caused the death were acting responsibly, the death would not have occurred. In deaths of this sort, survivors often struggle with the injustice of what has happened to their loved one.

7. It is common for survivors of a traumatic death to be preoccupied with what their loved one's final moments were like, and whether their loved one suffered. This is especially the case when the death resulted from a violent incident and when there was damage to the loved one's body.

Survivors of a loved one who dies of natural causes rarely encounter these problems. They constitute a special burden for those who experience a traumatic loss.

MOURNING

Mourning refers to the active processes of coping with a death and its implications. It is what a person does to contend with and adapt to the death, making necessary changes in order to accommodate or reconcile themselves to the loss. The active processes of mourning involve change, as well as remembering and integrating what was lost. They will have an impact on your relationship with your deceased significant other and with the world. Traumatic bereavement creates obstacles to these natural, active processes. This treatment is designed to help and support you through the mourning processes.

Because people suffering from traumatic bereavement must come to terms with the death of their significant other, as well as the manner in which it occurred, it can take longer than expected for the painful feelings and thoughts to diminish. As the initial shock of the death dissipates, there may be intervals when a survivor is able to focus on other issues and not feel the pain of the loss so intensely. Gradually, these intervals will become longer, and there will be good days and bad days. Over time, the proportion of good days to bad days typically increases. However, people can experience setbacks during the process. On a relatively good day, a bereaved person may encounter a reminder of the significant other—for example, hearing a favorite song of the loved one—and this may cause the reemergence of painful feelings of loss. People also have difficulty dealing with occasions such as holidays, birthdays, and the anniversary date of the death.

(continued)

WHAT CAN YOU DO TO HELP YOURSELF?

You and your therapist will focus on these issues when you meet. But there are some things you could do now. For example, because grief can affect physical health, it is important to maintain adequate nutrition, sleep, and physical exercise. If you have any chronic health problems (such as heart disease), it's especially important to stay in contact with your primary physician. Survivors are often preoccupied by their grief, and thus are prone to mishaps such as automobile accidents. So use extra care. Similarly, it may be best to avoid making any major decisions for 6–12 months after the death, if possible. As a result of everything that you have been through, your judgment may be compromised. Further life changes, even those you choose, can bring on additional stress. Now is a time to take a break from big decisions, if you can.

Most experts recommend that survivors confide in someone about the death. This can be a friend, a member of the clergy, or another person who has experienced a similar loss. It may take some trial and error to identify people who can be good listeners. Since many people do not know what to say or do to be helpful, they may say the "wrong" thing. Some survivors withdraw from social contact because of the possibility of such hurtful comments. This is unfortunate because it cuts them off from interactions that could be healing.

Mourning is a difficult process in part because it involves remembering what happened. The memories may be so upsetting that it can seem like more than you can bear. Hence it is important for you to learn strategies for calming yourself. You and your therapist can talk about this when you meet, but strategies others have found useful include taking a walk, exercising, listening to calming music, or meditating.

The kind of work you will do with your therapist is designed to support you through the mourning process. The treatment will help you process the traumatic elements of your loved one's death and find ways to learn to live with your loss, to work toward maintaining positive connections with your support system, and to learn coping strategies that will help you to move forward.

Orientation to the Treatment

This treatment will help you process the loss and develop coping strategies that will allow you to move forward.

WHAT THIS TREATMENT INCLUDES

➢ *Evidence-based approaches.* Each element of the treatment is based on research evidence showing that it can help people who have experienced a traumatic loss.

➢ *Psychoeducation.* Your therapist will share information with you about trauma, loss, mourning, and coping. In addition to discussions in sessions, your therapist will give you handouts that summarize important aspects of what you need for recovery.

➢ *Structure.* Your therapist may direct the treatment with a list of tasks the two of you will complete during each session. Alternatively, the two of you may collaborate in structuring each session.

➢ *Supported exposure.* The treatment provides opportunities for you to confront what you've found difficult to face, with lots of support. Your therapist will invite you to think, talk, and write about your loved one, the loved one's death, and how you have been affected by the loss. This probably sounds scary, but the treatment is designed so that you will be ready for those tasks when the time comes.

➢ *Developing skills and resources.* The treatment will help you develop coping skills (feelings skills, thinking skills, etc.), as well as techniques to address beliefs about yourself or the world that keep you stuck in your grief, and techniques for obtaining interpersonal or social support. The goal of this treatment is to help you develop skills that will be useful to you during the treatment and after it ends.

WHAT TO EXPECT OF YOUR THERAPIST

➢ *Preparation.* Your therapist will be familiar with the concepts and tasks that you will address during each session.

➢ *Direction.* Throughout the treatment, your therapist will serve as your guide, and also as a source of support.

➢ *Collaboration.* Your therapist is your partner in your recovery process.

➢ *Respect.* Although your therapist knows what helps people who have experienced sudden, traumatic losses, you are the expert on you.

(continued)

YOUR ROLE

➢ *Show up.* Come to each session ready to stay focused on the tasks.
➢ *Work between sessions.* This treatment requires you to engage in various activities between sessions. These independent activities are essential to the success of the treatment, and will also provide you with tools you can use in the future.

WHAT YOU'LL TAKE AWAY ("TOOLS FOR THE JOURNEY")

➢ New skills.
➢ Emotional freedom.
➢ A new orientation to your loved one and your loss.
➢ A sense of accomplishment and empowerment.
➢ Lots of handouts!

THINGS TO REMEMBER

➢ You are the best judge of how you're doing.
➢ Your therapist can only help with what you can share or discuss in sessions.
➢ You may feel worse before you feel better.
➢ Staying in treatment is a choice . . . but don't give up without giving it your best effort and letting your therapist help you through any rough patches.

Treatment Goals and Tools

This handout describes the primary goals of the treatment, the "R" processes that you will move through as you mourn, the treatment tools, and the independent activities.

TREATMENT GOALS

The *goals of the treatment* refer to where you are heading: the desired destination or endpoint of the treatment.

➤ To feel better.
➤ To honor your loved one and the relationship you had with this person.
➤ To move forward in your life in healthy, growth-promoting ways.

SIX "R" PROCESSES: STEPS TO MOVE THROUGH IN YOUR MOURNING

The *six "R" processes of mourning* are the steps that bereaved survivors take during the mourning process. These steps overlap, and you may find that you move through some of them more than once.

➤ *Recognize the loss.*
➤ *React to the separation.*
➤ *Recollect and reexperience your loved one and the relationship you had.*
➤ *Relinquish your old attachments to your loved one and your old assumptive world.*
➤ *Readjust to move adaptively into the new world without forgetting the old.* (This includes establishing a new, healthy relationship with your loved one, and integrating your particular loss so that you can move forward in a healthy way.)
➤ *Reinvest.*

TREATMENT TOOLS

Treatment tools are the techniques that you and your therapist will use to move through the six "Rs" and achieve your treatment goals. You will use these tools within sessions and you will practice with them outside of sessions, so that when the treatment is over, you'll be able to take them with you and use them on your own when needed. They include different types of activities, as described below.

(continued)

Resource-Building Activities

Resource-building activities will support you through the pain and challenges of mourning, processing the trauma, and moving through the treatment more generally. You may recognize these activities more generally as *coping activities*. You and your therapist will do some of these activities in session, and you will practice them outside sessions as well. They include the following:

➤ *Social support activities.* These involve building and maintaining positive connections with others.
➤ *Feelings skills and coping activities.* These involve learning new coping strategies that will assist you in managing strong or distressing feelings and taking care of yourself. You and your therapist will also address stressful bereavement-related problems (such as, coping with holidays, anniversaries, and birthdays).
➤ *Activities for goals, values, and meaning.* These include identifying your personal goals and values, exploring how the loss has changed you and your life, and allowing you to make conscious decisions about moving forward and honoring your loved one. These activities will also help you focus on what is meaningful in your life now, which can facilitate the healing process.

Trauma-Processing Activities

➤ *Cognitive processing.* This involves modifying distressing things that you say to yourself about the loss. You and your therapist will work together to notice and change the thoughts, beliefs, and interpretations that may be automatic for you, but that may inhibit the process of mourning your loss.
➤ *Emotional processing.* This entails experiencing your full range of feelings and memories about your loss. The treatment will enable you to experience and express feelings that, at an earlier point, were hard to face.

The six "R" processes are adapted from T. A. Rando (2014). *Coping with the sudden death of your loved one: A self-help handbook for traumatic bereavement.* Indianapolis, IN: Dog Ear. Used with permission.

Self-Care

Self-care means nurturing and caring for your body, mind, and spirit. It can also mean reducing the frequency of any harmful things that you do, such as overusing alcohol or other drugs. It involves working toward eating regular meals, exercising, getting enough rest, avoiding reliance on substances that compromise your health, taking time for yourself, and doing things that help you relax and restore your energy for the many tasks you are facing. Self-care requires *boundary setting*—saying yes to activities that help nurture and sustain you, and saying no to those that do not.

It is important that you recognize those things you already do to take care of yourself. The goal is to add self-care routines to your life in small steps. Making small changes that you can stick with is the key to long-lasting change. Many of the activities assigned in this treatment promote self-care.

INDEPENDENT ACTIVITY: SELF-CARE

Engage in one self-care activity this week, writing down this and any other activities you have done during the week in an effort to care for yourself.

Exploring the Impact of the Death

The goal of this exercise is for you to begin to think about what your loss means to you. Please write a statement about the impact that this loss has had on you. Some things to consider as you write include your understanding of why the death occurred and the effect it has had on your beliefs about yourself, others, and the world.

It is best to write during a time when you can experience your emotions fully. Try to find a time and place in which you can write without interruption. Try not to worry about whether your writing is neat or grammatically correct. Write as much as you want, but write at least one or two pages. You can use the blank space below to get started.

The Six "R" Processes of Mourning

The six "R" processes of mourning are an essential element of this treatment approach. We list them here in detail. After each "R" process, we list the subprocesses that promote healthy movement through the "Rs."

➢ *Recognize the loss.*
  • Acknowledge the death.
  • Understand the death.
➢ *React to the separation.*
  • Experience the pain.
  • Feel, identify, accept, and express your reactions to the loss.
  • Identify and mourn your secondary losses.
➢ *Recollect and reexperience your loved one and the relationship you had.*
  • Review and remember realistically.
  • Revive and reexperience the feelings.
➢ *Relinquish your old attachments to your loved one and your old assumptive world.*
  • Let go of your old attachments to the person who has died.
  • Let go of your old attachments to your assumptive world.
➢ *Readjust to move adaptively into the new world without forgetting the old.*
  • Revise your assumptive world.
  • Develop a new relationship with your loved one.
  • Adopt new ways of being in the world.
  • Form a new identity.
➢ *Reinvest.*

From T. A. Rando (2014). *Coping with the sudden death of your loved one: A self-help handbook for traumatic bereavement.* Indianapolis, IN: Dog Ear. Reprinted with permission.

Breathing Retraining

When people feel anxious, they often start to take in quick, shallow breaths. This rapid, shallow breathing (known as *chest breathing*) is associated with a number of uncomfortable sensations, including tightness or pressure in the throat or chest, dry mouth, dizziness, tingling in the fingers, and the sensation that one's heart is racing. All of these sensations contribute to an increase in feelings of fear or anxiety. Something as simple as learning to slow down your breathing can help you to stop feelings of anxiety as soon as they start.

INDEPENDENT ACTIVITY: BREATHING RETRAINING

This exercise will help you teach yourself to slow down your breathing so that you can relax and decrease your anxiety.

- ❖ Breathe in through your nose with your mouth closed, to a slow count of 4.
- ❖ Exhale slowly through your nose, to a slow count of 4.
- ❖ At the beginning of the exhale, say "calm" before counting to 4.
- ❖ After exhaling, count to 4 slowly before inhaling again.
- ❖ Repeat for 10 inhale–exhale–wait cycles at each practice session.

It is important to practice this exercise at least twice a day when you are feeling calm, especially when you first begin. Once this type of breathing has become familiar to you, you will often find it useful in stressful situations, both in session and between sessions.

Based on Foa and Rothbaum (1998).

Feelings Skills

Feelings skills are inner abilities that help people remain internally steady in times of distress. A loss often brings up strong emotions. For this reason, feelings skills are a foundational part of this treatment. Having specific skills to deal with intense or even overwhelming emotions will help you to experience your emotions more fully and with less discomfort or fear. These skills will help you throughout this treatment and recovery process.

There are three feelings skills that are essential to this internal steadiness: *inner connection* (which helps people to stay connected to images and memories of loved ones), *self-worth* (which helps people to maintain a generally positive and stable sense of being "good enough" individuals), and *feelings management* (which helps people to handle strong feelings). We describe each of these skills and ways to build them below.

INNER CONNECTION

Inner connection is the feelings skill that allows us all to carry images and memories of loved ones with us, even in their absence. When we wonder what a beloved grandparent, former teacher, or friend might say, we may hear words of love, comfort, or support that reflect a strong sense of inner connection with these "loving others." That connection can help us through challenging times, guiding us and enabling us to feel less lonely.

Why Is Developing or Maintaining Inner Connection Difficult?

People who didn't experience much love or affection when they were growing up may not have many positive or loving figures to draw on in times of distress. Even if you have had loving connections with others, you may feel sadness, guilt, or anger when you think of your deceased loved one. This can get in the way of feeling that person's love and support for you.

How Can You Develop or Maintain Inner Connection?

It's important to be creative in thinking about who your "loving others" are. Such a figure may be a friend or family member, a former teacher or clergyperson, a pet, an admired public person, or an imaginary character. The "other" doesn't have to be alive, and you may never have met.

If one of your "loving others" is deceased, thinking about that person may bring sorrow or other feelings. If so, you might want to try to allow yourself to feel the emotions and try to keep this person's love with you while reminding yourself of loving things the person would say to you and the special connections you had with each other.

(continued)

Exercises for Strengthening Inner Connection

You can strengthen your sense of inner connection with your "loving others" by practicing calling upon them in your imagination when you feel good. Then when you need support, it will be easier to draw on this resource.

INDEPENDENT ACTIVITY: INNER CONNECTION

❖ Find a quiet spot to sit where you can be comfortable and uninterrupted for at least 20 minutes.

❖ Write down the names of three positive figures (for example, people you know or have known; animals; figures from history, public life, religion, or fiction).

❖ Imagine one of these characters comforting, encouraging, or supporting you. What advice might this individual give you about yourself, your behaviors, your relationship with your loved one, and your life? How might this person demonstrate understanding or compassion for you?

❖ When you finish imagining, take one of these positive words or phrases and repeat it to yourself several times. Then practice using that phrase when you feel lonely or lost.

SELF-WORTH

Feeling worthy or deserving of life and good fortune even when times are difficult is a sign of positive *self-worth*. It comes from a *secure base* or deeply felt sense of security in childhood, where adults treat children with love, compassion, and respect. As children grow up, they take in that positive regard and come to feel "good enough" about themselves. It doesn't mean never having a bad day or feeling bad, but it does mean that even when people feel bad, they know (or can recall) that they are still reasonably good human beings. When they do something they know is wrong, they feel guilty. Guilt is a natural, and sometimes even useful, feeling. It's easy to confuse bad feelings about what you did or did not do (guilt) with bad feelings about yourself as a person.

Why Is Developing or Maintaining Self-Worth Difficult?

People who grew up in homes where adults or peers were unsupportive or harsh may have taken in negative messages about themselves. This makes it difficult for them to feel like "good enough" persons, especially when things go wrong. It may be natural to move to self-blame or feelings of worthlessness when bad things happen.

How Can You Develop or Maintain Self-Worth?

Associating with people who respect you, treat you with dignity, and bring out the best in you is an important way to develop a sense of self-worth. In addition, treating yourself with respect, doing things that are consistent with a positive self-image, and not doing things that diminish you in your

(continued)

own eyes can increase your self-worth. Acknowledging your mistakes, apologizing, and making amends when you do something wrong can help to build your sense of self-worth as well. Building skills and developing your knowledge and talents can also contribute. Finally, helping others and treating them with respect, compassion, and dignity can increase your own self-worth.

Exercises for Strengthening Self-Worth

The next time you are in the company of someone who likes you, ask yourself what that person values about you. You may also ask that person the same question.

Notice how you feel when you offer someone else assistance or support. What does that say about you as a person?

INDEPENDENT ACTIVITY: SELF-WORTH

❖ Make some notes about the kind of person you would like to be—your "best self." This is your *ego ideal*, something to which you aspire. When you consider various actions in advance, try to follow the path to your best self. As you act according to this path, your sense of value and self-respect will grow.

❖ Think about something you did (or did not do) about which you feel bad or guilty.

- Write for a few minutes about what happened, why you made the decision or acted as you did, and what your subsequent thoughts have been about your choices.
- Think about or write down a few things you might do to make up for your mistake.
- Identify one or two things that seem possible to do and not too challenging.
- Experiment by doing one of these things, and see whether you feel better about yourself.

FEELINGS MANAGEMENT

Feelings management refers to the ways people cope with emotions that are particularly challenging. (We use *feelings* and *emotions* interchangeably here.) When most people experience happiness, they will express it easily. An emotion such as anger may be more difficult for some people to express, especially if the anger is powerful. If they have trouble experiencing intense anger, they may "bury" it or try to pretend it's not there. Some people are so good at this that they aren't even aware that they are angry.

Emotions—even strong ones—help you to stay connected to yourself, to others, and to the world. This is important because emotions provide you with information about both the world around you and how you relate to that world. If you are feeling angry, for example, this feeling might reveal that there was an injustice or that someone wronged you. Your anger might be a way of recognizing and standing up to the injustice. If you are not aware of it, however, you will miss this connection.

There are four steps involved in feelings management, each of which will be important to you throughout this treatment and beyond. The steps are *recognizing, tolerating, modulating,* and *integrating* feelings.

(continued)

Recognizing Feelings

Recognizing feelings means being able to sense emotions as they arise in your body and to label or name them. You may find this step to be easy, difficult, or somewhere in between. You may also find that you are able to recognize some feelings more readily than others. Past experiences may help you to identify a specific emotion. You may know that a particular type of experience (such as loss) is often connected with a certain feeling (such as sadness). These links can be another pathway to recognizing your feelings.

INDEPENDENT ACTIVITIES: RECOGNIZING FEELINGS

1. **Create a feelings vocabulary.** Begin to create a feelings vocabulary by learning the names of feelings and beginning to attach those names to your bodily states. Below is a list of feelings that may help you begin to name your feelings. Use this list to check those you are aware of once or more per day.

___ angry	___ irritated	___ helpless
___ restless	___ numb	___ lonely
___ heartbroken	___ aching	___ vulnerable
___ enraged	___ regretful	___ detached
___ anxious	___ overwhelmed	___ in despair
___ ashamed	___ lost	___ crushed
___ preoccupied	___ exhausted	___ empty
___ isolated	___ annoyed	___ bitter
___ sorrowful	___ in agony	___ frustrated
___ sad	___ confused	___ guilty
___ depressed	___ hopeless	___ embarrassed
___ insecure	___ nervous	___ scared
___ proud	___ disgusted	___ hurt
___ excited	___ mad	___ panicky
___ happy	___ frightened	___ disappointed
___ cheerful	___ loving	___ eager
___ depleted	___ humiliated	___ calm
___ content		

2. **Link names of feelings with bodily sensations.** Once you become acquainted with names of feelings, you can pay attention to how each feeling is present in your body. For example, sorrow may feel like a pit in your stomach. Another person might feel sorrow as tightness in the throat.

3. **Create a feelings intensity scale.** That is, assign levels to each feeling state. For example, someone can feel frustrated, irked, annoyed, irritated, angry, or enraged—all of which are different intensities of the emotion often labeled *anger*.

4. **Differentiate feelings from actions.** Whereas *anger* is a feeling, *violence* is an action. *Sad* is a feeling that might go with the action of *withdrawing*. See whether you can create a list of actions you engaged in today, and then list some feelings that might go along with those actions.

(continued)

These associations or connections can vary from one day to the next. So being withdrawn today might have to do with feeling sad, while being withdrawn on another day might have to do with feeling lonely or angry.

5. **Pay attention to your body.** A tight throat or chest may signal anxiety or fear. Practicing labeling certain bodily sensations, and talking about this with your therapist or another person, will help you to learn which emotions go with different bodily sensations for you. You may find that it is difficult to notice your bodily sensations as you go through your day. The following exercises can help you slow down and focus enough to become aware of what your body feels.

❖ *Sit quietly and let your attention go to what you are currently feeling in your body.* Focus your attention on any place in your body where you notice a physical sensation. What is the name of the sensation (tightness, pain, ache, etc.)? Do this again for each place in your body where you have a sensation.

❖ *Notice your breath.* Attend to how the air feels coming in and out of your body. See whether you can feel the air entering your nostrils, lungs, and diaphragm. Notice how your body feels as the air moves in and out. Write down any names of emotions that come into your mind as you breathe.

❖ *Move your body.* First, move gently—standing up and swaying back and forth, dancing to some music, or bending and reaching. Stop and notice sensations in your body. Let your mind create some names of emotions that might match those sensations. Then try moving vigorously. Walk briskly around the block or do some jumping jacks. When you slow down and then stop, look again for physical sensations, and create emotion names to go with them.

❖ *Go back to the checklist above (see Activity 1 in this box) and check off the feelings that you are currently experiencing.* Circle the three that are most intense right now.

Tolerating Feelings

Tolerating feelings means being able to accept and work with emotions as they arise. The following exercises can help you learn to tolerate feelings.

INDEPENDENT ACTIVITY: TOLERATING FEELINGS

❖ *Name early associations (thoughts, images, memories) that you have to a particular emotion.* Understanding what might have made feelings *seem* negative or dangerous can be a helpful step toward tolerating them. This step will also be easier if you can step back from the emotion a bit and observe, name, and discuss it.

❖ *Understand what current situation triggered the emotion.* Once the emotion begins to make sense, you can recognize that it is here for a reason and move closer to accepting and even welcoming it.

(continued)

❖ *Try to name associations among feelings (your emotions), thoughts (ideas, things you tell your-self), and behaviors (things you do).* Observe any thoughts that accompany the feeling as well as any behaviors that seem to result from, express, or disguise it in some way.

❖ *Remind yourself that feelings provide useful information.* This acknowledgment helps to make them less scary and to remind you that your feelings make sense.

❖ *Know that emotions exist on a continuum of intensity and always run their course.* The next time you have a feeling that you can recognize, take a moment to notice where that feeling is located in your body. See whether you can identify a color, a shape, a sound or song, an animal, or an object that represents the feeling. Try to recall a time in the past when you felt this emotion. See whether you can recall how long the feeling lasted, what intensified or diminished it, and how it began to ebb.

Modulating Feelings

Modulating feelings entails being able to control the intensity of what you experience, rather than feeling as if the emotion is controlling you. The first step in modulating feelings is to notice that your feelings have *different levels of intensity*. For example, when you're upset, you may be very upset or just a little bit upset. Noticing what's going on in your body is one way of observing your levels of upset. The more intense your feelings are, the more likely you are to have strong bodily sensations. Of course, some people have learned not to feel, in which case numbing may be a sign of intense feelings.

INDEPENDENT ACTIVITIES: MODULATING FEELINGS

❖ *Breathe.* Breathing is a key to modulating strong feelings. The next time you are distressed, try to focus on your breath. After 10 long, slow breaths, see whether the intensity of your feeling has changed. You might also try the breathing retraining exercise described in Handout 7.

❖ *Name your feelings.* Being able to name feelings also helps in modulating them. For instance, if you know *that* you are sad, you may have some ideas about *why* you are sad and what may help you to regulate your sorrow.

❖ *Describe the intensity of the feeling.* The next time you are aware of an emotion, write down its intensity on a scale from 1 (very mild) to 10 (very strong). At the end of one of the following exercises, come back and rate the intensity of that emotion again.

❖ *Examine the emotion.* Choose an emotion that you experienced very recently. Try to figure out when you started feeling this way and what was going on around you, between you and other people, and within yourself.

  • Write down the name of the feeling, and then write down what happened and what you were thinking about just before you started feeling it.

  • Ask yourself, "What is this feeling trying to tell me?" and write down any responses that come up for you.

❖ *Choose a calming word or a phrase.* You can say this to yourself when you notice the impulse to run away from or bury a feeling. For example, it can be helpful to say, "Calm," "Breathe,"

(continued)

"It's only a feeling," "Feelings can't harm me," or "The name of this feeling is _____.
Its intensity is __ (1 to 10). That feeling is difficult for me because _____."

❖ *Imagine that your feeling is on a video or audio recording.* You can regulate the intensity of your feeling by turning the volume down, rewinding or fast-forwarding it, or letting it play more slowly. You can practice turning it up, down, off, or on.

❖ *Choose to do something constructive or soothing.* When you need help modulating a specific emotion, pick a soothing alternative activity and engage in it. This might include playing your favorite music, watching a favorite movie, going for a walk, praying, meditating, connecting with nature, reading poetry, working in the garden, or the like.

❖ *Connect with someone who cares.* Sometimes talking with a friend about what's going on for you can help you modulate your feelings. At other times, you may simply want to spend time with a friend or family member, not necessarily talking, so that you don't have to be alone with your feelings.

Integrating Feelings

Integrating feelings means connecting emotions with their context and incorporating them into the narrative or story of your life. You can learn to integrate your feelings by paying attention to the broad context of the feeling. Spend some time exploring a particular emotion within the context of your life story. This can happen within therapy, within an intimate relationship with a supportive other, or by yourself.

INDEPENDENT ACTIVITY: INTEGRATING FEELINGS

Journal writing (which is a way of speaking to yourself) can help enormously with integrating feelings. Try writing about a situation in which you noticed a particular feeling. Allow your writing to lead you, and try not to worry about whether the writing makes sense as you write. Choose a particular feeling that you had in the past day or two, and try to answer the following questions about that feeling:

❖ Where do you experience that particular feeling in your body?

❖ What was the context that gave rise to the feeling?

❖ What are some of your past experiences of the feeling?

❖ When do you remember experiencing this feeling before? What was going on then?

❖ Are you aware of a connection between this feeling and any physical or psychological needs you may have?

❖ With what information does this feeling provide you?

❖ What new thoughts or feelings come up for you now as you reflect on the context of this feeling?

❖ What does this feeling say about you as a person?

❖ Can you see how this feeling might fit into your identity and life in the future?

A Model for Change

The following diagram illustrates the model on which the next part of this treatment is based.

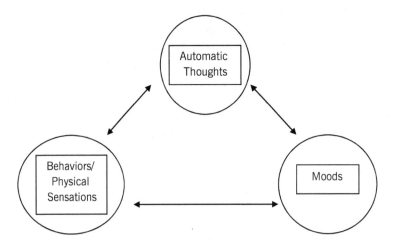

This model illustrates the idea that thoughts, moods, behaviors, and physical sensations all influence each other. You can learn to question the habitual or automatic thoughts that have a negative impact on your mood, behavior, and physical well-being. We call these *automatic thoughts* because you may not even be aware of having them. Automatic thoughts can become part of a negative loop in which a thought leads to negative emotions, uncomfortable physical reactions, and behaviors that create a vicious cycle. The process of identifying and challenging automatic thoughts is a very important part of breaking this cycle and getting through the loss of a loved one.

Automatic thoughts are particularly likely to cause problems after the sudden death of a significant other. These may be new since the loss, or they may be old thoughts that the traumatic death has amplified.

The diagram is based on Beck, Rush, Shaw, and Emery (1979).

What Are Automatic Thoughts?

The following is a list of 10 qualities that often describe automatic thoughts.

1. *They are usually abbreviated or brief ("can't go on," "alone," etc.).* They may actually appear as images, smells, sensations, or sounds instead of words. A thought may obviously relate to your loss, such as an image of destruction related to the death, or it may seem arbitrary, such as the smell of the cologne your significant other wore to a special event you attended together.

2. *They occur as if they were 100% true.* You usually believe them, no matter how unbelievable they are when you really examine them. For example, you may have the automatic thought that your significant other died to punish you. You may fully believe it each time the thought occurs to you, even though you know realistically that it isn't true.

3. *You experience them as spontaneous.* Part of the reason automatic thoughts are so believable is that they are automatic. We rarely question them because we hardly notice them.

4. *Automatic thoughts are often expressed as "shoulds."* The phrases "I should," "I ought," and "I must" often indicate automatic thoughts.

5. *They often seem to suggest catastrophe.* People refer to this type of thinking as *catastrophizing.* When you catastrophize, you tend to expect the worst.

6. *Automatic thoughts tend to be idiosyncratic.* Each interpretation of an event depends on the thinking, past experience, and worldview of the person doing the interpreting. Different people witnessing or experiencing the same event may have very different automatic thoughts about that event.

7. *Automatic thoughts are persistent and self-perpetuating.* They can be viewed as "habits of thought," and so they occur without notice and become a persistent part of your thinking. Each new occurrence of the thought reinforces the last.

8. *They are often more blunt and less intellectual than your normal statements.* Automatic thoughts tend to be much more harsh and extreme than what you might actually say to others. You might say, "I made an error in judgment" while thinking, "I've ruined everything." Automatic thoughts may occur simultaneously with other, more logical thoughts.

9. *Automatic thoughts can be grouped into themes.* For most people, automatic thoughts tend to run along themes that are associated with deeper core beliefs. For example, thoughts such as "she doesn't like me" or "I have no friends" may both be related to the deeper core belief "I'm not lovable." The thought "I'm going to be attacked" and "my children aren't safe walking to school" may both be related to the core belief that the world is a dangerous place. Thoughts related to the same theme tend to prompt the same emotion. Thoughts related to "I'm not lovable" would prompt sadness, while those related to the core belief that the world is dangerous would prompt fear.

10. *Automatic thoughts are often related more to the past than to the present.* Automatic thoughts can be triggered by events or emotions that remind us of the past. They may sound like

(continued)

something a young child would say (e.g., "I'm a loser," "I'm in trouble," "Nobody likes me"). When we look more closely at the thoughts, we may realize that they are "old" and have little to do with the current situation.

The following questions will give you a head start on learning to identify automatic thoughts—a skill you will be developing further in Handouts 11 and 13.

INDEPENDENT ACTIVITY: LEARNING TO IDENTIFY AUTOMATIC THOUGHTS

❖ What was I thinking just prior to the start of a negative emotion?

❖ What was I thinking as the situation progressed?

❖ What was I telling myself would happen?

❖ What was the worst thing that could happen?

❖ What was I saying about myself in this situation?

❖ What did I worry other people might think about me in this situation?

❖ What words, phrases, or images flashed through my head as I started to feel this way?

Adapted with permission from M. McKay, M. Davis, and P. Fanning (1997). *Thoughts and feelings: Taking control of your moods and your life*. Oakland, CA: New Harbinger.

Identifying Automatic Thoughts Worksheet

This worksheet is a tool to use as you continue learning to recognize problematic thoughts and the moods they cause. You and your therapist will use this and similar worksheets throughout the rest of the treatment process to help you identify and challenge those thoughts that are causing you distress and pain.

Situation	Moods	Automatic Thoughts (or Images)

Sample Automatic Thought Record

Situation: Who? What? When? Where?	Moods (rate 0–100%) What did you feel?	Automatic Thoughts (Images): What was going through your mind just before you started feeling this way? Circle the most distressing thought, if you had more than one.	Evidence That Supports the Automatic Thought	Evidence Against the Automatic Thought (use challenging questions)	Alternative/ Balanced Thoughts
Looking at old photo of my son.	Guilt (85%) Sadness (70%) Anger at self (80%)	If I hadn't taught him to care so much about work, he wouldn't have gone in so early, and he wouldn't have been killed.	I told him over and over when he was young that he should work hard at everything he tries. He was killed before work hours. I had a bad feeling that day and should have called him. I wouldn't feel this guilty if I hadn't done something wrong.	It is good to teach children to work hard. There is no evidence that going to work later (or on time) would have prevented this. I had no way to predict this. I feel sad that he's gone, so I'm blaming myself.	I did teach my son to work hard, but his work ethic was not what killed him. The accident did, and that could have happened at any time.

Adapted with permission from B. Thorn (2004). *Cognitive therapy for chronic pain: A step-by-step guide.* New York: Guilford Press.

Automatic Thought Record

Situation: Who? What? When? Where?	Moods (rate 0–100%) What did you feel?	Automatic Thoughts (Images): What was going through your mind just before you started feeling this way? Circle the most distressing thought, if you had more than one.	Evidence That Supports the Automatic Thought	Evidence Against the Automatic Thought (use challenging questions)	Alternative/ Balanced Thoughts

Adapted with permission from B. Thorn (2004). *Cognitive therapy for chronic pain: A step-by-step guide.* New York: Guilford Press.

Challenging Questions Worksheet

Is there an alternative interpretation of the situation, other than your automatic thought?

_____

_____

Is the automatic thought really accurate, or is it an overgeneralization? Is it true that this situation means that your automatic thought is true?

_____

_____

If someone who loves you knew you were thinking this thought, what would that person say to you? Would he or she suggest any evidence that your thought is not completely true?

_____

_____

Are there exceptions to this automatic thought? Can you think of examples of situations that suggest that this automatic thought is untrue or not entirely true?

_____

_____

_____

Are you taking all of the blame for this situation, even if you did not have complete control?

_____

_____

_____

Are there other circumstances that might soften negative aspects of the situation? Are there times when this type of situation has gone well for you? Are there other situations you feel good about?

_____

_____

_____

(continued)

Adapted with permission from M. McKay, M. Davis, and P. Fanning (1997). *Thoughts and feelings: Taking control of your moods and your life.* Oakland, CA: New Harbinger.

Challenging Questions Worksheet *(page 2 of 2)*

What are the likely consequences and outcomes of the situation? Can you differentiate between what you fear might happen and what you can reasonably expect will happen?

_____

_____

_____

Have you had this kind of thought before? If so, how often? How many of those times were you predicting the outcome accurately? Based on your history with this kind of thought or prediction, what are the real odds that what you fear happening in this situation will actually occur? For example, if you've had this type of thought about twice a month for 5 years (120 times) and you were only right once, your odds of being right this time are 1 in 120 (less than 1%).

_____

_____

_____

Could you create a plan to change the situation? Is there someone you know who might deal with this differently? If so, what would that person do?

_____

_____

_____

Do you have the social or problem-solving skills to handle the situation? If you need help handling it, can you think of people who could help you or ways you might help yourself?

_____

_____

_____

How are you likely to be thinking about this in a year? How would you think about it if you had been feeling good or sleeping enough?

_____

_____

_____

Are there objective facts that would contradict items in the "Evidence That Supports . . ." column of Handout 13? What are they?

_____

_____

_____

Processing the Loss

One of the most important goals of this treatment is to help you react to your significant other's death in a way that fits who you are and that is acceptable to you. Once you have identified, felt, and accepted your thoughts, feelings, and memories, you will be able to respond to them with more choice and freedom, and your emotions will become more manageable. This can be a painful process, although the goal is for you eventually to live with less pain. This process allows you to deal with your hurt. It also helps you accept that your significant other is truly gone, honor what the death means to you, and help you prepare to move forward in a healthy way.

Experiencing and integrating your full range of feelings is essential to working through your loss. Although most people tend to avoid feelings and thoughts about loss because they are painful, you may intuitively know that avoiding feelings, events, and reminders of the death doesn't make the pain go away in the end.

Unfortunately, the pain usually finds its way into your life in one way or another, as flashbacks, intrusive thoughts, intense distress, or nightmares. Avoidance just prolongs this pain. Research has shown that the more you avoid painful feelings, the more they will disturb your life. Your therapist wants to help you *not* to avoid the loss, trauma, or any feelings associated with your significant other's death. Experiencing the feelings is the path to recovery.

This treatment helps clients who have lost a loved one to experience emotions in a safe environment, with a lot of support. Throughout the treatment, you will work with your therapist to face your loss and your painful feelings. You will do this together in a safe environment. You will work to face the loss a little at a time, and you will be in charge of choosing what you feel you are ready to face. The activities you and your therapist will develop and work on are called *exposure exercises*. Your therapist will support and guide you through them.

Sticking with exposure alleviates pain. When you create a safe environment and allow yourself to confront the painful thoughts, memories, and emotions, the pain will gradually lessen. The pain does not diminish as quickly as it does when you escape it by avoiding (leaving the place that reminds you of your significant other, distracting yourself from thinking about your significant other, or working long hours to help keep your mind off of what happened), but the relief is permanent. Escape and avoidance may alleviate your discomfort in the moment, but when you escape by avoiding, the painful emotion comes back full force or even stronger the next time you encounter that situation, memory, or thought. However, when you purposely and repeatedly confront the situation, you will find that the painful emotions decrease more and more, until you can begin to move forward again.

This treatment involves exposure to the images of the death itself (witnessing the death, or vivid imagery of the death even if you did not witness it); exposure to the memory of finding out about the death; exposure to feelings about the loss and about your significant other; and exposure to current reminders of the death. You will work on this gradually through writing and other assignments.

The goal of all the exposure activities in this treatment is for you to think about and remember your significant other's death so that you can begin to confront the pain that you have been experiencing in a safe environment, rather than continuing to avoid (and thus prolong) the pain. Getting past this pain allows you to remember your loved one more fully.

(continued)

Your first assignment is to write about your loved one's death. You should write in a place where you feel comfortable and at a time when you will not be disturbed. Exposure works by allowing you to become used to your painful feelings, and by allowing you to experience them over time so that they gradually lessen. It is important to stick with your writing, even though it brings you in touch with your painful feelings.

Of course, it is important that you not feel retraumatized or overwhelmed. The feelings skills that you and your therapist have talked about should help you to feel safe. For example, if you begin to feel overwhelmed by your feelings, you can remind yourself, "This is a feeling, and it will pass. It is important for me to experience my feelings." You can know that once you are done with the assignment, you can practice the breathing exercise to help calm yourself, or you can practice a self-care activity in order to soothe yourself. The writing exercise will be most helpful if you complete it all at once, not taking any breaks unless it is necessary. We ask you not to use the breathing exercise during the assignment because that will allow you to escape from your feelings rather than experiencing them fully.

First Account of the Death

Please write an account of your significant other's death. Do this writing activity as soon as possible (ideally, today). Write your account by hand, and write it in the present tense. Try to include sensory and other details, including what you were thinking and feeling at the time you learned of your significant other's death. Also, include your current thoughts and feelings (that is, your thoughts and feelings as you are writing), in parentheses. Try to experience your emotions as fully as you can. If you need to stop writing at any point, please draw a line on the paper where you stop, and begin writing again when you can. Please read the account to yourself each day before the next session. Write as much as you want, but write at least one or two pages. You can use the blank space below to get started.

Secondary Losses[1]

Following the sudden, traumatic death of a loved one, most survivors experience a profound sense of loss. They often feel as though their world has been ripped apart. In understanding the ramifications of the loved one's death, it can be helpful to distinguish primary and secondary losses. A primary loss is the initial loss—in this case, the loved one's death.

Secondary losses are those losses that coincide with or develop because of the death. In most cases, mourners experience some secondary losses right away. For example, a widow may miss her husband's companionship immediately after his death. Yet it may take weeks, and perhaps months or even years, for survivors to become aware of the full range of secondary losses associated with the death. When tax season comes around, for example, a widower may recognize that he needs help with a task that his spouse had previously handled. He may be confused about whom he should contact for assistance. It is critically important for survivors to identify and mourn secondary losses. If these losses are not addressed, mourners often get stuck in the mourning process.

Bereaved individuals encounter secondary losses in many domains of their lives—for example, such losses may be emotional, physical, or financial. To aid you in identifying the losses you have experienced, we have listed some of the most common kinds of secondary losses below. In each case, we have provided examples of the types of losses that mourners typically encounter.

➤ *Emotional losses.* Emotional losses are numerous and can be difficult to put into words. With the loss of a significant other, a person experiences the loss of emotional support from that person— the loss of someone to listen, to provide support, and to comfort him when he is upset.

➤ *Physical losses.* Physical secondary losses are those physical things that are no longer available to a survivor since the death. Physical losses include the loss of the physical body of the loved one (which the survivor can no longer touch or be touched by), and the loss of physical objects such as a car or a house (which sometimes must be sold when the loved one dies).

➤ *Loss of identity.* Many survivors report feeling empty inside following the death of their loved one. They feel as though part of themselves has died. They often describe themselves as a "different person" as a result of the loss—someone who is less easygoing, less fun-loving, and more serious. It is also common for survivors to report a loss of self-confidence, and to struggle with feelings of inadequacy following the loss.

➤ *Loss of our beliefs about the world.* Sudden, traumatic losses make us recognize that the things that are most important can be taken away in an instant. As a result, feelings of safety, security, and trust can be shattered by a traumatic death. If a surgeon makes an error that contributes to a husband's death, this may cause the survivor to question the beliefs she held prior to the loss. Consequently, she may have great difficulty seeking the care of a physician, even when she is quite

(continued)

[1]Based on the following: S. Caplan and G. Lang (1995). *Grief's courageous journey: A workbook*. Oakland, CA: New Harbinger. A. Matsakis (1994). *Post-traumatic stress disorder: A complete treatment guide* (L. Tilley, Ed.). Oakland, CA: New Harbinger. T. A. Rando (1993). *Treatment of complicated mourning*. Champaign, IL: Research Press.

ill. If a doctor tells her that she or another close family member requires hospitalization, she is likely to experience intense anxiety.

➤ *Relational losses.* The secondary losses that follow a traumatic death are determined in large part by the role of relationship that was lost. Following the death of a spouse, the surviving spouse may struggle with a loss of identity, feeling as though a part of herself has died. She may also experience the loss of a caring presence day to day, the loss of her partner's participation in childrearing, and the destruction of her hopes and dreams for the future. When a child dies, parents must contend with the loss of their identity as parents, which is centered around caring for and nurturing the child. In many cases, they also lose a sense of meaning and purpose that was provided by the parental role. They are robbed of the satisfaction they would get from the child's milestones and accomplishments. In addition, children often embody the parents' hopes and dreams for the future, which are often shattered by the child's death.

The death of a parent is also associated with a unique set of secondary losses. These may include the loss of a life-long emotionally supportive relationship, and the loss of guidance and advice at important crossroads. Surviving children may also lose an important source of recognition and praise for their accomplishments and achievements. In some cases, they may lose a loving presence of a grandparent in the lives of their children.

➤ *Financial losses.* Many bereaved survivors suffer both direct and indirect financial losses because of the death of their significant other. One financial loss that often accompanies the loss of a spouse is the income formerly provided by the spouse. Another is the loss of health insurance. If the deceased is the one who carried health insurance for the family, this coverage typically ends with her death. This loss may trigger a host of additional losses, such as the inability of the surviving spouse to obtain the necessary medication for his child, who may have a chronic illness. Financial losses are also common following the death of a child. For example, as a result of the death of their only son, one couple felt that they could not bear to stay in the home where their son was raised. They also felt that it would be painful to live in the town, which had many reminders of things the family did together. They put their home on the market, but the only way they could sell it was to lower the price dramatically. This not only reduced the amount of money they had available, but also had an adverse effect on their credit rating.

➤ *Daily living losses.* Daily living losses are those secondary losses that affect a person's daily activities. Help with the dishes and other household chores, help raising the children, sharing a meal, going shopping with your significant other, and engaging in a conversation about how your day was are all examples of daily living losses. Daily living losses also include the difficulties of coping with special occasions, such as birthdays or holidays, without the loved one.

➤ *The loss of hopes and dreams for the future.* In many cases, the survivor envisions a future that includes the loved one. A couple may have planned to retire together and travel across the United States. As their children grow into adults, parents may anticipate a future that includes grandchildren. A future that survivors eagerly anticipated is now uncertain, and in some cases dreaded.

All secondary losses become part of the experience of grief and mourning and need to be mourned in their own right. Each of your own secondary losses will call forth unique reactions and responses. It is important to be able to recognize, label, and honor these losses, so that you can mourn them in your treatment. Knowing what these losses are and being able to name them can be an empowering

(continued)

experience and can help you to feel less overwhelmed by the enormity of your grief. We encourage you to begin this process by drawing from the material above.

INDEPENDENT ACTIVITY: LISTING YOUR SECONDARY LOSSES

Below, please list as many of the secondary losses resulting from your loved one's death as you can. The categories will help you to think about the different areas of your life that your loss has affected. If you're not sure which category a loss fits in, just write it under any heading. There is also space for you to include secondary losses that do not fit into any of the categories listed below.

Emotional losses: _____

_____

_____

Physical losses: _____

_____

_____

Loss of identity: _____

_____

_____

Loss of beliefs about the world: _____

_____

_____

Relational losses: _____

_____

_____

(continued)

Secondary Losses (page 4 of 4)

Financial losses: _____

_____

_____

Daily living losses: _____

_____

_____

Loss of hopes and dreams for the future: _____

_____

_____

Other secondary losses: _____

_____

_____

The Importance of Enhancing Social Support

Social support is the emotional and physical comfort that people may receive from others, including their family members, friends, co-workers, and neighbors. Social support may take many forms, such as empathy, concern, caring, willingness to listen, and help with practical tasks. If social support is effective, it helps people feel loved, cared for, valued, and understood.

Following a traumatic loss, social support is one of the most important resources for healing. Below are some reasons why it is important to work with your therapist to enhance the social support available to you.

➤ Survivors who feel supported are more likely to show a decrease in symptoms over time.

➤ Receiving support helps survivors see that there is still some good in the world. As a result, they may become more hopeful about the future.

➤ Support is important because it helps mourners to move forward in the healing process. For example, a survivor may recognize that she should get more exercise but have trouble actually doing so. By inviting her for a walk or accompanying her to the gym, a friend can help her get on the right track.

➤ Social contact with others can help to provide a respite from the difficult work of mourning.

➤ Supportive relationships can help survivors begin investing in the future by exposing them to new people, ideas, and activities.

➤ Despite the benefits of support, research indicates that in many cases, those in the survivor's social network are unable to provide effective support. Some people are uncomfortable relating to survivors of a traumatic death, and may therefore avoid you and your family. Others may wish to help, but do not know what to say or do. Survivors are often disappointed and hurt by others' comments. Some of the most common types of remarks people make that the bereaved generally regard as unhelpful include the following: Asking questions (e.g., "Was there a lot of blood?" "What are you going to do with his tools?"); giving advice (e.g., "You should not be going to the cemetery every day," "It's time to move on"); minimizing the loss (e.g., "At least he's not a vegetable," "You're young enough to have another child"); inappropriate identification with feelings (e.g., "I know how you feel; my dog was run over by a car"); providing a philosophical or religious perspective (e.g., "Life goes on," "God needed him more than you did").

- Not having the energy or motivation to make contact with others.
- Feeling self-conscious: "I felt that everyone was looking at me."
- Feeling guilty, or worrying that others believe the survivors are responsible for the death.
- Not wanting to encounter unhelpful support attempts.
- Feeling afraid that they will make others uncomfortable, or seen as a "wet blanket."
- Feeling uncomfortable with conversations about everyday things. Such conversations may seem trivial or meaningless.
- For bereaved parents, feeling uncomfortable when other people talk about their children's accomplishments and future plans.
- Difficulty dealing with others' complaints about their loved ones.

Your therapist can help you develop strategies for dealing with these situations, and for developing supportive ties that are beneficial to you.

Building Social Support

Social support is important to your recovery. This includes reaching out to people who can help you with specific tasks, finding good listeners, and staying connected to those people in your life who are positive sources of emotional support. This can be challenging, but it is also extremely important to the process of healing. The independent activities below will help you to explore any difficulties you may have had finding or receiving social support since your loved one's death, and to think of ways you can build support.

INDEPENDENT ACTIVITY: ASSESSING YOUR SOCIAL SUPPORT NETWORK

Consider the following questions in assessing your social support network. You may want to jot down some notes as you consider these questions.

❖ What does your social support network look like now? Who is in it?

❖ Socially, what or whom have you lost?

❖ How has your support changed since the loss? For example, have some people you thought were good friends stayed away since your loved one's death? Have some people who were just acquaintances been more helpful than you might have expected?

❖ Have some friends who rallied around you after your loved one's death become less available?

❖ Have you bonded with any new friends since the loss?

❖ How have your relationships with old friends changed?

❖ How do you understand any changes in your support?

❖ What are some situations in which you had the experience of feeling misunderstood or not heard? What types of comments have others made that have left you feeling misunderstood? What other feelings have you experienced upon hearing these comments?

❖ Are there ways in which you have experienced a loss of connection with others? For example, are you spending more time at home? Are you getting together with people less often than you did before the loss? Are you turning down social invitations, and/or neglecting to initiate contact or maintain social ties?

(continued)

INDEPENDENT ACTIVITY: BEGINNING TO SET SOCIAL SUPPORT GOALS

Your answers to the following questions will help you begin to think of small goals that involve relating to others.

❖ Whom can you turn to for emotional support?

❖ Whom do you know who is a good (nonjudgmental, supportive) listener, and who might be available to you if you feel like talking about your significant other's death?

❖ Are there people in your social network who have invited you to do something, whom you have turned them down because you did not feel up to getting together?

❖ Who could help you with daily tasks?

❖ What are the attitudes of the important people in your life about asking for help? For example, do they support you in asking? Encourage it? Discourage it?

❖ What cultural or religious influences in your life affect your ability or willingness to reach out to others?

Second Account of the Death

Please write an account of when your significant other died. Do this writing activity as soon as possible (ideally, today). This time, focus on _____ . Include sensory and other details. Also, include your current thoughts and feelings (that is, your thoughts and feelings as you are writing), in parentheses.

    As with the first account of the death (Handout 16), write in the present tense, write the account by hand, and write where and when you have enough time and privacy. Allow yourself to experience your emotions fully. If you need to stop writing at any point, please draw a line on the paper where you stop, and resume writing when you can. Please read the account to yourself each day before the next session. Write as much as you want, but write at least one or two pages. You can use the blank space below to get started.

Values*

The sudden, traumatic death of a loved one can drain your life of purpose, meaning, and vitality. One of the comments we have heard most often from survivors of traumatic loss is that nothing seems to matter anymore. These exercises will help you clarify your values—that is, things that you still care about, despite everything that has happened. They will also help you make some decisions about how you want to live the rest of your life.

In many cases, survivors' core values and their goals for the future are shattered by what has happened. For example, a mourner may place great value on education. Prior to the loss, she may have decided to go back to school and earn an advanced degree. Following the death of her loved one, she may have to abandon this plan because she is unable to concentrate on her studies. Another survivor may have rated religion and his relationship with God as his most important value. If he loses his child in a needless accident, he may feel betrayed by God and turn against his faith.

For many reasons, you may not feel ready to think about your goals for the future. However, evidence suggests that taking even the smallest steps toward identifying future goals, and developing plans for reaching them, can facilitate the healing process.

Below, we first ask you to complete some exercises that will help you to identify your most important values at this time. Next, we provide information to help you to differentiate among *values*, which are the principles by which you live your life; *goals*, which are tasks you can accomplish in the service of your values; and *action plans*, which are the specific steps you take to reach your goals. Finally, we show you how to set goals and develop action plans that are feasible for your situation.

Some mourners believe that it is inappropriate to think about values and future goals when they are still in so much pain. In fact, values work can be very helpful for people in this situation. Working on values and goals does not require people to give up their pain; it gives them something to focus on in addition to their pain.

Mourners are often reluctant to become engaged in work on values and goals because they believe it is disloyal to their lost loved one. If you feel this way, you might consider the following question: What would your loved one recommend that you do? Most people feel that their loved ones not only would support them, but would actively encourage them to develop goals for the future and to carry them out. The Independent Activity that follows will help you to gain a greater understanding of working with values and goals.

(continued)

---

*This is one of two handouts focusing on values and goals. The second, Handout S1, Personal Goal Setting, is on the book's website (*www.guilford.com/pearlman-materials*). Both handouts are designed to help you clarify and prioritize your values. Both guide you through the process of developing goals that are consonant with your values, and identifying action steps that will help you reach your goals. This handout provides a more comprehensive analysis of how to develop goals and action plans. It also addresses ways to overcome barriers that may keep us from reaching our goals.

INDEPENDENT ACTIVITY: PRIORITIZING YOUR VALUES AND SETTING GOALS

The purpose of this exercise is to identify those values that are most important to you. Below is a list of values or life domains; some of these may be very important to you, while others may be insignificant or irrelevant to your situation. Please look through the list below and check off the five values that are most important to you at this point in your life. We want to emphasize that there are no right or wrong values. Only you can know what is most important to you.

____ Health/physical well-being   ____ Spirituality/religion

____ Marital or couple relationship   ____ Education/training/personal growth

____ Parenting   ____ Service to others

____ Extended family (parents, siblings) ____ Recreation/leisure/fun

____ Friendships/social life   ____ Financial security

____ Work/career   ____ Other (specify) _____

Now please list the values you have checked off in the spaces below. List these in any order. You don't have to rank them.

Next, look over the five values that you selected. In so doing, please ask yourself the following questions: What are the real priorities in my life at this time? What do I care about most?

Now go through your top five values again and, keeping these questions in mind, cross off three of the values, leaving the two that are most important to you now. Some people find it difficult to eliminate values they care about. You should keep in mind that once you have made progress on the values you selected, you can begin working on other values.

Experts have found that in doing work with values and goals, clients usually make more progress if they focus on one value at a time. For this reason, this exercise has been designed to help you identify the value that you would like to work on now. Focusing on one of your two remaining values, ask yourself the following question: What would it mean for me to live that value, and what would it mean if I didn't? *Living a value* means making day-to-day decisions that are consistent with that value. For example, suppose the value you select is health. What it would mean to live that value is to make day-to-day decisions such as exercising regularly, avoiding unhealthy foods, and cutting back on alcohol consumption or smoking.

Now focus on the remaining value and ask the same question. On the basis of your answers, select the value that you would like to work on at this time. You will be setting goals and developing action plans that will help you live the value you have chosen. In all likelihood, you will feel a sense of accomplishment and pride that you have been able to make choices that will help you move forward.

Below, please write in the value you would like to work on now.

(continued)

GOAL SETTING

Now it is time to select a goal that reflects the value you have chosen. Goals help us to focus our energy, and to behave in ways that are consistent with our values. Goals are empowering because they can show us what we are capable of.

Unlike a value, a goal is something you plan to accomplish. Goals are specific, realistic, and concrete. There should be some way of determining or measuring whether you have achieved your goal. To provide an example, "being a good friend" might be your most important value. "Getting together with one of my good friends each week" is a goal that supports your value.

Here are some examples that will help you differentiate between values and goals:

❖ If your value is financial security, your goal might be to find a financial planner.
❖ If your value is extended family, your goal might be to plan a birthday party for your sister.
❖ If your value is your marital or couple relationship, your goal might be to arrange a "date" with your spouse or partner once per week.

In selecting a goal, it can be helpful to raise the following question: What goal could I pursue in the service of my value that is feasible for my situation now? Realistically, do I have the time, energy, and resources to reach that goal?

We would like you to select one goal to work on at the present time. Make sure that the goal you select will help you to live in accordance with the value you have chosen. In deciding on which goal to pursue at this time, select one a goal that is realistic. Your goal should also be measurable—you should be able to determine whether you are reaching your goal or not. We strongly recommend that you discuss your initial selection of values and goals with your therapist.

Once you have identified a goal that meets the criteria described above, please write it here:

_____

_____

INDEPENDENT ACTIVITY: GOALS AND ACTION PLANS

Now that you have chosen the value and goal you want to pursue at this time, the next task is to identify the specific, small steps or actions you will need to complete in order to reach your goal. The most common reason people don't reach their goals is that they do not have an action plan. An action plan helps you to make steady progress toward your goal, step by step. Here are some examples that will help you differentiate between goals and action plans:

(continued)

❖ If your goal is to find a financial planner, steps in your action plan might include:

- Asking friends, coworkers, or members of your congregation for recommendations.
- Doing research to learn more about certifications for a financial planner, and deciding on the level of expertise you need.
- Making an appointment to consult with at least one financial planner during the next 2 weeks.

❖ If your goal is to throw a birthday party for your sister, steps in your action plan might include:

- Selecting a date and time for the party, after checking with other family members and friends.
- Making a guest list and contacting potential guests.
- Planning the menu and ordering a cake.
- Arranging for the house to be cleaned the day before the party.

❖ If your goal is to arrange a "date" with your spouse, your action steps might include:

- Reading movie reviews to identify a film you and your spouse would both enjoy.
- Selecting a restaurant and making a reservation.
- Arranging for a babysitter.
- Doing extra work at the office on the day before the date, so that you can arrive home on time the day of the date.

In formulating your goals and action steps, it is important to attach a time frame to each one. For example, you might give yourself 1 week to select a date and time for the party, or you might give yourself 4 days to ask people for recommendations for a financial planner. Research has shown that without specific time frames, most people are not able to achieve their goals.

Please list three to five specific actions, behaviors, or steps you plan to take toward reaching your goal. Try to identify a time frame when you will engage in each behavior. Check off each action step once you have completed it. Feel free to add more action steps that will help you reach your goal if you wish.

Specific action steps toward goal: Time frame:

1. _____   _____

2. _____   _____

3. _____   _____

4. _____   _____

5. _____   _____

Additional actions:

1. _____   _____

2. _____   _____

3. _____   _____

Please remember to check these off as you complete them.

(continued)

We recommend that you discuss the exercises in this handout with your therapist before attempting to carry out your goal. Your therapist may be able to provide feedback on the values, goals, and action steps you have developed—for example, whether they are realistic and are attainable for you at this time.

Before you attempt the assignment, you can also talk about potential barriers to reaching your goals. You can write down any feelings or beliefs that might prevent you from completing your goal. Then talk with your therapist about what you might do to ensure that you will be able to complete your action steps and achieve your goal.

BARRIERS TO REACHING YOUR GOALS AND ACTION PLANS

On some occasions, you may find that even though you worked hard to reach your goal or complete your action steps, something got in the way. For example, maybe one of your action plans involved asking your neighbor for help, and you were just not able to do it. Perhaps you thought your request would be annoying to your neighbor. In discussing these issues with your therapist, you can develop some strategies that will help you the next time you are in a similar situation.

Survivors are often surprised by how they react to working with goals. As one woman who lost a child expressed it, "I didn't think I could pull off throwing a birthday party for my sister, but I did it. She was so happy that despite everything that has happened, it made me happy too."

Third Account of the Death

Please write an account of when your significant other died. Do this writing activity as soon as possible (ideally, today). This time, focus on _____. Include sensory and other details. Also, include your thoughts and feelings as you are writing, in parentheses.

As with the earlier accounts of the death (Handouts 16 and 20), write in the present tense, write the account by hand, and write where and when you have enough time and privacy. Allow yourself to experience your emotions fully. If you need to stop writing at any point, please draw a line on the paper where you stop, and resume writing when you can. Please read the account to yourself each day before the next session. Write as much as you want, but write at least one or two pages. You can use the blank space below to get started.

Psychological Needs

SAFETY

A sense of *safety* (or *security*) is fundamental to all of us. We all need to feel that we are safe and reasonably invulnerable to harm, and that the people we care about are safe. Without these basic beliefs, it's hard to feel comfortable. The sudden, traumatic death of your significant other has probably disrupted your sense of safety. Because something sudden and unexpected happened to your loved one, it's easy to think that something awful could happen to you or someone else you love. You may become extremely anxious if another significant person is late coming home, or if you receive a phone call late at night.

Disrupted safety beliefs can get in the way of activities or relationships. Concerns about becoming close to people when they are vulnerable to harm (because you don't want to lose someone you're close to again) can prevent you from seeking relationships. Similarly, you may fear that anyone you love may be endangered simply because of being close to you; you may be using the loss of your loved one as "evidence" for this fear.

INDEPENDENT ACTIVITY: SAFETY

Think about how your beliefs about your own safety and that of your surviving significant others have changed since the death. Complete an Automatic Thought Record (Handout 13) about one of those safety beliefs.

TRUST

Trusting Oneself

Self-trust is the belief that you can rely on your own perceptions and judgments. A sudden, traumatic death may challenge these beliefs. It is common (although it may not be rational) for survivors to focus on decisions they made before the significant other died and to imagine that things would have turned out differently if they had made different decisions. This can lead to self-statements like "If only I had [or had not] done [or said] X, Y, or Z, the accident would not have happened." These statements can then lead the survivors to doubt their judgment: "If I did X before and things turned out so badly, how can I ever trust myself to make good decisions?"

Of course, in all relationships, there are many choices and things we could have done differently. In typical daily life, we don't have any reason to focus on these small things. We make dozens of decisions every day (including what to wear, what to eat, where to park the car, etc.), generally without questioning our judgment. When something goes terribly wrong, it's natural to look for reasons for

(continued)

---

what happened and to question our behavior and judgment. That search naturally takes us into areas of self-doubt.

When your self-trust is disrupted, you may doubt yourself, feel overcautious, or have difficulty making decisions.

Trusting Others

Other-trust is the belief that you can count on others to be there for you when you need them—that people will keep their promises. One of the earliest tasks of childhood is developing trust. Everyone needs to learn a healthy balance of trust and mistrust, and learn when each is appropriate. Sudden, traumatic loss can affect your trust in others in a variety of ways. If the significant other was someone who was always there for you, it's easy to decide that the way to avoid feeling bad in the future is to avoid forming trusting relationships. This might mean not getting close to others out of fear that close-ness might lead to trust, dependency, and then more loss. You may go to extremes to avoid relying on others.

If important people betrayed you early in life, you may have developed the belief "No one can be trusted." The sudden death of a significant other may serve to confirm this belief. If you had par-ticularly good experiences growing up, you may have developed the belief "Generally, people can be trusted." The sudden, traumatic death of a significant other can shatter this belief.

If the people you counted on and trusted were distant, unsupportive, or judgmental of you and your family after your loved one's death, your belief in their trustworthiness may also have been shat-tered.

When other-trust beliefs are disrupted, you may experience a pervasive sense of disillusionment or disappointment in others, fear of betrayal or abandonment, anger and rage at betrayers, fear of rela-tionships (new or old), and general suspicion of others. New relationships may create anxiety because as trust develops, you may feel frightened about the possibility that someone will again abandon or betray you.

INDEPENDENT ACTIVITY: TRUST

Think about how your beliefs about trust have changed since the death of your significant other. Complete an Automatic Thought Record (Handout 13) about one of those trust beliefs.

CONTROL

Self-Control

Self-control refers to your beliefs about your ability to feel in charge of your own thoughts, feelings, and behaviors. A sudden, traumatic loss can lead to feeling out of control. This can be frightening, especially if the feelings seem particularly intense or if they lead you to say or do things that don't feel comfortable or familiar. A sudden, traumatic death can change your beliefs about what you think

(continued)

you are able to control. If, for example, you grew up believing that you could control what happens in your life, the realization that there are important things you cannot control can feel overwhelming.

After a sudden, traumatic death, survivors often find themselves with less control over their own behaviors. That can be scary, especially if they are behaving in destructive ways, like drinking too much, pushing people away, not showing up for work, or behaving aggressively toward others.

Other-Control

Other-control refers to your beliefs about your ability to influence those around you. Many sudden, traumatic deaths leave people feeling guilty. For example, if someone did something that resulted in the death of someone you love, it's easy to feel as if you should have been able to prevent it. Other types of losses—such as those resulting from industrial or transportation accidents, homicides, terrorist attacks like 9/11, and suicides—can also stimulate a sense of having no control or influence over anything or anyone. When you are upset, your emotions become more intense, and you may generalize from the thought that you had no control over one person in a particular situation to a belief that you cannot control or influence anyone.

INDEPENDENT ACTIVITY: CONTROL

Think about how your beliefs about both self-control and other-control have changed since the death. Complete an Automatic Thought Record (Handout 13) about one of those beliefs.

ESTEEM

Self-Esteem

Self-esteem refers to your beliefs about your own value and the value of what you think, feel, do, and believe. It's natural for survivors to feel some responsibility for the death of a significant other, or to feel that they could or should have done something differently. Even if groundless, this guilt is a common outcome of traumatic loss. Although doing so is irrational, it's not a difficult next step for survivors to devalue themselves—to feel bad, unworthy, ashamed, or inadequate. Some people even come to believe that their very presence in the loved one's life was toxic. This is especially true for people whose self-esteem wasn't strong before the loss—for example, some survivors of early traumatic experiences. These individuals may have a chronically low sense of self-esteem and may be more susceptible to feeling that way after the death of a loved one. For them, the current loss can become just another example of their inadequacy or unworthiness.

Problems with self-esteem can also arise during the process of trying to make sense of what happened. It is natural to try to find someone to blame for a sudden, traumatic death. Especially when there is no obvious target, survivors may blame themselves. In most relationships, we all sometimes do things that we don't feel good about, such as speaking sharply to the other person or in some way failing to respond to the other person's needs. If the person dies in a sudden, traumatic incident, we may then focus on these small failures and use them as proof that we are bad. Guilt is a natural

(continued)

response to loss, and we may have legitimate regret over failures or neglected aspects of our relationships. However, it is important to challenge self-blaming beliefs and thoughts that may be exaggerated. Guilt and self-blame that are out of proportion to the actual relationship are especially likely to emerge if we were having problems with the lost loved one, or had a bad interaction with this person shortly before the death.

People may also experience problems with self-esteem because the challenges that follow traumatic death, such as feeling overwhelmed, difficulty concentrating, or feeling exhausted, can make it hard to function well at work or school or when relating to family members and friends. This can further erode self-esteem.

Finally, feelings of grief often include feeling bad for oneself. Unfortunately, it's easy to go from feeling bad *for* oneself to feeling bad *about* oneself.

Other-Esteem

Other-esteem refers to your beliefs that others are valuable and worthy of respect. If a significant other has died in some way that involves another person (e.g., a violent death, an industrial or transportation accident, or a terrorist attack), it's natural to blame the other people involved, who truly may be responsible. From there, it's easy to generalize to the belief that no one is worthy of respect, people are incompetent, or people are evil.

INDEPENDENT ACTIVITY: ESTEEM

Think about your beliefs about self-esteem and other-esteem. Have they changed since the death? Complete an Automatic Thought Record (Handout 13) about one of those esteem-related beliefs.

INTIMACY

Self-Intimacy

Self-intimacy refers to your beliefs about your ability to feel connected to your inner experience, including your thoughts and feelings. After a major loss, survivors often don't want to feel their pain, anger, terror, grief, sorrow, loneliness, or longing. Although they know that avoiding these feelings is, paradoxically, the thing that keeps the feelings alive and hurting them, avoidance is a natural human tendency—one that takes effort to overcome. Grief often brings fatigue with it, which makes it difficult to exert effort. It may often feel easier for you to have a drink, keep busy, sleep, lose yourself in work, or think and talk about anything other than the death. However, these strategies also separate you from your inner life—from your awareness of who you are and what you need.

Other-Intimacy

Other-intimacy refers to the belief that you can feel close and connected to other people. A sudden, traumatic death can seriously challenge those beliefs. Survivors often feel that their pain after the

(continued)

death relates to the depth of the connection with the significant other, and thus that connection is something to avoid in the future. They may think they have lost the one person who really knew or understood them. This belief may lead to withdrawal from others, with the intention of not investing in other relationships in order to avoid that kind of loss in the future. That decision and behavior can then lead to loneliness.

INDEPENDENT ACTIVITY: INTIMACY

Think about how your beliefs about self-intimacy or other-intimacy, and/or your behaviors regarding intimacy, have changed since the death of your significant other. Complete an Automatic Thought Record (Handout 13) about one of those intimacy beliefs.

Positive and Negative Aspects of Your Relationship with Your Significant Other

YOUR RELATIONSHIP

All relationships have positive and negative aspects. Below, please identify at least three positive and at least three negative or less positive aspects of your relationship. Feel free to list more of either if you would like.

Positive aspects of your relationship:

1. _____

_____

2. _____

_____

3. _____

_____

Less positive, or negative, aspects of your relationship:

1. _____

_____

2. _____

_____

3. _____

_____

(continued)

PERSONAL QUALITIES OF YOUR LOVED ONE

When we think about people we care about, it is usually possible to identify some qualities we really like, as well as some qualities that are not so positive. Below, please identify at least three positive qualities of your loved one, and at least three not-so-positive or negative qualities.

Positive qualities of your loved one (that is, things you loved, admired, or appreciated about this person):

1. _____

_____

2. _____

_____

3. _____

_____

Not-so-positive or negative qualities of your loved one (that is, things you did not like or things you found irritating or annoying):

1. _____

_____

2. _____

_____

3. _____

_____

Fear and Avoidance Hierarchy Form

Situation/Activity | Distress Rating (0–100)

1. _____ _____

2. _____ _____

3. _____ _____

4. _____ _____

5. _____ _____

6. _____ _____

7. _____ _____

8. _____ _____

9. _____ _____

10. _____ _____

11. _____ _____

12. _____ _____

13. _____ _____

14. _____ _____

15. _____ _____

Based on Foa and Rothbaum (1998).

Account of Your Relationship with Your Significant Other

Write an account of your relationship with your significant other, focusing on the time right before the death. Do this writing activity as soon as possible (ideally, today). Include in your account regrets or unfinished business that you may have had with the deceased, and things you wished you could have done or said before your significant other died. Feel free to include aspects of the relationship that you have not yet remembered fully, as discussed at the opening of this session. Also, include your thoughts and feelings as you are writing, in parentheses. As in earlier writing assignments, write in the present tense, hand write the account, and write where and when you have enough time and privacy. Allow yourself to experience your emotions fully. If you need to stop writing at any point, draw a line on the paper where you stop, and begin writing again when you can. Please read the account to yourself each day before the next session. Write as much as you want, but write at least one or two pages. You can use the blank space below to get started.

Guilt, Regret, and Sudden, Traumatic Death

GUILT

One common response to sudden, traumatic death is feeling guilty. As mentioned in earlier handouts, survivors sometimes blame themselves, either directly or indirectly, for what happened. Or they might blame themselves for things that happened or did not happen when their loved ones were alive—things about which they now feel bad or responsible. As defined by *Webster's New World College Dictionary* (2005), *guilt* is "a painful feeling of self-reproach resulting from a belief that one has done something wrong or immoral." To feel guilty means to feel as though one is responsible for a wrongdoing.

Given this definition, we could say that guilt is appropriate when a person has done something wrong. Sometimes this is appropriate: the survivor may have been the one who was driving the car when it crashed. More commonly, survivors feel guilty about innocent acts that set the stage for the death. For example, a parent may berate himself for allowing his teenage daughter to ride in the car with a friend who was speeding and failed to negotiate a turn. Survivors may feel sorry about what happened and wish that they had done things differently with regard to their loved ones. However, wishing that things were different and blaming oneself for these things are not the same. Of course, a survivor may also experience appropriate guilt and misguided guilt at the same time. For example, a person who harassed a sibling consistently may feel guilty when that sibling dies in a workplace explosion. The guilt for the harassment may be appropriate, but the guilt for the death is not.

Guilt can also result from the violation of a personal standard that a person holds either consciously or unconsciously. An example of this would be a father who feels he should be able to protect his child from all harm or pain, and then feels guilty when the child dies, regardless of the circumstances. This is a common state of affairs; the wish to protect one's child is natural, although the belief that one can protect children from all harm is not a realistic expectation. When guilt arises from the violation of a personal standard, as opposed to arising from objective wrongdoing, we need to ask whether that personal standard was realistic in the first place.

How Can You Make Sense of Guilt Feelings?

No one can tell whether guilt is appropriate or not merely by how it feels; inappropriate guilt feels just as bad as appropriate guilt. If you are feeling guilty, it is a good idea to check in with your therapist about the legitimacy of your guilt. In other words, what would an objective or neutral person say about whether you committed a wrongdoing? What would a friend, a colleague, or your therapist say about whether you are actually responsible for what happened? Alternatively, if someone you cared about were feeling guilty about the same thing you are—in other words, if this person were in the same position as you—what would you say to that person? Would you hold the person responsible for the action, event, or situation? Looking at your situation from different perspectives can help you to determine whether the guilt you are feeling is appropriate.

(continued)

If you are feeling guilty, it is also important to ask yourself whether you feel you have violated a personal standard. Again, it can be helpful to explore this question with your therapist or a trusted friend, especially if you are not fully aware of the standards you hold for yourself. For instance, if you feel guilt because you occasionally became angry with your loved one and believe that you violated your personal standard of never being angry with those you love, you need to examine this standard. In fact, this unrealistic standard can never be met in a close relationship.

REGRET

The concept of regret provides an alternative to guilt as a way of understanding painful feelings about a loss. *Regret* means "to feel sorry about or mourn for (a person or thing gone, lost, etc.) . . . [or] to feel troubled or remorseful over (something that has happened, one's own acts, etc.)" (*Webster's New World College Dictionary*, 2005). Regret is an inherent part of loss. All of us make choices in life all the time. When we choose X, we are saying no to Y and Z. All choices, therefore, involve loss, and some may involve regret. Regret is part of life, and it is certainly part of death. We cannot do everything, and we cannot be all things to all people.

Conflict occurs in all intimate relationships. It's natural to feel bad about disagreements, arguments, differences, or harsh words, especially after a loved one dies. If that death was unexpected, there wasn't an opportunity to say goodbye, to finish the "unfinished business," or to place the conflicts in a broader context. Although it is painful, this type of regret is a normal part of unexpected loss.

In a time of sorrow and distress, it can be easy to misinterpret regret as guilt, and this can happen for a variety of reasons.

> ➤ We may feel a strong need to explain the death. If explanations are not readily available, then we may blame ourselves, partly as an effort to make sense of the death.
>
> ➤ All of us need to have some control over our lives. A sudden, traumatic loss challenges this need. In an effort to reestablish a sense of control, we may blame ourselves for things we did or did not do, thereby believing (on some level) that we could have prevented the death if only we had done X or hadn't done Y.
>
> ➤ If we grew up in families that readily and wrongly placed blame (because of stress, fear, anger, or frustration), then we may have internalized these messages, believing that "everything is my fault."
>
> ➤ Modern Western culture is litigious. We often seek to blame someone for something that happened. If someone is responsible, then it is not just an accident—not just something about which to feel disappointed, helpless, or regretful, which people often find easier.

After the death of a significant other, hindsight bias comes into play. *Hindsight bias* means judging something in the past on the basis of knowledge that we have now but did not have then. This belief gives rise to the common saying "Hindsight is 20/20." Most of us make the best decisions and choices that we can, given what we know and the resources available to us at the time. After the fact, if we gain new knowledge or if circumstances change, we may wish we had done things differently; we may feel as if what we did was wrong when in fact we did the best we could.

(continued)

HOW CAN YOU ADDRESS GUILT AND REGRET?

The first step in addressing guilt and regret is distinguishing one from the other. Again, you may be able to do this best with another person who can offer a more objective view of the situation. It is also important not only to distinguish guilt from regret, but also to distinguish guilt resulting from an objective wrongdoing from guilt resulting from the violation of an unrealistic personal standard.

If you are still feeling guilty about a wrongdoing or a violation of your personal standards, it will be important to practice compassion toward yourself and to work to forgive yourself eventually.

Later in the treatment, you will address this issue in more detail and talk about ways of transforming your guilt or regret. For now, it is important to be aware of any guilt or regret that you are carrying, and to find the time and space to express your thoughts and feelings.

Anger and Sudden, Traumatic Death

Webster's New World College Dictionary (2005) defines *anger* as "a feeling of displeasure resulting from injury, mistreatment, opposition, etc., and usually showing itself in a desire to fight back at the supposed cause of this feeling." The English language has many words to indicate feelings related to anger, including upset, furious, or annoyed; this large vocabulary is a clue to the many levels, sources, and presentations of anger among people. Each survivor's anger experience is unique, as is the person's ability to cope with the emotion.

For some survivors, anger is an easily recognizable feeling. For others, anger is a very difficult emotion to feel; they may not have a lot of experience with anger, given their family, cultural, or social background, and so feelings of anger might feel "foreign" or unfamiliar. These same people, however, may be aware of feelings of irritability, frustration, negativity, or bitterness. It is fine to insert these words for the word *anger* throughout this handout if they are a better fit with your own experience.

IS IT NATURAL TO FEEL ANGRY AFTER A TRAUMATIC DEATH?

After the death of a significant other, it's quite common to feel angry. You may feel angry that what happened to your loved one was unfair, that you are deprived of someone you value, that you don't feel heard or understood, or that your needs aren't being met. You may feel angry with God for allowing this to happen. You may feel angry at the person or people who brought about the death or those who did not do enough to prevent it. You may feel angry that your loved one didn't have the opportunity to live out a full life, or that you didn't have a chance to say goodbye.

You may even feel angry with your significant other. And you may wonder, "How can I feel angry with someone who has died? Does it mean I didn't or don't really love this person?" Not at all. Anger can arise in an intimate relationship, for example, when an important expectation isn't met, including the expectation or assumption that the person would be with you for the rest of your life. In this case and others, it is natural to feel disappointed and angry.

WHAT ARE SOME REASONS FOR BEING ANGRY AFTER A TRAUMATIC DEATH?

You may feel angry after the death of a significant other for many reasons:

> ➤ It is common to feel anger toward those who caused or brought about the death of your significant other, or toward those who failed to prevent the tragedy. You may experience thoughts or fantasies of revenge toward the perpetrator, if there is one. You may also feel that both you and your loved one were cheated by what happened.

> ➤ You may also feel angry if the death was preventable in some way. This may be particularly the case if you believe that someone is responsible for the death, but this person is not held accountable for what has happened.

(continued)

➤ Anger is also a natural response to abandonment. You may have felt that your loved one was the one person who really understood you, and that now you are truly on your own. Even if your significant other had no control over when or how the death occurred, you may feel deserted or left behind.

➤ Sometimes anger takes the place of other feelings or masks other feelings that are harder to tolerate. In some situations, anger can be empowering, whereas other feelings may confront you with your vulnerability. For example, anger—though legitimate in its own right—may also camouflage grief, sorrow, hurt, regret, anxiety, fear, loneliness, and other feelings and responses. It may be easier to experience anger than grief or fear, for example.

➤ Another reason you may feel angry is because of unfinished business with your loved one. You may have been chronically disappointed or unhappy in your relationship with this person. You may feel angry because you didn't have a chance to say something important—negative or positive—to the loved one. There may have been something (for example, a disagreement or separation) going on at the time of the death that now cannot be addressed or resolved.

➤ Anger is also a natural response to secondary losses. You may feel angry about all of the consequences of the primary loss, such as losing your sense of optimism, your financial security (if you are suffering financial consequences), or your social life (if the primary loss has affected it).

➤ As a survivor of traumatic death, you may also suffer *secondary victimization*. That is, you may sometimes be let down or hurt by those you turn to for help, such as the courts, the mental health system, or even your own family members or friends. For example, a friend may tell you that it's already been 2 years since the death and it's time to move on. Such comments can precipitate anger.

➤ In addition to feeling angry with God, the perpetrator (if there is one), and the loved one, you may feel angry with others after the loss. As noted above, it's common to feel angry with others for their lack of understanding, apparent insensitivity, or inability to meet your needs. It is also common to be angry that their lives are progressing normally while yours is not. Sometimes your anger may "leak out" in relationships with friends, family members, or co-workers. You may find that you have become more irritable and less patient with others because of the loss.

WHY IS ANGER SCARY?

People are often afraid of their anger, and this may be the case for you. There are multiple reasons for that fear, many of which have a lot to do with how your family of origin handled anger. Anger may be unfamiliar if you grew up in a family that suppressed it. It can be a very strong feeling, and strong feelings in general may seem scary if you didn't learn how to recognize, tolerate, modulate, and integrate them while you were growing up. In some homes, anger (a feeling) quickly turns into violence (a behavior). Growing up with people who expressed their anger in violent words or acts, or by drinking alcohol or running away, doesn't teach constructive anger management.

(continued)

USING ANGER CONSTRUCTIVELY

Anger is a natural feeling that you can use constructively. Anger provides information. For example, it can signal a place where you are stuck in coping with the death, a problem in a relationship, or a need or expectation that isn't being met. Anger may also signal an injustice and a need or desire to stand up against that injustice.

Using anger constructively means being able to understand it, and to choose how to respond to the feelings of anger and the situations that evoked them. Therefore, using your anger constructively entails taking time out to reflect on exactly what is making you angry. Being aware of the situations in which anger arises, other feelings that may be present with it, and thoughts or beliefs that accompany it can be a useful way of becoming aware of what is making you angry.

Using anger constructively involves tolerating the emotion by learning to sit with it. It also requires making a choice about how to respond to the feeling itself, to the situation that evoked the feeling, and to others with whom you are angry. Talking over your options with your therapist or another person; writing about your anger and other possible reactions; and taking a "time out" to reflect, to experience the emotion, and to think about potential responses may all help you to use your anger constructively.

If you experience your anger as "energy"—that is, if you're feeling "wound up" or "charged," or feel as if you might "explode"—then physical exercise can be a useful way of managing anger. In addition, the independent activity below provides ways for you to gain awareness of and insight into your anger, as well as to use your anger constructively.

INDEPENDENT ACTIVITY: ANGER

When you feel or remember a time when you felt angry, choose two or more of the questions below and write your responses.

With whom am I angry?

_____

_____

What other feelings (such as, loss, fear, vulnerability, guilt, sorrow, or grief) might underlie the anger?

_____

_____

(continued)

Is fear or another feeling underlying my anger in some way?

_____

_____

Do I feel guilty about something that may be related to my anger?

_____

_____

What do I need that I don't believe I can get?

_____

_____

Are any of my expectations of other people unrealistic? If so, how can I work to modify them?

_____

_____

Are there other ways I can meet my needs so I'll feel less angry?

_____

_____

Letter to Your Significant Other

Think about the conversation you had with your loved one during the empty-chair exercise. Then write a letter to your significant other expressing anything else that you would like to say. You may wish to express gratitude, regret, or simply tell the loved one how you are doing in the treatment or in your life. You can also ask for this person's support as you continue your life. Use self-care and coping skills as necessary before and after (but not during) the exercise to provide support for yourself in this activity. Write as much as you want, but write at least one or two pages. You can use the blank space below to get started.

Exploring the Meaning of the Loss

For this assignment, please consider what this loss has meant to you. Please find a quiet time and place where you can write freely. Try to write as many meanings as come to you, and try not to edit any out for any reason. When you have finished, read what you've written and circle several meanings you feel you could explore further with Handout 13, the Automatic Thought Record. Choose the one that you think about most often or find most troubling. You can use the blank space below to get started.

Spirituality

As human beings, we all need to make sense of our experiences, to assimilate or fit them into our view of the world, and/or to revise our assumptions to accommodate our new experiences. Our spiritual beliefs are a significant aspect of our assumptive world and reflect our ways of making meaning.

The term *spirituality* refers to those aspects of one's life in which one is connected with something beyond oneself. This may include one's connection with God, nature, history, and/or humanity. It is not limited to religious practice. For one person, spirituality can describe his commitment to awareness of the beauty in nature. For another person, spirituality may mean a connection with animals that provides her with a sense of meaning and hope. For many of us, our spirituality can be a source of sustenance in difficult times.

Some people are able to find comfort in their religious or spiritual beliefs following a traumatic death—for example, envisioning the significant other in a better place. However, traumatic losses often lead people to question their spiritual beliefs, or to feel angry, betrayed, or confused. They may wonder, "If such a tragedy could happen, how could there be a loving God?" Practices that once felt restorative such as walking in the woods may no longer work for them. In addition, sudden, traumatic death often robs the survivors of a sense of purpose or meaning. Often the bereaved seek to find meaning for a death that seems to have none. People often simply cannot comprehend why the significant other had to die.

Disruptions in spirituality after a traumatic event are normal. Unfortunately, these disruptions can prevent you from being aware of a larger context and may create another, secondary loss—the loss of a past or potential spiritual connection. Please think about your sense of spirituality and any disruptions you have noticed since the loss. Also, spend some time thinking about how you might redirect, develop, or renew your connection to your spirituality.

INDEPENDENT ACTIVITY: SPIRITUALITY

Creating or reaffirming spirituality after a loss may seem too difficult. You may have to create situations in which you can "hear" your spirituality a number of times before you begin to feel connected to it. Some ideas about ways to begin to renew or create a new spiritual connection are listed below.

- ❖ Watching a sunrise or sunset and meditating on it.
- ❖ Going to see a choir perform, especially children singing.
- ❖ Lying down, closing your eyes, and listening to music (Gregorian chant, Native American flute, etc.).
- ❖ Journaling outside, sitting on the grass or near a body of water.

Please try one of these exercises, or something else that appeals to you, as an independent activity for this week. If this feels too difficult, you might complete an Automatic Thought Record (Handout 13) on your beliefs about spirituality or about how the world works.

Final Impact Statement

Write a statement about the impact that this loss has had on you. Write as much as you want about what the loss means to you. Consider the effects that the loss has had on your beliefs about yourself, your beliefs about others, and your beliefs about the world. Include a description of how you account for this loss having happened—in other words, your understanding of why it happened. Write as much as you want, but write at least one or two pages. You can use the blank space below to get started.

References

Abraham, K. (1927). A short study of the development of the libido, viewed in the light of mental disorders. In *Selected papers of Karl Abraham, M.D.* London: Hogarth Press and the Institute of Psycho-Analysis. (Original work published 1924)

Adams, S. A., & Riggs, S. A. (2008). An exploratory study of vicarious trauma among therapist trainees. *Training and Education in Professional Psychology, 2*(1), 26–34.

Aderka, I. M., Gillihan, S. J., McLean, C. P., & Foa, E. B. (2013). The relationship between posttraumatic and depressive symptoms during prolonged exposure with and without cognitive restructuring for the treatment of posttraumatic stress disorder. *Journal of Consulting and Clinical Psychology, 81*(3), 375–382.

Adolfsson, A., Larsson, P. G., Wijma, B., & Berterö, C. (2004). Guilt and emptiness: Women's experiences of miscarriage. *Health Care for Women International, 25*(6), 543–560.

Allen, J. G. (2001). *Traumatic relationships and serious mental disorders.* New York: Wiley.

Allen, J. G. (2013). *Restoring mentalizing in attachment relationships: Treating trauma with plain old therapy.* Arlington, VA: American Psychiatric Publishing.

Allumbaugh, D. L., & Hoyt, W. T. (1999). Effectiveness of grief therapy: A meta-analysis. *Journal of Counseling Psychology, 46,* 370–380.

American Psychiatric Association. (2013). *Diagnostic and statistical manual of mental disorders* (5th ed.). Arlington, VA: Author.

Amick-McMullan, A., Kilpatrick, D. G., Veronen, L. J., & Smith, S. (1989). Family survivors of homicide victims: Theoretical perspectives and an exploratory study. *Journal of Traumatic Stress, 2,* 21–35.

Amstadter, A. B., Broman-Fulks, J., Zinzow, H., Ruggiero, K. J., & Cercone, J. (2009). Internet-based interventions for traumatic stress-related mental health problems: A review and suggestion for future research. *Clinical Psychology Review, 29*(5), 410–420.

Archer, J. (1999). *The nature of grief: The evolution and psychology of reactions to loss.* New York: Routledge.

Armour, M. (2003). Meaning making in the aftermath of homicide. *Death Studies, 27*(6), 519–540.

Armour, M. (2006). Violent death: Understanding the context of traumatic and stigmatized grief. *Journal of Human Behavior in the Social Environment, 14*(4), 53–90.

Arnold, D., Calhoun, L. G., Tedeschi, R., & Cann, A. (2005). Vicarious posttraumatic growth in psychotherapy. *Journal of Humanistic Psychology, 45,* 239–263.

Attig, T. (1996). *How we grieve: Relearning the world.* New York: Oxford University Press.

Auster, T., Moutier, C., & Lanouette, N. (2008). Bereavement and depression: Implications for diagnosis and treatment. *Psychiatric Annals, 38*(10), 655–661.

Badenoch, B. (2008). *Being a brain-wise therapist: A practical guide to interpersonal neurobiology.* New York: Norton.

Bailley, S. E., Kral, M. J., & Dunham, K. (1999). Survivors of suicide do grieve differently: Empirical support for a common sense proposition. *Suicide and Life-Threatening Behavior, 29*(3), 256–271.

Barrett, C. J., & Schneweis, K. M. (1981). An empirical search for stages of widowhood. *Omega: Journal of Death and Dying, 11*(2), 97–104.

Barsky, A. E. (2012). *Clinicians in court: A guide to subpoenas, depositions, testifying, and everything else you need to know* (2nd ed.). New York: Guilford Press.

Bartholomew, K., & Horowitz, L. M. (1991). Attachment styles among young adults: A test of a four-category model. *Journal of Personality and Social Psychology, 61*, 226–244.

Batson, C. D., Fultz, J., & Schoenrade, P. A. (1987). Distress and empathy: Two qualitatively distinct vicarious emotions with different motivational consequences. *Journal of Personality, 55*(1), 19–39.

Beck, A. T., Rush, A. J., Shaw, B. F., & Emery, G. (1979). *Cognitive therapy of depression*. New York: Guilford Press.

Becker, G., Xander, C. J., Blum, H. E., Lutterbach, J., Gysels, M., & Higginson, I. J. (2007). Do religious or spiritual beliefs influence bereavement?: A systematic review. *Palliative Medicine, 21*, 207–217.

Becker, C. B., Zayfert, C., & Anderson, E. (2004). A survey of psychologists' attitudes towards and utilization of exposure therapy for PTSD. *Behaviour Research and Therapy, 42*, 277–292.

Bell, H., Kulkarni, S., & Dalton, L. (2003). Organizational prevention of vicarious trauma. *Social Work Practice Today, 84*(4), 463–470.

Bennett, K. M., & Bennett, G. (2000–2001). "And there's always this great hole inside that hurts": An empirical study of bereavement in later life. *Omega: Journal of Death and Dying, 42*(3), 237–251.

Blanchard, E. B., Hickling, E. J., Barton, K. A., Taylor, A. E., Loos, R., & Jones-Alexander, J. (1996). One-year prospective follow-up of motor vehicle accident victims. *Behaviour Research and Therapy, 34*, 775–786.

Blanchard, E. B., Hickling, E. J., Devineni, T., Veazy, C. H., Galovski, T. E., Mundy, E., et al. (2003). A controlled evaluation of cognitive behavioral therapy for posttraumatic stress in motor vehicle accident survivors. *Behaviour Research and Therapy, 421*, 79–96.

Bober, T., & Regehr, C. (2006). Strategies for reducing secondary or vicarious trauma: Do they work? *Brief Treatment and Crisis Intervention, 6*(1), 1–9.

Boelen, P. A. (2006). Cognitive-behavioral therapy for complicated grief: Theoretical underpinnings and case descriptions. *Journal of Loss and Trauma, 11*(1), 1–30.

Boelen, P. A., de Keijser, J., van den Hout, M., & van den Bout, J. (2007). Treatment of complicated grief: A comparison between cognitive-behavioral therapy and supportive counseling. *Journal of Consulting and Clinical Psychology, 75*(2), 277–284.

Boelen, P. A., & Prigerson, H. G. (2013). Prolonged grief disorder as a new diagnostic category in DSM-5. In M. S. Stroebe, H. Schut, & J. van den Bout (Eds.), *Complicated grief: Scientific foundations for health care professionals* (pp. 85–94). New York: Routledge.

Boelen, P. A., van den Hout, M. A., & van den Bout, J. (2006). A cognitive-behavioral conceptualization of complicated grief. *Clinical Psychology: Science and Practice, 13*, 109–128.

Boelen, P. A., Van den Hout, M., & van den Bout, J. (2013). Prolonged grief disorder: Cognitive-behavioral theory and therapy. In M. Stroebe, H. Schut, & J. van den Bout (Eds.), *Complicated grief: Scientific foundations for health care professionals* (pp. 221–234). New York: Routledge/Taylor Francis.

Bonanno, G. A. (2001). Grief and emotion: A social-functional perspective. In M. S. Stroebe, R. O. Hansson, W. Stroebe, & H. Schut (Eds.), *Handbook of bereavement research: Consequences, coping, and care* (pp. 493–515). Washington, DC: American Psychological Association.

Bonanno, G. A., & Kaltman, S. (1999). Toward an integrative perspective on bereavement. *Psychological Bulletin, 125*, 760–786.

Bonanno, G. A., & Keltner, D. (1997). Facial expressions of emotion and the course of conjugal bereavement. *Journal of Abnormal Psychology, 106*, 126–137.

Bonanno, G. A., Moskowitz, J. T., Pappa, A., & Folkman, S. (2005). Resilience to loss in bereaved spouses, bereaved parents, and bereaved gay men. *Journal of Personality and Social Psychology, 88*(5), 827–843.

Bonanno, G. A., Neria, Y., Mancini, A., Coifman, K. G., Litz, B., & Insel, B. (2007). Is there more to complicated grief than depression and posttraumatic stress disorder?: A test of incremental validity. *Journal of Abnormal Psychology, 116*(2), 342–351.

Bonanno, G. A., Wortman, C. B., Lehman, D., Tweed, R., Haring, M., Sonnega, J., et al. (2002). Resilience to loss, chronic grief, and their pre-bereavement predictors. *Journal of Personality and Social Psychology, 83*, 1150–1164.

Botkin, A. L., Hogan, C., & Moody, R. A. (2005). *Induced after-death communication: A new therapy for healing grief and trauma*. Newburyport, MA: Hampton Road.

Bower, B. (2010). Humans: Seeing body aids bereaved relatives: Viewing the death can give comfort in cases of sudden loss. *Science News, 177*(12), 10.

Bowlby, J. (1969). *Attachment and loss: Vol. 1. Attachment.* New York: Basic Books.

Bowlby, J. (1973). *Attachment and loss: Vol. 2. Separation: Anxiety and anger.* New York: Basic Books.

Bowlby, J. (1980). *Attachment and loss: Vol. 3. Loss: Sadness and depression.* New York: Basic Books.

Bowlby, J. (1988). *A secure base: Clinical applications of attachment theory.* London: Routledge.

Bowlby, J., & Parkes, C. M. (1970). Separation and loss. In E. J. Anthony & C. Koupernik (Eds.), *International yearbook of child psychiatry and allied professions: Vol. 1. The child and his family* (pp. 197–216). New York: Wiley.

Bradburn, N. M. (1969). *The structure of psychological well-being.* Chicago: Aldine.

Bradley, R., Greene, J., Russ, E., Dutra, L., & Westen, D. (2005). A multidimensional meta-analysis of psychotherapy for PTSD. *American Journal of Psychiatry, 162*(2), 214–227.

Breen, L. J. (2010–2011). Professionals' experiences of grief counseling: Implications for bridging the gap between research and practice. *Omega: Journal of Death and Dying, 62*(3), 285–303.

Breen, L. J., & O'Connor, M. (2007). The fundamental paradox in the grief literature: A critical reflection. *Omega: Journal of Death and Dying, 55*(3), 199–218.

Bremner, J. D. (2006). Traumatic stress: Effects on the brain. *Dialogues in Clinical Neuroscience, 8,* 445–461.

Bremner, J. D., Randall, P., Scott, T. M., Bronen, R. A., Seibyl, J. P., Southwick, S. M., et al. (1995). MRI-based measurement of hippocampal volume in patients with combat-related posttraumatic stress disorder. *American Journal of Psychiatry, 152*(7), 973–981.

Bremner, J. D., Staib, L. H., Kaloupek, D., Southwick, S. M., Soufer, R., & Charney, D. S. (1999). Neural correlates of exposure to traumatic pictures and sound in Vietnam combat veterans with and without posttraumatic stress disorder: A positron emission tomography study. *Biological Psychiatry, 45,* 806–816.

Bremner, J. D., Vythilingam, M., Vermetten, E., Southwick, S. M., McGlashan, T., Nazeer, A., et al. (2003). MRI and PET study of deficits in hippocampal structure and function in women with childhood sexual abuse and posttraumatic stress disorder. *American Journal of Psychiatry, 160,* 924–932.

Brent, D. A., Perper, J., Moritz, G., Allman, C., Friend, A., Schweers, J., et al. (1992). Psychiatric effects of exposure to suicide among the friends and acquaintances of adolescent suicide victims. *Journal of the American Academy of Child and Adolescent Psychiatry, 31*(4), 629–639.

Bride, B. E. (2004). The impact of providing psychosocial services to traumatized populations. *Stress, Trauma, and Crisis, 7*(1), 29–46.

Briere, J. (1996a). A self-trauma model for treating adult survivors of severe child abuse. In J. Briere, L. Berliner, J. A. Bulkley, C. Jenny, & T. Reid (Eds.), *The APSAC handbook on child maltreatment* (pp. 140–157). Thousand Oaks, CA: Sage.

Briere, J. (1996b). *Therapy for adults molested as children: Beyond survival* (2nd ed.). New York: Springer.

Briere, J. (2002). Treating adult survivors of severe childhood abuse and neglect: Further development of an integrative model. In J. E. B. Myers, L. Berliner, J. Briere, C. T. Hendrix, T. Reid, & C. Jenny (Eds.), *The APSAC handbook on child maltreatment* (2nd ed., pp. 1–26). Thousand Oaks, CA: Sage.

Briere, J., & Runtz, M. (2002). The Inventory of Altered Self Capacities (IASC): A standardized measure of identity, affect regulation, and relationship disturbance. *Assessment, 9*(3), 230–239.

Briere, J., & Scott, C. (2006). *Principles of trauma therapy: A guide to symptoms, evaluation, and treatment.* Thousand Oaks, CA: Sage.

Brock, K. J., Pearlman, L. A., & Varra, E. M. (2006). Child maltreatment, self capacities, and trauma symptoms: Psychometric properties of the Inner Experience Questionnaire. *Journal of Emotional Abuse, 6,* 103–125.

Brom, D., & Kleber, R. (2000). On coping with trauma and coping with grief: Similarities and differences. In R. Malkinson, S. S. Rubin, & E. Wiztum (Eds.), *Traumatic and nontraumatic loss and bereavement: Clinical theory and practice* (pp. 41–66). Madison, CT: Psychosocial Press.

Buchi, S. M., Hanspeter, S., Jenewein, U., Hepp, J., Jina, U., Neuhaus, E., et al. (2007). Grief and posttraumatic growth in parents 2–6 years after the death of their extremely premature baby. *Psychotherapy and Psychosomatics, 76*(2), 106–114.

Buckle, J. L., & Fleming, S. J. (2011). Parenting challenges after the death of a child. In R. A. Neimeyer, D. L. Harris, H. R. Winokuer, & G. F. Thornton (Eds.), *Grief and bereavement in contemporary society: Bridging research and practice* (pp. 93–106). New York: Routledge.

Cahill, S. P., Foa, E. B., Hembree, E. A., Marshall, R. D., & Nacash, N. (2006). Dissemination of exposure therapy in the treatment of posttraumatic stress disorder. *Journal of Traumatic Stress, 19*(5), 597–610.

Cahill, S. P., Rothbaum, B. O., Resick, P. A., & Follette, V. M. (2009). Cognitive-behavioral therapy for adults. In E. B. Foa, T. M. Keane, M. J. Friedman, & J. A. Cohen (Eds.), *Effective treatments for PTSD: Practice guidelines from the International Society for Traumatic Stress Studies* (2nd ed., pp. 139–222). New York: Guilford Press.

Caplan, S., & Lang, G. (1995). *Grief's courageous journey: A workbook*. Oakland, CA: New Harbinger.

Carr, D. (2008). Factors that influence late-life bereavement: Considering data from the Changing Lives of Older Couples study. In M. Stroebe, R. O. Hansson, H. Schut, & W. Stroebe (Eds.), *Handbook of bereavement research and practice: Advances in theory and intervention* (pp. 417–440). Washington, DC: American Psychological Association.

Carr, D., House, J. S., Kessler, R. C., Nesse, R. M., Sonnega, J., & Wortman, C. (2000). Marital quality and psychological adjustment to widowhood among older adults: A longitudinal analysis. *Journal of Gerontology: Series B. Psychological Sciences and Social Sciences, 55B*, S197–S207.

Chapple, A., Swift, C., & Ziebland, S. (2011). The role of spirituality and religion for those bereaved due to a traumatic death. *Mortality, 16*(1), 1–19.

Chapple, A., & Ziebland, S. (2010). Viewing the body after bereavement due to a traumatic death: Qualitative study in the UK. *British Medical Journal, 340*, c2032.

Christ, G. H., Kane, D., & Horsley, H. (2011). Grief after terrorism: Toward a family-focused intervention. In R. A. Neimeyer, D. L. Harris, H. R. Winokuer, & G. F. Thornton (Eds.), *Grief and bereavement in contemporary society: Bridging research and practice* (pp. 203–222). New York: Routledge.

Cleiren, M. P. H. D. (1991). *Adaptation after bereavement: A comparative study of the aftermath of death from suicide, traffic accident, and illness for next of kin*. Leiden, the Netherlands: DSWO Press.

Cleiren, M. P. H. D. (1993). *Bereavement and adaptation: A comparative study of the aftermath of death*. Washington, DC: Hemisphere.

Cleiren, M. P. H. D., Diekstra, R., Kerkhof, A., & van der Wal, J. (1994). Mode of death and kinship in bereavement: Focusing on "who" rather than "how." *Crisis, 15*(1), 22–36.

Cloitre, M., Cohen, L. R., & Koenen, K. C. (2006). *Treating survivors of childhood abuse: Psychotherapy for the interrupted life*. New York: Guilford Press.

Cloitre, M., Koenen, K. C., Cohen, L. R., & Han, H. (2002). Skills training in affective and interpersonal regulation followed by exposure: A phase-based treatment for PTSD related to childhood abuse. *Journal of Clinical and Consulting Psychology, 70*, 1067–1074.

Cloitre, M., & Rosenberg, A. (2006). Sexual revictimization: Risk factors and prevention. In V. M. Follette & J. I. Ruzek (Eds.), *Cognitive-behavioral therapies for trauma* (2nd ed., pp. 321–361). New York: Guilford Press.

Cloitre, M., Stovall-McClough, K. C., Nooner, K., Zorbas, P., Cherry, S., Jackson, C. L., et al. (2010). Treatment for PTSD related to childhood abuse: A randomized controlled trial. *American Journal of Psychiatry, 167*(8), 915–924.

Courtois, C. A. (2010). *Healing the incest wound: Adult survivors in therapy* (2nd ed.). New York: Norton.

Courtois, C. A., & Ford, J. D. (Eds.). (2009). *Treating complex traumatic stress disorders: An evidence-based guide*. New York: Guilford Press.

Cowchock, F. S., Lasker, J. N., Toedter, L. J., Skumanich, S. A., & Koenig, H. G. (2010). Religious beliefs affect grieving after pregnancy loss. *Journal of Religion and Health, 49*(4), 485–497.

Currier, J. M., Holland, J. M., & Neimeyer, R. A. (2006). Sense-making, grief, and the experience of violent loss: Toward a mediational model. *Death Studies, 30*(5), 403–428.

Currier, J. M., Mallot, J., Martinez, T. E., Sandy, C., & Neimeyer, R. A. (2012). Bereavement, religion, and posttraumatic growth: A matched control group investigation. *Psychology of Religion and Spirituality, 4*(2), 108–122.

Currier, J. M., Neimeyer, R. A., & Berman, J. S. (2008). The effectiveness of psychotherapeutic interventions for bereaved persons: A comprehensive quantitative review. *Psychological Bulletin, 134*, 648–661.

Dalenberg, C. J. (2000). *Countertransference and the treatment of trauma*. Washington, DC: American Psychological Association.

Danieli, Y. (1994). Countertransference, trauma, and training. In J. P. Wilson & J. D. Lindy (Eds.), *Countertransference in the treatment of PTSD* (pp. 368–388). New York: Guilford Press.

Dass-Brailsford, P. (Ed.). (2010). *Crisis and disaster counseling: Lessons learned from Hurricane Katrina and other disasters*. Thousand Oaks, CA: Sage.

Davis, C. G. (2001). The tormented and the transformed: Understanding response to loss and trauma. In R. A. Neimeyer (Ed.), *Meaning reconstruction and the experience of loss* (pp. 137–155). Washington, DC: American Psychological Association.

Davis, C. G., Wortman, C. B., Lehman, D. R., & Silver, R. C. (2000). Searching for meaning in loss: Are clinical assumptions correct? *Death Studies, 24*, 497–540.

Derogatis, L. R. (1977). *SCL-90: Administration, scoring and procedures manual–I for the revised version*. Baltimore: Johns Hopkins University School of Medicine.

Deutsch, H. (1937). Absence of grief. *Psychoanalytic Quarterly, 6*, 12–22.

Doka, K. J., & Martin, T. L. (2010). *Grieving beyond gender: Understanding the way men and women mourn*. New York: Routledge.

Dominick, S. A., Blair, I. A., Beauchamp, N., Seeley, J. R., Nolen-Hoeksema, S., Doka, K. J., et al. (2009–2010). An Internet tool to normalize grief. *Omega: Journal of Death and Dying, 60*(1), 71–87.

Dull, V. T., & Skokan, L. A. (1995). A cognitive model of religion's influence on health. *Journal of Social Issues, 51*(2), 49–64.

Dyregrov, A., & Matthiesen, S. B. (1987). Similarities and differences in mothers' and fathers' grief following the death of an infant. *Scandinavian Journal of Psychology, 28*, 1–15.

Dyregrov, K. (2002). Assistance from local authorities versus survivors' needs for support after suicide. *Death Studies, 26*(8), 647–668.

Dyregrov, K. (2003–2004). Micro-sociological analysis of social support following traumatic bereavement: Unhelpful and avoidant responses from the community. *Omega: Journal of Death and Dying, 48*(1), 23–44.

Dyregrov, K. (2005–2006). Experiences of social networks supporting traumatically bereaved. *Omega: Journal of Death and Dying, 52*(4), 339–358.

Dyregrov, K., Nordanger, D., & Dyregrov, A. (2003). Predictors of psychosocial distress after suicide, SIDS and accidents. *Death Studies, 27*(2), 143–165.

Eifert, G. H., & Forsyth, J. P. (2005). *Acceptance and commitment therapy for anxiety disorders: A practitioner's treatment guide to using mindfulness, acceptance, and values-based behavior change strategies*. Oakland, CA: New Harbinger.

Elwood, L. S., Mott, J., Lohr, J. M., & Galovski, T. E. (2011). Secondary trauma symptoms in clinicians: A critical review of the construct, specificity, and implications for trauma-focused treatment. *Clinical Psychology Review, 31*(1), 25–36.

Emmons, R. A., & Mishra, A. (2011). Why gratitude enhances well-being: What we know, what we need to know. In K. M. Sheldon, T. B. Kashdan, & M. F. Steger (Eds.), *Designing positive psychology: Taking stock and moving forward* (pp. 248–262). New York: Oxford University Press.

Engel, G. L. (1961). Is grief a disease? *Psychosomatic Medicine, 23*, 18–22.

Eth, S., & Pynoos, R. (1985). Developmental perspective on psychic trauma in childhood. In C. R. Figley (Ed.), *Trauma and its wake: The study and treatment of post-traumatic stress disorder* (pp. 36–52). New York: Brunner/Mazel.

Eth, S., & Pynoos, R. S. (1994). Children who witness the homicide of a parent. *Psychiatry: Interpersonal and Biological Processes, 57*(4), 287–306.

Fawcett, J. (Ed.). (2003). *Stress and trauma handbook: Strategies for flourishing in demanding environments*. Monrovia, CA: World Vision International.

Fearon, J. C. (2011). *The technology of grief: Social networking sites as a modern death ritual*. Unpublished doctoral dissertation, Antioch University New England.

Fearon, J. C. (2012). The technology of grief: Social networking sites as a modern death ritual. *Dissertation Abstracts International: Section B: The Sciences and Engineering, 72*(12-B), 7741.

Feigelman, W., Jordan, J., McIntosh, J., & Feigelman, B. (2012). *Devastating losses: How parents cope with the death of a child to suicide or drugs*. New York: Springer.

Field, N. P. (2008). Whether to relinquish or maintain a bond with the deceased. In M. S. Stroebe, R. O. Hansson, H. Schut, & W. Stroebe (Eds.), *Handbook of bereavement research and practice: Advances in theory and intervention* (pp. 113–132). Washington, DC: American Psychological Association.

Field, N. P., & Wogrin, C. (2011). The changing bond in therapy for unresolved loss: An attachment theory perspective. In R. A. Neimeyer, D. L. Harris, H. R. Winokuer, & G. F. Thornton (Eds.), *Grief and bereavement in contemporary society: Bridging research and practice* (pp. 37–46). New York: Routledge.

Figley, C. R. (1995). *Compassion fatigue: Coping with secondary traumatic stress disorders in those who treat the traumatized*. New York: Brunner/Mazel.

Figley, C. R. (1998). *The traumatology of grieving*. Philadelphia: Brunner/Mazel.

Figley, C. R., Bride, B. E., & Mazza, N. (1997). *Death and trauma: The traumatology of grieving*. Washington, DC: Taylor & Francis.

Finkbeiner, A. K. (1996). *After the death of a child: Living with loss through the years.* Baltimore, MD: Johns Hopkins University Press.

Foa, E. B., Dancu, C. V., Hembree, E. A., Jaycox, L. H., Meadows, E. A., & Street, G. P. (1999). A comparison of exposure therapy, stress inoculation training, and their combination for reducing posttraumatic stress disorder in female assault victims. *Journal of Consulting and Clinical Psychology, 67*(2), 194–200.

Foa, E. B., Davidson, J. R. T., & Frances, A. (Eds.). (1999). The expert consensus guideline series: Treatment of posttraumatic stress disorder. *Journal of Clinical Psychiatry, 60*(Suppl. 16), 4–76.

Foa, E. B., Hembree, E. A., Cahill, S. P., Rauch, S. A. M., Riggs, D. S., Feeny, N. C., et al. (2005). Randomized trial of prolonged exposure for posttraumatic stress disorder with and without cognitive restructuring: Outcome at academic and community clinics. *Journal of Consulting and Clinical Psychology, 73*(5), 953–964.

Foa, E. B., Hembree, E. A., & Rothbaum, B. O. (2007). *Prolonged exposure therapy for PTSD: Emotional processing of traumatic experiences: Therapist guide.* New York: Oxford University Press.

Foa, E., Keane, T., & Friedman, M. (Eds.). (2000). *Effective treatments for PTSD: Practice guidelines from the International Society for Traumatic Stress Studies.* New York: Guilford Press.

Foa, E. B., Keane, T. M., Friedman, M. J., & Cohen, J. A. (Eds.). (2009). *Effective treatments for PTSD: Practice guidelines from the International Society for Traumatic Stress Studies* (2nd ed.). New York: Guilford Press.

Foa, E. B., & Kozak, M. J. (1991). Emotional processing: Theory, research, and clinical implications for anxiety disorders. In J. D. Safran & L. S. Greenberg (Eds.), *Emotion, psychotherapy, and change* (pp. 21–49). New York: Guilford Press.

Foa, E. B., & Rothbaum, B. O. (1998). *Treating the trauma of rape: Cognitive-behavioral therapy for PTSD.* New York: Guilford Press.

Foa, E. B., Rothbaum, B. O., Riggs, D. S., & Murdock, T. B. (1991). Treatment of posttraumatic stress disorder in rape victims: A comparison between cognitive-behavioral procedures and counseling. *Journal of Consulting and Clinical Psychology, 59*(5), 715–723.

Foa, E. B., Zoellner, L. A., Feeny, N. C., Hembree, E. A., & Alvarez-Conrad, J. (2002). Does imaginal exposure exacerbate PTSD symptoms? *Journal of Consulting and Clinical Psychology, 70*(4), 1022–1028.

Folkman, S. (1997a). Introduction to the special section: Use of bereavement narratives to predict well-being in gay men whose partner died of AIDS—Four theoretical perspectives. *Journal of Personality and Social Psychology, 72,* 851–854.

Folkman, S. (1997b). Positive psychological states and coping with severe stress. *Social Science and Medicine, 45,* 1207–1221.

Folkman, S. (2001). Revised coping theory and the process of bereavement. In M. S. Stroebe, R. O. Hansson, W. Stroebe, & H. Schut (Eds.), *Handbook of bereavement research: Consequences, coping, and care* (pp. 563–584). Washington, DC: American Psychological Association.

Folkman, S. (2008). The case for positive emotions in the stress process. *Anxiety, Stress and Coping, 21*(1), 3–14.

Folkman, S., & Moskowitz, J. T. (2000). Stress, positive emotion, and coping. *Current Directions in Psychological Science, 9,* 115–118.

Follette, V. M., Polusny, M. M., & Milbeck, K. (1994). Mental health and law enforcement professionals: Trauma history, psychological symptoms, and impact of providing services to child sexual abuse survivors. *Professional Psychology: Research and Practice, 25,* 275–282.

Fraley, R. C., & Bonanno, G. A. (2004). Attachment and loss: A test of three competing models on the association between attachment-related avoidance and adaptation to bereavement. *Personality and Social Psychology Bulletin, 30,* 878–890.

Fraley, R. C., & Shaver, P. R. (1999). Loss and bereavement: Attachment theory and recent controversies concerning "grief work" and the nature of detachment. In J. Cassidy & P. R. Shaver (Eds.), *Handbook of attachment: Theory, research, and clinical applications* (pp. 735–759). New York: Guilford Press.

Fredrickson, B. L. (2001). The role of positive emotions in positive psychology: The broaden-and-build theory of positive emotions. *American Psychologist, 56,* 218–226.

Fredrickson, B. L., Tugade, M. M., Waugh, C. E., & Larkin, G. R. (2003). What good are positive emotions?: A prospective study of resilience and emotions following the terrorist attacks on the United States on September 11, 2001. *Journal of Personality and Social Psychology, 84,* 365–376.

Freud, S. (1957). Mourning and melancholia. In J. Strachey (Ed. & Trans.), *The standard edition of the complete works of Sigmund Freud* (Vol. 14, pp. 237–260). London: Hogarth Press. (Original work published 1917)

Gamino, L. A., Hogan, N. S., & Sewell, K. W. (2002).

Feeling the absence: A content analysis from the Scott and White grief study. *Death Studies, 26*(10), 793–813.

Gamino, L. A., & Sewell, K. W. (2004). Meaning constructs as predictors of bereavement adjustment: A report from the Scott & White grief study. *Death Studies, 28*, 397–421.

George, A. J., Elliott, A., Jennings, J., Cleland, K., & Brown, M. (2009). Grief support group for spouses of deceased Iraq war veterans. *Praxis, 9*, 70–86.

Gilbert, K. R., & Horsley, G. C. (2011). Technology and grief support in the twenty-first century: A multimedia platform. In R. A. Neimeyer, D. L. Harris, H. R. Winokuer, & G. F. Thornton (Eds.), *Grief and bereavement in contemporary society: Bridging research and practice* (pp. 365–373). New York: Routledge.

Glick, I. O., Weiss, R. S., & Parkes, C. M. (1974). *The first year of bereavement*. New York: Wiley.

Green, B. L., Goodman, L. A., Krupnick, J. L., Corcoran, C. B., Petty, R. M., Stockton, P., et al. (2000). Outcomes of single versus multiple trauma exposure in a screening sample. *Journal of Traumatic Stress, 13*(2), 271–286.

Green, B. L., Krupnick, J. L., Stockton, P., Goodman, L., Corcoran, C., & Petty, R. (2005). Effects of adolescent trauma exposure on risky behavior in college women. *Psychiatry, 68*(4), 363–378.

Handsley, S. (2001). "But what about us?": The residual effects of sudden death on self-identity and family relationships. *Mortality, 6*(1), 9–29.

Harrington-Lamorie, J., & McDevitt-Murphy, M. E. (2011). Traumatic death in the United States military: Initiating the dialogue on war-related loss. In R. A. Neimeyer, D. L. Harris, H. R. Winokuer, & G. F. Thornton (Eds.), *Grief and bereavement in contemporary society: Bridging research and practice* (pp. 261–272). New York: Routledge.

Harrison, R. L., & Westwood, M. J. (2009). Preventing vicarious traumatization of mental health therapists: Identifying protective practices. *Psychotherapy: Theory, Research, Practice, and Training, 46*(2), 203–219.

Harvey, A. G., Bryant, R. A., & Tarrier, N. (2003). Cognitive behaviour therapy for posttraumatic stress disorder. *Clinical Psychology Review, 23*(3), 501–522.

Harvey, M. R. (1996). An ecological view of psychological trauma and trauma recovery. *Journal of Traumatic Stress, 9*(1), 3–23.

Hayes, S. C. (2004). Acceptance and commitment therapy, relational frame theory, and the third wave of behavioral and cognitive therapies. *Behavior Therapy, 35*(4), 639–665.

Hayes, S. C. (with Smith, S.). (2005). *Get out of your mind and into your life*. Oakland, CA: New Harbinger.

Hays, J. C., & Hendrix, C. C. (2008). The role of religion in bereavement. In M. S. Stroebe, R. O. Hansson, H. Schut, & W. Stroebe (Eds.), *Handbook of bereavement research and practice: Advances in theory and intervention* (pp. 327–348). Washington, DC: American Psychological Association.

Heim, C., & Nemeroff, C. B. (2009). Neurobiology of posttraumatic stress disorder. *CNS Spectrum, 14*(1), 13–24.

Hernandez, P., Gangsei, D., & Engstrom, D. (2007). Vicarious resilience: A new concept in work with those who survive trauma. *Family Process, 46*(2), 229–241.

Heron, M. (2012). Deaths: Leading causes for 2009. *National Vital Statistics Reports, 61*(7). Available at *www.cdc.gov/nchs/data/nvsr/nvsr61/ nvsr61_07.pdf*.

Hibberd, R., Elwood, L. S., & Galovski, T. E. (2010). Risk and protective factors for posttraumatic stress disorder, prolonged grief and depression in survivors of the violent death of a loved one. *Journal of Loss and Trauma, 15*, 426–447.

Holland, J. M., Currier, J. M., & Neimeyer, R. A. (2006). Meaning reconstruction in the first two years of bereavement: The role of sense-making and benefit-finding. *Omega: Journal of Death and Dying, 53*, 175–191.

Holland, J. M., & Neimeyer, R. A. (2010). An examination of stage theory of grief among individuals bereaved by natural and violent causes: A meaning-oriented contribution. *Omega: Journal of Death and Dying, 61*(12), 103–120.

Holland, J. M., & Neimeyer, R. A. (2011). Separation and traumatic distress in prolonged grief: The role of cause of death and relationship to the deceased. *Journal of Psychopathology and Behavioral Assessment, 33*(2), 254–263.

Hollon, S. D., Stewart, M. O., & Strunk, D. (2006). Enduring effects for cognitive behavior therapy in the treatment of depression and anxiety. *Annual Review of Psychology, 57*, 285–315.

Holman, E. A., Perisho, J., Edwards, A., & Mlakar, N. (2010). The myths of coping with loss in undergraduate psychiatric nursing books. *Research in Nursing and Health, 33*(6), 486–499.

Horowitz, M. J. (1997). Cognitive psychodynamics: The clinical use of states, person schemas, and defensive control process theories. In D. J. Stein (Ed.), *Cognitive science and the unconscious* (pp. 189–205). Washington, DC: American Psychiatric Association.

Horowitz, M. J., Siegel, B., Holen, A., Bonanno, G. A., Milbrath, C., & Stinson, C. H. (1997). Diagnostic criteria for complicated grief. *American Journal of Psychiatry, 154*(7), 904–910.

Houben, L. M. (2012). *Counseling Hispanics through loss, grief, and bereavement: A guide for mental health professionals.* New York: Springer.

Huggard, P., Stamm, B. H., & Pearlman, L. A. (2013). Physician stress: Compassion satisfaction, compassion fatigue and vicarious traumatization. In C. R. Figley, P. Huggard, & C. Rees (Eds.), *First do no self-harm: Understanding and promoting physician stress resilience* (pp. 127–145). New York: Oxford University Press.

Humphrey, G. M., & Zimpfer, D. G. (1996). *Counseling for grief and bereavement* (pp. 127–145). Thousand Oaks, CA: Sage.

Jacobs, S., Mazure, C., & Prigerson, H. (2000). Diagnostic criteria for traumatic grief. *Death Studies, 24*(3), 185–199.

Jacobson, N. S., & Gortner, E. T. (2000). Can depression be de-medicalized in the 21st century: Scientific revolutions, counter-revolutions and the magnetic field of normal science. *Behaviour Research and Therapy, 38*, 103–117.

Jaeger, J. A., Echiverri, A., Zoellner, L., Post, L., & Feeny, N. C. (2010). Factors associated with choice of exposure therapy for PTSD. *International Journal of Behavioral Consultation and Therapy, 5*(3–4), 294–310.

Jaffe, J., & Diamond, M. O. (2011). Grieving a reproductive loss. In J. Jaffe & M. O. Diamond (Eds.), *Reproductive trauma: Psychotherapy with infertility and pregnancy loss clients* (pp. 91–111). Washington, DC: American Psychological Association.

Janoff-Bulman, R. (1988). Victims of violence. In S. Fisher & J. Reason (Eds.), *Handbook of life stress, cognition, and health* (pp. 101–113). Chichester, UK: Wiley.

Janoff-Bulman, R. (1992). *Shattered assumptions: Toward a new psychology of trauma.* New York: Free Press.

Johannesson, K. B., Lundin, T., Hultman, C. M., Frojd, T., & Michel, P. (2011). Prolonged grief among traumatically bereaved relatives exposed and not exposed to a tsunami. *Journal of Traumatic Stress, 24*(4), 456–464.

Johnson, D. C., Polusny, M. A., Erbes, C. R., King, D. W., King, L. A., Litz, B. T., et al. (2011). Development and initial validation of the Response to Stressful Experiences Scale. *Military Medicine, 176*(2), 161–169.

Johnson, J. G., Zhang, B., Greer, J. A., & Prigerson, H. G. (2007). Parental control, partner dependency, and complicated grief among widowed adults in the community. *Journal of Nervous and Mental Disease, 195*(1), 26–30.

Johnson, J. G., Zhang, B., & Prigerson, H. G. (2008). Investigation of a developmental model of risk for depression and suicidality following spousal bereavement. *Suicide and Life-Threatening Behavior, 38*(1), 1–12.

Jordan, J. R. (1991). Cumulative loss, current stress, and the family: A pilot investigation of individual and systematic effects. *Omega: Journal of Death and Dying, 24*(4), 309–332.

Jordan, J. R. (2001). Is suicide bereavement different?: A reassessment of the literature. *Suicide and Life-Threatening Behavior, 31*(1), 91–102.

Jordan, J. R., & McIntosh, J. L. (2010). *Grief after suicide: Understanding the consequences and caring for the survivors.* New York: Taylor & Francis.

Jordan, J. R., & McIntosh, J. L. (2011). Is suicide bereavement different?: Perspectives from research and practice. In R. A. Neimeyer, D. L. Harris, H. R. Winokuer, & G. F. Thornton (Eds.), *Grief and bereavement in contemporary society: Bridging research and practice* (pp. 223–234). New York: Routledge.

Jordan, J. R., & Neimeyer, R. A. (2003). Does grief counseling work? *Death Studies, 27*, 765–786.

Jordan, J. V., Kaplan, A. G., Miller, J. B., Stiver, I. P., & Surrey, J. L. (1991). *Women's growth in connection: Writings from the Stone Center.* New York: Guilford Press.

Jordan, K. (2010). Vicarious trauma: Proposed factors that impact clinicians. *Journal of Family Psychotherapy, 21*(4), 225–237.

Kahn, L. (2006). The understanding and treatment of betrayal trauma as a traumatic experience of love. *Journal of Trauma Practice, 5*(3), 57–72.

Kaltman, S., & Bonanno, G. A. (2003). Trauma and bereavement: Examining the impact of sudden and violent deaths. *Journal of Anxiety Disorders, 17*(2), 131–147.

Kastenbaum, R. (1969). Death and bereavement in later life. In A. Kutscher (Ed.), *Death and bereavement* (pp. 28–54). Springfield, IL: Thomas.

Kato, P. M., & Mann, T. (1999). A synthesis of psychological interventions for the bereaved. *Clinical Psychology Review, 19*, 275–296.

Kazantzis, N., & Deane, F. (1999). Psychologists' use of homework assignments in clinical practice. *Professional Psychology: Research and Practice, 30*(6), 581–585.

Kazantzis, N., Deane, F., Ronan, K. R., & L'Abate, L. (Eds.). (2005). *Using homework assignments in cognitive behavior therapy*. New York: Routledge.

Kazantzis, N., Whittington, C., & Dattilio, F. (2010). Meta-analysis of homework effects in cognitive and behavioral therapy: A replication and extension. *Clinical Psychology Science and Practice, 17*, 144–156.

Keesee, N. J., Currier, J. M., & Neimeyer, R. A. (2008). Predictors of grief following the death of one's child: The contribution of finding meaning. *Journal of Clinical Psychology, 64*(10), 1145–1163.

Kelley, M. M., & Chan, K. T. (2012). Assessing the role of attachment to God, meaning and religious coping as mediators in the grief experience. *Death Studies, 36*, 199–227.

Keltner, D., & Bonanno, G. A. (1997). A study of laughter and dissociation: Distinct correlates of laughter and smiling during bereavement. *Journal of Personality and Social Psychology, 73*, 687–702.

Kersting, A., Kroker, K., Schlicht, S., Baust, K., & Wagner, B. (2011). Efficacy of cognitive behavioral Internet-based therapy in parents after the loss of a child during pregnancy: pilot data from a randomized controlled trial. *Archive of Women's Health, 14*, 465–477.

Killian, K. (2008). Helping till it hurts?: A multimethod study of compassion fatigue, burnout, and self-care in clinicians working with trauma survivors. *Traumatology, 14*(2), 32–44.

Klass, D., & Chow, A. Y. M. (2011). Culture and ethnicity in experiencing, policing, and handling grief. In R. A. Neimeyer, D. L. Harris, H. R. Winokuer, & G. F. Thornton (Eds.), *Grief and bereavement in contemporary society: Bridging research and practice* (pp. 341–353). New York: Routledge.

Klass, D., Silverman, P. R., & Nickman, S. L. (Eds.). (1996). *Continuing bonds: New understandings of grief*. Washington, DC: Taylor & Francis.

Klass, D., & Walter, J. (2001). Processes of grieving: How bonds are continued. In M. S. Stroebe, R. O. Hansson, W. Stroebe, & H. Schut (Eds.), *Handbook of bereavement research: Consequences, coping, and care* (pp. 431–448). Washington, DC: American Psychological Association.

Klugman, C. M. (2006). Dead men talking: Evidence of post death contact and continuing bonds. *Omega: Journal of Death and Dying, 53*(3), 249–262.

Korn, D. M., & Leeds, A. M. (2002). Preliminary evidence of efficacy for EMDR resource development and installation in the stabilization phase of treatment of complex posttraumatic stress disorder. *Journal of Clinical Psychology, 58*, 1465–1487.

Kristensen, P., & Pereira, M. (2011). Bereavement and disasters: Research and clinical intervention. In R. A. Neimeyer, D. L. Harris, H. R. Winokuer, & G. F. Thornton (Eds.), *Grief and bereavement in contemporary society: Bridging research and practice* (pp. 189–201). New York: Routledge.

Kristensen, P., Weisaeth, L., & Heir, T. (2009). Psychiatric disorders among disaster bereaved: An interview study of individuals directly or not directly exposed to the 2004 tsunami. *Depression and Anxiety, 26*, 1127–1133.

Kristensen, P., Weisaerth, L., & Heir, T. (2012). Bereavement and mental health after sudden and violent losses: A review. *Psychiatry, 75*(1), 76–97.

Kubany, E. S., Hill, E. E., & Owens, J. A. (2003). Cognitive trauma therapy for battered women with PTSD: Preliminary findings. *Journal of Traumatic Stress, 16*(1), 81–91.

Kübler-Ross, E. (1969). *On death and dying*. New York: Macmillan.

Kübler-Ross, E., & Kessler, D. (2005). *On grief and grieving: Finding the meaning of grief through the five stages of loss*. New York: Scribner.

Larson, D. G., & Hoyt, W. T. (2007). What has become of grief counseling? An evaluation of the empirical foundations of the new pessimism. *Professional Psychology: Research and Practice, 38*, 347–355.

Lazarus, R. S., & Folkman, S. (1984). *Stress, appraisal and coping*. New York: Springer.

Lazarus, R. S., Kanner, A. D., & Folkman, S. (1980). Emotions: A cognitive-phenomenological analysis. In R. Plutchik & H. Kellerman (Eds.), *Emotions: Theory, research, and experience* (Vol. 1, pp. 189–217). New York: Academic Press.

Leahy, J. M. (1992). A comparison of depression in women bereaved of a spouse, child, or a parent. *Omega: Journal of Death and Dying, 26*(3), 207–217.

Lehman, D. R., Ellard, J. H., & Wortman, C. B. (1986). Social support for the bereaved: Recipients' and providers' perspectives on what is helpful. *Journal of Consulting and Clinical Psychology, 54*, 438–446.

Lehman, D. R., Wortman, C. B., & Williams, A. F. (1987). Long-term effects of losing a spouse or child in a motor vehicle crash. *Journal of Personality and Social Psychology, 52*, 218–231.

Levine, P. (2010). *In an unspoken voice: How the body releases trauma and restores goodness*. Berkeley, CA: North Atlantic Books.

Lewis, L. H., & Hoy, W. G. (2011). Bereavement rituals and the creation of legacy. In R. W. Neimeyer, D. L. Harris, H. R. Winokuer, & G. F. Thornton

(Eds.), *Grief and bereavement in contemporary society: Bridging research and practice* (pp. 315–323). New York: Routledge.

Li, J., Laursen, T. M., Precht, D. H., Olsen, J., & Mortensen, P. B. (2005). Hospitalization for mental illness among parents after the death of a child. *New England Journal of Medicine, 352*(12), 1190–1196.

Li, J., Precht, D. H., Mortensen, P. B., & Olsen, J. (2003). Mortality in parents after death of a child in Denmark: A nationwide follow-up study. *Lancet, 361*, 363–367.

Lichtenthal, W. G. (2012). Schema therapy for the lost relationship. In R. A. Neimeyer (Ed.), *Techniques of grief therapy: Creative practices for counseling the bereaved* (pp. 139–141). New York: Routledge/Taylor & Francis.

Lichtenthal, W. G., Cruess, D. G., & Prigerson, H. G. (2004). A case for establishing complicated grief as a distinct mental disorder in DSM-V. *Clinical Psychology Review, 24*(6), 637–662.

Lichtenthal, W. G., Currier, J. M., Neimeyer, R. A., & Keesee, N. J. (2010). Sense and significance: A mixed methods examination of meaning making after the loss of one's child. *Journal of Clinical Psychology, 66*(7), 791–812.

Lifton, R. (1976). *Death in life: Survivors of Hiroshima*. New York: Touchstone.

Lindy, J. (1986). An outline for the psychoanalytic psychotherapy of post-traumatic stress disorder. In C. Figley (Ed.), *Trauma and its wake: Vol. 2. Traumatic stress theory, research and intervention* (pp. 195–212). New York: Brunner/Mazel.

Linehan, M. M. (1993). *Cognitive-behavioral treatment of borderline personality disorder*. New York: Guilford Press.

Litz, B. T., Stein, N., Delaney, E., Lebowitz, L., Nash, W. P., Silva, C., et al. (2009). Moral injury and moral repair in war veterans: A preliminary model and intervention strategy. *Clinical Psychology Review, 29*, 695–706.

Lobb, E. A., Kristjanson, L. J., Aoun, S. M., Monterosso, L., Halkett, G. K. B., & Davies, A. (2010). Predictors of complicated grief: A systematic review of studies. *Death Studies, 34*(8), 673–698.

Londono, E. (2013, January 14). Military suicides rise to a record 349, topping number of troops killed in combat. *Washington Post*. Available at *http://articles.washingtonpost.com/2013-01-14/world/36343832_1_military-suicides-rise-suicide-rate-active-duty-suicides*.

Lopata, H. Z. (1979). *Women as widows: Support systems*. New York: Elsevier.

Lynn, C., & Rath, A. (2012). GriefNet: Creating and maintaining an Internet bereavement community. In C. J. Sofka, I. N. Cupit, & K. R. Gilbert (Eds.), *Dying, death, and grief in an online universe: For counselors and educators* (pp. 87–102). New York: Springer.

Lyons-Ruth, K., Dutra, L., Schuder, M., & Bianchi, I. (2006). From infant attachment disorganization to adult dissociation: Relational adaptations or traumatic experiences? *Psychiatric Clinics of North America, 29*, 63–86.

Maciejewski, P. K., Zhang, B., Block, S. D., & Prigerson, H. G. (2007). An empirical examination of the stage theory of grief. *Journal of the American Medical Association, 297*(7), 716–723.

Mahler, M. (1975). *The psychological birth of the human infant: Symbiosis and individuation*. New York: Basic Books.

Malkinson, R. (2010). Cognitive-behavioral grief therapy: The ABC model of rational-emotion behavior therapy. *Psychological Topics, 19*(2), 289–305.

Malkinson, R., & Bar-Tur, L. (1999). The aging of grief in Israel: A perspective of bereaved parents. *Death Studies, 23*(5), 413–431.

Malkinson, R., Rubin, S. S., & Witztum, E. (Eds.). (2000). *Traumatic and nontraumatic loss and bereavement: Clinical theory and practice*. Madison, CT: Psychosocial Press.

Mancini, A. D., Robinaugh, D., Shear, K., & Bonanno, G. A. (2009). Does attachment avoidance help people cope with loss?: The moderating effects of relationship quality. *Journal of Clinical Psychology, 65*(10), 1127–1136.

Marris, P. (1975). *Loss and change*. Garden City, NY: Anchor Press/Doubleday.

Marshall, B., & Davies, B. (2011). Bereavement in children and adults following the death of a sibling. In R. A. Neimeyer, D. L. Harris, H. R. Winokuer, & G. F. Thornton (Eds.), *Grief and bereavement in contemporary society: Bridging research and practice* (pp. 107–116). New York: Routledge.

Martin, T. L., & Doka, K. (2000). *Men don't cry . . . women do: Transcending gender stereotypes of grief*. Philadelphia: Brunner/Mazel.

Martin, T. L., & Doka, K. J. (2011). The influence of gender and socialization on grieving styles. In R. A. Neimeyer, D. L. Harris, H. R. Winokuer, & G. F. Thornton (Eds.), *Grief and bereavement in contemporary society: Bridging research and practice* (pp. 69–77). New York: Routledge.

Marwit, S. J., & Carusa, S. S. (1998). Communicated support following loss: Examining the experiences of parental death and parental divorce in adolescence. *Death Studies, 22*, 237–255.

Marwit, S. J., & Klass, D. (1996). Grief and the role of the inner representation of the deceased. In D. Klass, P. R. Silverman, & S. L. Nickman (Eds.), *Continuing bonds: New understandings of grief* (pp. 297–309). Washington, DC: Taylor & Francis.

Matsakis, A. (1994). *Post-traumatic stress disorder: A complete treatment guide* (L. Tilley, Ed.). Oakland, CA: New Harbinger.

McCann, I. L., & Pearlman, L. A. (1990a). Constructivist self-development theory as a framework for assessing and treating victims of family violence. In S. M. Stith, M. B. Williams, & K. H. Rosen (Eds.), *Violence hits home: Comprehensive treatment approaches to domestic violence*. New York: Springer.

McCann, I. L., & Pearlman, L. A. (1990b). *Psychological trauma and the adult survivor: Theory, therapy, and transformation*. New York: Brunner/Mazel.

McCann, I. L., & Pearlman, L. A. (1990c). Vicarious traumatization: A framework for understanding the psychological effects of working with victims. *Journal of Traumatic Stress, 3*(1), 131–149.

McDevitt-Murphy, M. E., Neimeyer, R. A., Burke, L. A., Williams, J. L., & Lawson, K. (2012). The toll of traumatic loss in African Americans bereaved by homicide. *Psychological Trauma: Theory, Research, Practice, and Policy, 4*(3), 303–311.

McEwen, B. S., & Gianaros, P. J. (2011). Stress- and allostasis-induced brain plasticity. *Annual Review of Medicine, 62*(5), 431–445.

McIntosh, D., Silver, R., & Wortman, C. B. (1993). Religion's role in adjustment to a negative life event: Coping with the loss of a child. *Journal of Personality and Social Psychology, 65*, 812–821.

McKay, M., Davis, M., & Fanning, P. (1997). *Thoughts and feelings: Taking control of your moods and your life*. Oakland, CA: New Harbinger.

Mehren, E. (1997). *After the darkest hour, the sun will shine again*. New York: Simon & Schuster.

Mikulincer, M., & Shaver, P. R. (2008). An attachment perspective on bereavement. In M. S. Stroebe, R. O. Hansson, H. Schut, & W. Stroebe (Eds.), *Handbook of bereavement research and practice: Advances in theory and intervention* (pp. 87–112). Washington, DC: American Psychological Association.

Miller, E., & Wortman, C. B. (2002). Gender differences in mortality and morbidity following a major stressor: The case of conjugal bereavement. In G. Weidner, S. M. Kopp, & M. Kristenson (Eds.), *Heart disease: Environment, stress and gender* (pp. 251–266). Washington, DC: IOS Press.

Morina, N., von Lersner, U., & Prigerson, H. G. (2011). War and bereavement: Consequences for mental and physical distress. *PLoS ONE, 6*(7), e22140.

Moskowitz, J. T., Folkman, S., & Acree, M. (2003). Do positive psychological states shed light on recovery from bereavement?: Findings from a 3-year longitudinal study. *Death Studies, 27*, 471–500.

Munroe, J. F., Shay, J., Fisher, L., Makary, C., Rapperport, K., & Zimering, R. (1995). Preventing compassion fatigue: A team treatment model. In C. R. Figley (Ed.), *Compassion fatigue: Secondary traumatic stress disorder from treating the traumatized* (pp. 209–231). New York: Brunner/Mazel.

Murphy, S. A. (2008). The loss of a child: Sudden death and extended illness perspectives. In M. Stroebe, R. O. Hansson, H. Schut, & W. Stroebe (Eds.), *Handbook of bereavement research and practice: Advances in theory and intervention* (pp. 373–416). Washington, DC: American Psychological Association.

Murphy, S. A., Chung, I. J., & Johnson, L. C. (2002). Patterns of mental distress following the violent death of a child and predictors of change over time. *Research in Nursing and Health, 25*(6), 425–437.

Murphy, S. A., Das Gupta, A., Cain, K. C., Johnson, L. C., Lohan, J., Wu, L., et al. (1999). Changes in parents' mental distress after the violent death of an adolescent or young adult child: A longitudinal prospective analysis. *Death Studies, 23*, 129–159.

Murphy, S. A., Johnson, L. C., Chung, I. J., & Beaton, R. D. (2003). The prevalence of PTSD following the violent death of a child and predictors of change 5 years later. *Journal of Traumatic Stress, 16*, 17–25.

Murphy, S. A., Johnson, L. C., & Lohan, J. (2003a). Challenging the myths about parents' adjustment after the sudden, violent death of a child. *Journal of Nursing Scholarship, 35*(4), 359–364.

Murphy, S. A., Johnson, L. C., & Lohan, J. (2003b). Finding meaning in a child's violent death: A five-year prospective analysis of parents' personal narratives and empirical data. *Death Studies, 27*(5), 381–404.

Murphy, S. A., Johnson, L. C., Wu, L., Fan, J., & Lohan, J. (2003). Bereaved parents' outcome 4 to 60 months after their children's death by accident, suicide, or homicide. A comparative study demonstrating differences. *Death Studies, 27*(1), 39–61.

Murphy, S. A., Lohan, J., Dimond, M., & Fan, J. (1998). Network and mutual support for parents bereaved following the violent deaths of their 12- to 28-year-old children: A longitudinal, prospective analysis. *Journal of Loss and Trauma, 3*, 303–333.

Nader, K. O. (1997). Treating traumatic grief in systems. In C. R. Figley, B. E. Bride, & N. Mazza (Eds.), *Death and trauma: The traumatology of grieving* (pp. 159–192). Philadelphia: Taylor & Francis.

Najavits, L. M. (2002). *Seeking safety: A treatment manual for PTSD and substance abuse*. New York: Guilford Press.

Najavits, L. M. (2005). Substance abuse. In N. Kazantzis, F. Deane, K. R. Ronan, & L. L'Abate (Eds.), *Using homework assignments in cognitive behavior therapy* (pp. 263–282). New York: Routledge.

Neimeyer, R. A. (1998). *Lessons of loss: A guide to coping*. Boston: McGraw-Hill.

Neimeyer, R. A. (2000a). Narrative disruptions in the construction of self. In R. A. Neimeyer & J. Raskin (Eds.), *Constructions of disorder* (pp. 207–242). Washington, DC: American Psychological Association.

Neimeyer, R. A. (2000b). Searching for the meaning of meaning: Grief therapy and the process of reconstruction. *Death Studies, 24*(6), 541–558.

Neimeyer, R. A. (Ed.). (2001). *Meaning reconstruction and the experience of loss*. Washington, DC: American Psychological Association.

Neimeyer, R. A. (2012). Reconstructing the self in the wake of loss: A dialogical contribution. In H. J. M. Herman & T. Geiser (Eds.), *Handbook of dialogical self theory* (pp. 374–389). New York: Cambridge University Press.

Neimeyer, R. A., Burke, L. A., Mackay, M. M., & van Dyke Stringer, J. G. (2010). Grief therapy and the reconstruction of meaning: From the principles to practice. *Journal of Contemporary Psychotherapy, 40*, 73–83.

Neimeyer, R. A., & Harris, D. L. (2011). Building bridges in bereavement research and practice: Some concluding reflections. In R. A. Neimeyer, D. L. Harris, H. R. Winokuer, & G. F. Thornton (Eds.), *Grief and bereavement in contemporary society: Bridging research and practice* (pp. 403–418). New York: Routledge.

Neimeyer, R. A., Harris, D. L., Winokuer, H. R., & Thornton, G. F. (Eds.). (2011). *Grief and bereavement in contemporary society: Bridging research and practice*. New York: Routledge.

Neimeyer, R. A., & Sands, D. C. (2011). Meaning reconstruction in bereavement: From principles to practice. In R. A. Neimeyer, D. L. Harris, H. R. Winokuer, & G. F. Thornton (Eds.), *Grief and bereavement in contemporary society: Bridging research and practice* (pp. 9–22). New York: Routledge.

Neria, Y., & Litz, B. T. (2004). Bereavement by traumatic means: The complex synergy of trauma and grief. *Journal of Loss and Trauma, 9*(1), 73–87.

Neumann, D. A., & Pearlman, L. A. (1992). *Toward a psychological language for spirituality*. Unpublished manuscript.

Nolen-Hoeksema, S. (2001). Ruminative coping and adjustment to bereavement. In M. S. Stroebe, R. O. Hansson, W. Stroebe, & H. Schut (Eds.), *Handbook of bereavement research: Consequences, coping, and care* (pp. 545–562). Washington, DC: American Psychological Association.

Nolen-Hoeksema, S., & Larson, J. (1999). *Coping with loss*. Mahwah, NJ: Erlbaum.

Norcross, J. C. (2000). Psychotherapist self-care: Practitioner-tested, research-informed strategies. *Professional Psychology: Research and Practice, 31*(6), 710–735.

Normand, C. L., Silverman, P. R., & Nickman, S. L. (1996). Bereaved children's changing relationships with the deceased. In D. Klass, P. R. Silverman, & S. L. Nickman (Eds.), *Continuing bonds: New understandings of grief* (pp. 87–111). Washington, DC: Taylor & Francis.

Ott, C. H. (2003). The impact of complicated grief on mental and physical health at various points in the bereavement process. *Death Studies, 27*(3), 249–272.

Pargament, K. I., & Park, C. L. (1995). Merely a defense?: The variety of religious means and ends. *Journal of Social Issues, 51*, 13–32.

Park, C. L., & Cohen, L. H. (1993). Religious and nonreligious coping with the death of a friend. *Cognitive Therapy and Research, 17*, 561–577.

Park, C. L., & Halifax, R. J. (2011). Religion and spirituality in adjusting to bereavement: Grief as burden, grief as gift. In R. A. Neimeyer, D. L. Harris, H. R. Winokuer, & G. F. Thornton (Eds.), *Grief and bereavement in contemporary society: Bridging research and practice* (pp. 355–364). New York: Routledge.

Parkes, C. M. (1971). Psycho-social transitions: A field for study. *Social Science and Medicine, 5*, 101–115.

Parkes, C. M. (1972). Health after bereavement: A controlled study of young Boston widows and widowers. *Psychosomatic Medicine, 34*(5), 449–461.

Parkes, C. M. (2001). A historical overview of the scientific study of bereavement. In M. S. Stroebe, R. O. Hansson, W. Stroebe, & H. Schut (Eds.), *Handbook of bereavement research: Consequences, coping, and care* (pp. 25–45). Washington, DC: American Psychological Association.

Parkes, C. M. (2009). *Love and loss: The roots of grief and its complications.* East Sussex, UK: Routledge.

Parkes, C. M., & Weiss, R. S. (1983). *Recovery from bereavement.* New York: Basic Books.

Payne, L. A. (2008). *Unsettling accounts: Neither truth nor reconciliation in confessions of state violence.* Durham, NC: Duke University Press.

Pearlman, L. A. (1998). Trauma and the self: A theoretical and clinical perspective. *Journal of Emotional Abuse, 1,* 7–25.

Pearlman, L. A. (2001). Treatment of persons with complex PTSD and other trauma-related disruptions of the self. In J. P. Wilson, M. J. Friedman, & J. D. Lindy (Eds.), *Treating psychological trauma and PTSD* (pp. 205–236). New York: Guilford Press.

Pearlman, L. A. (2003). *Trauma and Attachment Belief Scale (TABS) manual.* Los Angeles: Western Psychological Services.

Pearlman, L. A., & Caringi, J. (2009). Living and working self-reflectively to address vicarious trauma. In C. A. Courtois & J. D. Ford (Eds.), *Treating complex traumatic stress disorders: An evidence-based guide* (pp. 202–224). New York: Guilford Press.

Pearlman, L. A., & Courtois, C. A. (2005). Clinical applications of the attachment framework: Relational treatment of complex trauma. *Journal of Traumatic Stress, 18,* 449–460.

Pearlman, L. A., & Mac Ian, P. S. (1995). Vicarious traumatization: An empirical study of the effects of trauma work on trauma therapists. *Professional Psychology: Research and Practice, 26*(6), 558–565.

Pearlman, L. A., & McCann, I. L. (1994). Integrating structured and unstructured approaches to taking a trauma history. In M. B. Williams & J. F. Sommer, Jr. (Eds.), *Handbook of post-traumatic therapy* (pp. 38–48). Westport, CT: Greenwood Press.

Pearlman, L. A., & Saakvitne, K. W. (1995). *Trauma and the therapist: Countertransference and vicarious traumatization in psychotherapy with incest survivors.* New York: Norton.

Pearlman, L. A., & Saakvitne, K. W. (in press). Strategies for transforming vicarious traumatization and compassion fatigue. In C. R. Figley (Ed.), *Compassion fatigue: Coping with secondary traumatic stress disorder in those who treat the traumatized* (2nd ed.). New York: Brunner/Mazel.

Pelcovitz, D., van der Kolk, B., Roth, S., Mandel, F., Kaplan, S., & Resick, P. (1997). Development of a criteria set and a Structured Interview for Disorders of Extreme Stress (SIDES). *Journal of Traumatic Stress, 10*(1), 3–16.

Pietrzak, R. H., Morgan, C. A., & Southwick, S. M. (2010). Sleep quality in treatment-seeking veterans of Operations Enduring Freedom and Iraqi Freedom: The role of cognitive coping strategies and unit cohesion. *Journal of Psychosomatic Research, 69*(5), 441–448.

Porges, S. W. (2011). *The polyvagal theory: Neurophysiological foundations of emotions, attachment, communication, and self-regulation.* New York: Norton.

Powell, S., Butollo, W., & Hagl, M. (2010). Missing or killed: The differential effect on mental health in women in Bosnia and Herzegovina of the confirmed or unconfirmed loss of their husbands. *European Psychologist, 15*(3), 185–192.

Powers, M. B., Halpern, J. M., Ferenschak, M. P., Gillihan, S. J., & Foa, E. B. (2010). A meta-analytic review of prolonged exposure for posttraumatic stress disorder. *Clinical Psychology Review, 30*(6), 635–641.

Prigerson, H. G., Frank, E., Kasl, S. V., Reynolds, C. F., Anderson, B., Zubenko, G. S., et al. (1995). Complicated grief and bereavement-related depression as distinct disorders: Preliminary empirical validation in elderly bereaved spouses. *American Journal of Psychiatry, 152*(1), 22–30.

Prigerson, H. G., Horowitz, M. J., Jacobs, S. C., Parkes, C. M., Asian, M., Goodkin, K., et al. (2009). Prolonged grief disorder: Psychometric validation of criteria proposed for DSM-V and ICD-11. *PLoS Medicine, 6*(8), e100021.

Prigerson, H. G., Maciejewski, P. K., Reynolds, C. F., Bierhals, A. J., Newsom, J. T., Fasiczka, A., et al. (1995). Inventory of Complicated Grief: A scale to measure maladaptive symptoms of loss. *Psychiatry Research, 59,* 65–79.

Prigerson, H. G., Maciejewski, P. K., & Rosenheck, R. A. (2000). Preliminary explorations of the harmful interactive effects of widowhood and marital harmony on health, health service use, and health care costs. *The Gerontologist, 40*(3), 349–357.

Prigerson, H. G., Shear, M. K., Frank, E., & Beery, L. C. (1997). Traumatic grief: A case of loss-induced trauma. *American Journal of Psychiatry, 154*(7), 1003–1009.

Prigerson, H. G., Shear, M. K., Jacobs, S. C.,

Reynolds, C. F., Maciejewski, P. K., Davidson, J. R., et al. (1999). Consensus criteria for traumatic grief. *British Journal of Psychiatry, 174,* 67–73.

Prigerson, H. G., Vanderwerker, L. C., & Maciejewski, P. K. (2008). A case for inclusion of prolonged grief disorder in DSM-V. In M. S. Stroebe, R. O. Hansson, H. Schut, & W. Stroebe (Eds.), *Handbook of bereavement research and practice: Advances in theory and intervention* (pp. 165–186). Washington, DC: American Psychological Association.

Pryce, J. G., Shackelford, K. K., & Pryce, D. H. (2007). *Secondary traumatic stress and the child welfare professional.* Chicago: Lyceum Books.

Rachman, S. (1980). Emotional processing. *Behaviour Research and Therapy, 18*(1), 51–60.

Ramsay, R. W., & Happee, J. A. (1977). The stress of bereavement: Components and treatment. *Stress and Anxiety, 4,* 53–64.

Rando, T. A. (Ed.). (1986). *Parental loss of a child.* Champaign, IL: Research Press.

Rando, T. A. (1993). *Treatment of complicated mourning.* Champaign, IL: Research Press.

Rando, T. A. (1997). Foreword. In C. R. Figley, B. E. Bride, & N. Mazza (Eds.), *Death and trauma: The traumatology of grieving* (pp. xv–xix). Washington, DC: Taylor & Francis.

Rando, T. A. (2000). On the experience of traumatic stress in anticipatory and postdeath mourning. In T. A. Rando (Ed.), *Clinical dimensions of anticipatory mourning: Theory and practice in working with the dying, their loved ones, and their caregivers* (pp. 155–222). Champaign, IL: Research Press.

Rando, T. A. (2013). On achieving clarity regarding complicated grief: Lessons from clinical practice. In M. S. Stroebe, H. Schut, & J. van den Bout (Eds.), *Complicated grief: Scientific foundations for health care professionals* (pp. 40–54). New York: Routledge.

Rando, T. A. (2014). *Coping with the sudden death of your loved one: A self-help handbook for traumatic bereavement.* Indianapolis, IN: Dog Ear.

Rando, T. A., Doka, K. J., Fleming, S., Franco, M. H., Lobb, E. A., Parkes, C. M., et al. (2012). A call to the field: Complicated grief in the DSM-5. *Omega: Journal of Death and Dying, 65*(4), 251–255.

Raphael, B. (1983). *The anatomy of bereavement.* New York: Basic Books.

Raphael, B. (1986). *When disaster strikes: How individuals and communities cope with catastrophes.* New York: Basic Books.

Raphael, B., & Martinek, N. (1997). Assessing traumatic bereavement and posttraumatic stress disorder. In J. P. Wilson & T. M. Keane (Eds.), *Assessing psychological trauma and PTSD* (pp. 373–395). New York: Guilford Press.

Rauch, S. A., Defever, E., Favorite, T., Duroe, A., Garrity, A., Martis, B., et al. (2009). Prolonged exposure for PTSD in a Veterans Health Administration PTSD clinic. *Journal of Traumatic Stress, 22*(1), 60–64.

Redmond, L. (1989). *Surviving: When someone you loved was murdered.* Clearwater, FL: Psychological Consultation and Educational Services.

Resick, P. A., Galovski, T. E., Uhlmansick, M. O., Scher, C. D., Clum, G. A., & Young-Xu, Y. (2008). A randomized clinical trial to dismantle components of cognitive processing therapy for posttraumatic stress disorder in female victims of interpersonal violence. *Journal of Consulting and Clinical Psychology, 76*(2), 243–258.

Resick, P. A., & Schnicke, M. K. (1992). Cognitive processing therapy for sexual assault survivors. *Journal of Consulting and Clinical Psychology, 60,* 748–756.

Resick, P. A., & Schnicke, M. K. (1993). *Cognitive processing therapy for rape victims: A treatment manual.* Newbury Park, CA: Sage.

Resick, P. A., & Schnicke, M. K. (1996). *Cognitive processing therapy for rape victims: A treatment manual.* Newbury Park, CA: Sage.

Resick, P. A., Williams, L. F., Suvak, M. K., Monson, C. M., & Gradus, J. L. (2012). Long-term outcomes of cognitive-behavioral treatments for posttraumatic stress disorder among female rape survivors. *Journal of Consulting and Clinical Psychology, 80*(2), 201–210.

Richards, T., Acree, M., & Folkman, S. (1999). Spiritual aspects of loss among partners of men with AIDS: Postbereavement follow-up. *Death Studies, 23*(2), 105–127.

Richards, T. A., & Folkman, S. (1997). Spiritual aspects of loss at the time of partner's death from AIDS. *Death Studies, 21*(6), 527–552.

Richardson, V. E. (2010). The dual process model of coping with bereavement: A decade later. *Omega: Journal of Death and Dying, 61*(4), 269–271.

Riches, G., & Dawson, P. (1998). Spoiled memories: Problems of grief resolution in families bereaved through murder. *Mortality, 3*(2), 143–159.

Riggs, D. S., Cahill, S. P., & Foa, E. B. (2006). Prolonged exposure treatment of posttraumatic stress disorder. In V. M. Follette & J. I. Ruzek (Eds.), *Cognitive-behavioral therapies for trauma* (2nd ed., pp. 65–95). New York: Guilford Press.

Riley, L. P., LaMontagne, L. L., Hepworth, J. T., &

Murphy, B. A. (2007). Parental grief responses and personal growth following the death of a child. *Death Studies, 31*(4), 277–299.

Robinson, T., & Marwit, S. J. (2006). An investigation of the relationship of personality, coping and grief intensity among bereaved mothers. *Death Studies, 30*(7), 677–696.

Rogers, C. H., Floyd, F. J., Seltzer, M. M., Greenberg, J., & Hong, J. (2008). Long-term effects of the death of a child on parents' adjustment in midlife. *Journal of Family Psychology, 22*(2), 203–211.

Rosenblatt, P. C. (2008). Grief across cultures: A review and research agenda. In M. S. Stroebe, R. O. Hansson, H. Schut, & W. Stroebe (Eds.), *Handbook of bereavement research and practice: Advances in theory and intervention* (pp. 207–222). Washington, DC: American Psychological Association.

Rosenblatt, P. C., & Wallace, B. R. (2005). Narratives of grieving African-Americans about racism in the lives of deceased family members. *Death Studies, 29*(3), 217–235.

Rosenbloom, D. J., Pratt, A. C., & Pearlman, L. A. (1995). Helpers' responses to trauma work: Understanding and intervening in an organization. In B. H. Stamm (Ed.), *Secondary traumatic stress: Self-care issues for clinicians, researchers, and educators* (pp. 65–79). Lutherville, MD: Sidran Press.

Rosof, B. D. (1994). *The worst loss: How families heal from the death of a child.* New York: Holt.

Rothschild, B. (2000). *The body remembers: The psychophysiology of trauma and trauma treatment.* New York: Norton.

Rothschild, B. (2006). *Help for the helper: The psychophysiology of compassion fatigue and vicarious trauma.* New York: Norton.

Rubin, S. (1990). Death of the future: An outcome study of bereaved parents in Israel. *Omega: Journal of Death and Dying, 20,* 323–339.

Rubin, S. (1992). Adult child loss and the two-track model of bereavement. *Omega: Journal of Death and Dying, 24,* 183–202.

Rubin, S. S., Malkinson, R., & Witztum, E. (1999). The pervasive impact of war-related loss and bereavement in Israel. *International Journal of Group Tensions, 28*(1–2), 137–153.

Rudestam, K. E. (1987). Public perceptions of suicide survivors. In E. Dunne, J. L. McIntosh, & K. Dunne-Maxim (Eds.), *Suicide and its aftermath: Understanding and counseling the survivors* (pp. 31–44). New York: Norton.

Ryan, W. (1976). *Blaming the victim.* New York: Vintage Books.

Rynearson, E. K. (1987). Bereavement after unnatural dying. In S. Zisook (Ed.), *Advances in bereavement* (pp. 77–93). Washington, DC: American Psychiatric Press.

Rynearson, E. K. (2001). *Retelling violent death.* New York: Brunner-Routledge.

Rynearson, E. K. (2005). The narrative labyrinth of violent dying. *Death Studies, 29*(4), 351–360.

Rynearson, E. K. (2010). The clergy, the clinician, and the narrative of violent death. *Pastoral Psychology, 59,* 179–189.

Rynearson, E. K., & Geoffrey, R. (1999). Bereavement after homicide: Its assessment and treatment. In C. R. Figley (Ed.), *Traumatology of grieving: Conceptual, theoretical and treatment foundations* (pp. 109–130). Philadelphia: Brunner/Mazel.

Rynearson, E. K., Johnson, T. A., & Correa, F. (2006). The horror and helplessness of violent death. In R. S. Katz & T. A. Johnson (Eds.), *When professionals weep: Emotional and countertransference responses in end-of-life care* (pp. 139–155). New York: Routledge.

Rynearson, E. K., & McCreery, J. M. (1993). Bereavement after homicide: A synergism of trauma and loss. *American Journal of Psychiatry, 150*(2), 258–261.

Rynearson, E. K., & Salloum, A. (2011). Restorative retelling: Revising the narrative of violent death. In R. A. Neimeyer, D. L. Harris, H. R. Winokuer, & G. F. Thornton (Eds.), *Grief and bereavement in contemporary society: Bridging research and practice* (pp. 177–188). New York: Routledge.

Rynearson, E. K., Schut, H., & Stroebe, M. (2013). Complicated grief after violent death: Identification and intervention. In M. S. Stroebe, H. Schut, & J. van den Bout (Eds.), *Complicated grief: Scientific foundations for health care professionals* (pp. 278–292). New York: Routledge/Taylor & Francis.

Saakvitne, K. W., Gamble, S. G., Pearlman, L. A., & Lev, B. T. (2000). *Risking connection: A training curriculum for working with survivors of childhood abuse.* Lutherville, MD: Sidran Press.

Saakvitne, K. W., Pearlman, L. A., & the Staff of the Traumatic Stress Institute. (1996). *Transforming the pain: A workbook on vicarious traumatization.* New York: Norton.

Sanders, C. M. (1989). *Grief: The mourning after.* New York: Wiley.

Sanders, C. M. (1993). Risk factors in bereavement outcome. In M. Stroebe, W. Stroebe, & R. O. Hansson (Eds.), *Handbook of bereavement: Theory, research and intervention* (pp. 255–267). New York: Cambridge University Press.

Sands, D. C., Jordan, J. R., & Neimeyer, R. A. (2011). The meanings of suicide: A narrative approach to healing. In J. R. Jordan & J. L. McIntosh (Eds.), *Grief after suicide: Understanding the consequences and caring for the survivors* (pp. 249–282). New York: Routledge.

Sanger, M. (2008–2009). When clients sense the presence of loved ones who have died. *Omega: Journal of Death and Dying, 59,* 69–89.

Schauben, L. J., & Frazier, P. A. (1995). Vicarious trauma: The effects on female counselors of working with sexual violence survivors. *Psychology of Women Quarterly, 19*(1), 49–64.

Schore, A. N. (1994). *Affect regulation and the origin of the self: The neurobiology of emotional development.* Hillsdale, NJ: Erlbaum.

Schore, A. N. (2001). The effects of early relational trauma on right brain development, affect regulation, and infant mental health. *Infant Mental Health Journal, 22*(1–2), 201–269.

Schut, H., Stroebe, M. S., van den Bout, J., & de Keijser, J. (1997). Intervention for the bereaved: Gender differences in the efficacy of two counseling programmes. *British Journal of Clinical Psychology, 36,* 63–72.

Schut, H., Stroebe, M. S., van den Bout, J., & Terheggen, M. (2001). The efficacy of bereavement interventions: Determining who benefits. In M. S. Stroebe, R. O. Hansson, W. Stroebe, & H. Schut (Eds.), *Handbook of bereavement research: Consequences, coping, and care* (pp. 705–737). Washington, DC: American Psychological Association.

Shapiro, F. F., & Forrest, M. S. (2004). *EMDR: The breakthrough therapy for overcoming anxiety, stress, and trauma.* New York: Basic Books.

Sharpless, B. A., & Barber, J. P. (2011). A clinician's guide to PTSD treatments for returning veterans. *Professional Psychology: Research and Practice, 42*(1), 8–15.

Shaver, P. R., & Tancredy, C. M. (2001). Emotion, attachment, and bereavement: A conceptual commentary. In M. S. Stroebe, R. O. Hansson, W. Stroebe, & H. Schut (Eds.), *Handbook of bereavement research: Consequences, coping, and care* (pp. 63–88). Washington, DC: American Psychological Association.

Shear, M. K. (2010). Exploring the role of experiential avoidance from the perspective of attachment theory and the dual process model. *Omega: Journal of Death and Dying, 61*(4), 357–369.

Shear, M. K., Boelen, P. A., & Neimeyer, R. A. (2011). Treating complicated grief: Converging approaches. In R. A. Neimeyer, D. L. Harris, H.

R. Winokuer, & G. F. Thornton (Eds.), *Grief and bereavement in contemporary society: Bridging research and practice* (pp. 139–162). New York: Routledge.

Shear, M. K., & Frank, E. (2006). Treatment of complicated grief: Integrating cognitive-behavioral methods with other treatment approaches. In V. M. Follette & J. I. Ruzek (Eds.), *Cognitive-behavioral therapies for trauma* (2nd ed., pp. 290–320). New York: Guilford Press.

Shear, M. K., Frank, E., Houck, P. R., & Reynolds, C. F. (2005). Treatment of complicated grief: A randomized controlled trial. *Journal of the American Medical Association, 293*(21), 2601–2608.

Shear, M. K., Gorscak, B., & Simon, N. (2006). Treatment of complicated grief following violent death. In E. K. Rynearson (Ed.), *Violent death: Resilience and intervention beyond the crisis* (pp. 157–174). New York: Routledge/Taylor & Francis.

Shear, M. K., & Shair, H. (2005). Attachment, loss, and complicated grief. *Developmental Psychobiology, 47*(3), 253–267.

Shear, M. K., Simon, N., Wall, M., Zisook, S., Neimeyer, R. A., Duan, N., et al. (2011). Complicated grief and related bereavement issues for DSM-5. *Depression and Anxiety, 28,* 103–117.

Shin, L. M., Rauch, S. L., & Pitman, R. K. (2006). Amygdala, medial prefrontal cortex, and hippocampal function in PTSD. *Annals of the New York Academy of Sciences, 1071,* 67–79.

Shipherd, J. C., Street, A. E., & Resick, P. A. (2006). Cognitive therapy for posttraumatic stress disorder. In V. M. Follette & J. I. Ruzek (Eds.), *Cognitive-behavioral therapies for trauma* (2nd ed., pp. 96–116). New York: Guilford Press.

Shmotkin, D. (1999). Affective bonds of adult children with living versus deceased parents. *Psychology and Aging, 14,* 473–482.

Siegel, D., & Solomon, M. (Eds.). (2003). *Healing trauma: Attachment, mind, body and brain.* New York: Norton.

Silver, R. C., Wortman, C. B., & Crofton, C. (1990). The role of coping in support provision: The self-presentational dilemma of victims of life crises. In B. R. Sarason, I. G. Sarason, & G. R. Pierce (Eds.), *Social support: An interactional view* (pp. 397–426). New York: Wiley.

Silverman, G. K., Johnson, J. G., & Prigerson, H. G. (2001). Preliminary explorations of the effects of prior trauma and loss on risk for psychiatric disorders in recently widowed people. *Israel Journal of Psychiatry, 38,* 202–215.

Sofka, C. J., Cupit, I. N., & Gilbert, K. R. (Eds.).

(2012). *Dying, death, and grief in an online universe: For counselors and educators*. New York: Springer.

Solomon, R. M., & Rando, T. A. (2007). Utilization of EMDR in the treatment of grief and mourning. *Journal of EMDR Practice and Research, 1*(2), 109–117.

Solomon, R. M., & Shapiro, F. (1997). Eye movement desensitization and reprocessing: A therapeutic tool for trauma and grief. In C. R. Figley, B. E. Bride, & N. Mazza (Eds.), *Death and trauma: The traumatology of grieving* (pp. 231–247). Washington, DC: Taylor & Francis.

Sormanti, M., & August, J. (1997). Parental bereavement: An exploration of parents' spiritual connections with their deceased children. *American Journal of Orthopsychiatry, 67*(3), 460–469.

Southwick, S. M., Litz, B., Charney, D., & Friedman, M. J. (Eds.). (2011). *Resilience and mental health: Challenges across the lifespan*. New York: Cambridge University Press.

Sprang, G. (2001). The use of eye movement desensitization and reprocessing (EMDR) in the treatment of traumatic stress and complicated mourning: Psychological and behavioral outcomes. *Research on Social Work Practice, 11*, 300–329.

Stamm, B. H. (2005). *The Professional Quality of Life Scale: Compassion satisfaction, burnout and compassion fatigue/secondary trauma scales*. Lutherville, MD: Sidran Press.

Stein, N., Folkman, S., Trabasso, T., & Richards, T. A. (1997). Appraisal and goal processes as predictors of psychological well-being in bereaved caregivers. *Journal of Personality and Social Psychology, 72*(4), 872–884.

Stroebe, M. S. (1992–1993). Coping with bereavement: A review of the grief work hypothesis. *Omega: Journal of Death and Dying, 26*, 19–42.

Stroebe, M. S., & Schut, H. (1999). The dual process model of coping with bereavement: Rationale and description. *Death Studies, 23*, 197–224.

Stroebe, M. S., & Schut, H. (2001a). Meaning making in the dual process model of coping with bereavement. In R. A. Neimeyer (Ed.), *Meaning reconstruction and the experience of loss* (pp. 55–73). Washington, DC: American Psychological Association.

Stroebe, M. S., & Schut, H. (2001b). Models of coping with bereavement: A review. In M. S. Stroebe, R. O. Hansson, W. Stroebe, & H. Schut (Eds.), *Handbook of bereavement research: Consequences, coping, and care* (pp. 375–403). Washington, DC: American Psychological Association.

Stroebe, M. S., Schut, H., & Finkenauer, C. (2001). The traumatization of grief?: A conceptual framework for understanding the trauma-bereavement interface. *Israel Journal of Psychiatry and Related Sciences, 38*, 185–201.

Stroebe, M. S., & Schut, H. (2005). To continue or relinquish bonds: A review of consequences for the bereaved. *Death Studies, 29*, 477–494.

Stroebe, M. S., & Schut, H. (2010). The dual process model of coping with bereavement: A decade on. *Omega: Journal of Death and Dying, 61*(4), 273–289.

Stroebe, M. S., Schut, H., & Stroebe, W. (2005). Attachment in coping with bereavement: A theoretical integration. *Review of General Psychology, 9*(1), 48–66.

Stroebe, M. S., Schut, H., & van den Bout, J. (Eds.). (2013). *Complicated grief: Scientific foundations for health care professionals*. New York: Routledge.

Stroebe, M. S., & Stroebe, W. (1991). Does "grief work" work? *Journal of Consulting and Clinical Psychology, 59*, 479–482.

Stroebe, M. S., Stroebe, W., & Schut, H. (2001). Gender differences in adjustment to bereavement: An empirical and theoretical review. *Review of General Psychology, 5*, 62–83.

Stroebe, M. S., Stroebe, W., Schut, H. A. W., & van den Bout, J. (1998). Bereavement. In H. Friedman, N. Adler, & R. D. Parke (Eds.), *Encyclopedia of mental health* (pp. 235–246). San Diego, CA: Academic Press.

Stroebe, M. S., van der Houwen, K., & Schut, H. (2008). Bereavement support, intervention, and research on the Internet: A critical review. In M. S. Stroebe, R. O. Hansson, H. Schut, & W. Stroebe (Eds.), *Handbook of bereavement research and practice: Advances in theory and intervention* (pp. 551–574). Washington, DC: American Psychological Association.

Stroebe, W., Stroebe, M., Abakoumkin, G., & Schut, H. (1996). The role of loneliness and social support in adjustment to loss: A test of attachment versus stress theory. *Journal of Personality and Social Psychology, 70*, 1241–1249.

Stroebe, W., Zech, E., Stroebe, M. S., & Abakoumkin, G. (2005). Does social support help in bereavement? *Journal of Social and Clinical Psychology, 24*(7), 1030–1050.

Sveen, C. A., & Walby, F. A. (2008). Suicide survivors' mental health and grief reactions: A systematic review of controlled studies. *Suicide and Life-Threatening Behavior, 38*, 13–29.

Symonds, M. (1980). The "second injury" to victims. In L. Kivens (Ed.), *Evaluation and change: Services for survivors* (pp. 36–38). Minneapolis, MN: Minneapolis Medical Research Foundation.

Tedeschi, R. G., & Calhoun, L. G. (2006). Time of change?: The spiritual challenges of bereavement and loss. *Omega: Journal of Death and Dying, 53*(1–2), 105–116.

Tedeschi, R. G., & Calhoun, L. G. (2008). Beyond the concept of recovery: Growth and the experience of loss. *Death Studies, 32*(1), 27–39.

Terr, L. C. (1995). Childhood traumas: An outline and overview. In G. S. Everly, Jr., & J. M. Lating (Eds.), *Psychotraumatology: Key papers and core concepts in posttraumatic stress* (pp. 301–320). New York: Plenum Press.

Thoits, P. A. (1995). Identity-relevant events and psychological symptoms: A cautionary tale. *Journal of Health and Social Behavior, 36*(1), 72–82.

Thompson, M. P., & Vardaman, P. J. (1997). The role of religion in coping with the loss of a family member to homicide. *Journal for the Scientific Study of Religion, 36*(1), 44–51.

Thorn, B. (2004). *Cognitive therapy for chronic pain: A step-by-step guide.* New York: Guilford Press.

Tompkins, M. A. (2004). *Using homework in psychotherapy: Strategies, guidelines, and forms.* New York: Guilford Press.

Tosone, C. (2006). Therapeutic intimacy—a post-9/11 perspective. *Smith College Studies in Social Work, 76*(4), 89–98.

Umberson, D. (1987). Family status and health behaviors: Social control as a dimension of social integration. *Journal of Health and Social Behavior, 28*, 306–319.

Umberson, D. (1992). Gender, marital status and the social control of health behavior. *Social Science and Medicine, 34*, 907–917.

Umberson, D. (2003). *Death of a parent.* New York: Cambridge University Press.

Valentine, C. (2006). Academic constructions of bereavement. *Mortality, 11*(1), 57–78.

Van Baarsen, B., Smit, J. H., Snijders, T. A. B., & Knipscheer, K. P. M. (1999). Do personal conditions and circumstances surrounding partner loss explain loneliness in newly bereaved older adults? *Ageing and Society, 19*(4), 441–469.

van der Houwen, K., Stroebe, M., Stroebe, W., Schut, H., van den Bout, J., & Wijngaards-de Meij, L. (2010). Risk factors for bereavement outcome: A multivariate approach. *Death Studies, 34*, 195–220.

van der Kolk, B. A. (2006). Clinical implications of neuroscience research in PTSD. *Annals of the New York Academy of Sciences, 1071*, 277–293.

Vanderwerker, L. C., Jacobs, S. C., Parkes, C. M., & Prigerson, H. G. (2006). An exploration of associations between separation anxiety in childhood and complicated grief in later-life. *Journal of Nervous and Mental Disease, 194*, 121–123.

van Doorn, C., Kasl, S. V., Beery, L. C., Jacobs, S. C., & Prigerson, H. G. (1998). The influence of marital quality and attachment styles on traumatic grief and depressive symptoms. *Journal of Nervous and Mental Disease, 186*(9), 566–573.

Volkan, V. (1971). A study of a patient's 're-grief work' through dreams, psychological tests and psychoanalysis. *Psychiatric Quarterly, 45*(2), 244–273.

Wagner, B. (2013). Internet-based bereavement interventions and support: An overview. In M. Stroebe, H. Schut, & J. van den Bout (Eds.), *Complicated grief: Scientific foundations for health care professionals* (pp. 235–247). New York: Routledge/Taylor & Francis.

Wagner, B., Knaevelsrud, C., & Maercker, A. (2006). Internet-based cognitive-behavioral therapy for complicated grief: A randomized controlled trial. *Death Studies, 30*(5), 429–453.

Walliss, J. (2001). Continuing bonds: Relationships between the living and the dead within contemporary spiritualism. *Mortality, 6*(2), 127–145.

Walser, R. D., & Westrup, D. (2007). *Acceptance and commitment therapy for the treatment of post-traumatic stress disorder and trauma-related problems: A practitioner's guide to using mindfulness and acceptance strategies.* Oakland, CA: New Harbinger.

Waskowic, T. D., & Chartier, B. M. (2003). Attachment and the experience of grief following the loss of a spouse. *Omega: Journal of Death and Dying, 47*(1), 77–91.

Weiner, B. (2006). *Social motivation, justice, and the moral emotions: An attributional approach.* Mahwah, NJ: Erlbaum.

Wheaton, B. (1990). Life transitions, role histories, and mental health. *American Sociological Review, 55*, 209–223.

Wickie, S. K., & Marwit, S. J. (2000–2001). Assumptive world views and the grief reactions of parents of murdered children. *Omega: Journal of Death and Dying, 42*(2), 101–113.

Wijngaards-de Meij, L., Stroebe, M., Schut, H., Stroebe, W., van den Bout, J., van der Heijden, P., et al. (2005). Couples at risk following the death of their child: Predictors of grief versus depression. *Journal of Consulting and Clinical Psychology, 73*(4), 617–623.

Williams, A. L., & Merten, M. J. (2009). Adolescents' online social networking following the death of a peer. *Journal of Adolescent Research, 24*(1), 67–90.

Wilson, J. P., Friedman, M. J., & Lindy, J. D. (Eds.). (2002). *Treating psychological trauma and PTSD.* New York: Guilford Press.

Wilson, J. P., & Lindy, J. D. (1994). *Countertransference in the treatment of PTSD.* New York: Guilford Press.

Wilson, J. P., & Moran, T. A. (1998). Psychological trauma: Posttraumatic stress disorder and spirituality. *Journal of Psychology and Theology, 26*(2), 168–178.

Wilson, J. P., & Thomas, R. B. (2004). *Empathy in the treatment of trauma and PTSD.* New York: Brunner-Routledge.

Wittouck, C., Autreve, S. V., Jaegere, E. D., Portzky, G., & van Herringen, K. (2011). The prevention and treatment of complicated grief: A meta-analysis. *Clinical Psychology Review, 31,* 69–78.

Wolterstorff, N. (1987). *Lament for a son.* Grand Rapids, MI: Eerdmans.

Worden, J. W. (2009). *Grief counseling and grief therapy: A handbook for the mental health practitioner* (4th ed.). New York: Springer.

Worden, J. W., & Winokuer, H. R. (2011). A task-based approach for counseling the bereaved. In R. A. Neimeyer, D. L. Harris, H. R. Winokuer, & G. F. Thornton (Eds.), *Grief and bereavement in contemporary society: Bridging research and practice* (pp. 57–67). New York: Routledge.

Wortman, C. B. (2004). Posttraumatic growth: Progress and problems. *Psychological Inquiry, 15,* 81–90.

Wortman, C. B., Battle, E., & Lemkau, J. P. (1997). Coming to terms with the sudden traumatic death of a spouse or child. In A. J. Lurigio, W. G. Skogan, & R. C. Davis (Eds.), *Victims of crime: Problems, policies and programs* (2nd ed., pp. 108–133). Thousand Oaks, CA: Sage.

Wortman, C. B., & Boerner, K. (2007). Beyond the myths of coping with loss: Prevailing assumptions versus scientific evidence. In H. S. Friedman & R. C. Silver (Eds.), *Foundations of health psychology* (pp. 285–324). New York: Oxford University Press.

Wortman, C. B., & Boerner, K. (2011). Beyond the myths of coping with loss: Prevailing assumptions versus scientific evidence. In H. Friedman (Ed.), *Oxford handbook of health* (pp. 438–476). New York: Oxford University Press.

Wortman, C. B., Pearlman, L., Feuer, C., Farber, C., & Rando, T. (2012). Traumatic bereavement. In C. Figley (Ed.), *Encyclopedia of trauma* (pp. 750–754). Thousand Oaks, CA: Sage.

Wortmann, J. H., & Park, C. L. (2008). Religion and spirituality in adjustment following bereavement: An integrative review. *Death Studies, 32*(8), 703–736.

Wortmann, J. H., & Park, C. L. (2009). Religion/spirituality and change in meaning after bereavement: Qualitative evidence for the meaning making model. *Journal of Loss and Trauma, 14*(1), 17–34.

Zayfert, C., DeViva, J. C., Becker, C. B., Pike, J. L., Gillock, K. L., & Hayes, S. A. (2005). Exposure utilization and completion of cognitive behavioral therapy for PTSD in a "real world" clinical practice. *Journal of Traumatic Stress, 18*(6), 637–645.

Zech, E., & Arnold, C. (2011). Attachment and coping with bereavement: Implications for therapeutic interventions with the insecurely attached. In R. A. Neimeyer, D. L. Harris, H. R. Winokuer, & G. F. Thornton (Eds.), *Grief and bereavement in contemporary society: Bridging research and practice* (pp. 23–35). New York: Routledge.

Zettle, R. D. (2007). *ACT for depression: A clinician's guide to using acceptance and commitment therapy in treating depression.* Oakland, CA: New Harbinger.

Zhang, B., El-Jawahri, A., & Prigerson, H. G. (2006). Update on bereavement research: Evidence-based guidelines for the diagnosis and treatment of complicated bereavement. *Journal of Palliative Medicine, 9*(5), 1188–1203.

Zisook, S., Chentsova-Dutton, Y., & Schuchter, S. R. (1998). PTSD following bereavement. *Annals of Clinical Psychiatry, 10*(4), 157–163.

Zisook, S., & Shuchter, S. R. (1993). Uncomplicated bereavement. *Journal of Clinical Psychiatry, 54*(10), 365–372.

Index

Page references in *italic* refer to tables, figures, and handouts

354 Index

Professional Quality of Life Scale,
    256–257
Prolonged exposure (PE), 123–125, 128
Prolonged grief disorder (PGD),
    119–120
Psychic numbing, 74
Psychics, 222–224
Psychoeducation
    challenges of, 235
    in structured sessions, 156, 159
    in traumatic bereavement
        treatment, 14
Psychological needs
    defined, 26, 28
    importance to clients in treatment,
        28–29
Psychological Needs Handout,
    313–317
Psychological trauma
    CSDT framework for
        understanding, 25–26, 36
    defined, 25
    factors affecting the experience
        of, 25
    loss of meaning and, 255
    problematic responses to traumatic
        events, 25
    processing of, 31–33
    symptoms of, 134
    See also Posttraumatic stress
        disorder
Psychosocial loss, 19
PTSD treatment
    integrating grief and trauma
        research, 126–128
    prolonged exposure and CBT,
        123–125
    research on, 121–123
    strengthening self capacities, 125–126
    versus treatment for complicated
        grief, 120

Rage, 5
Random deaths, 73–74, 79
React to the Separation, 211–215
Readjusting to Move Adaptively
    into the New World without
    Forgetting the Old, 218–225
Recognize the Loss, 209–211
Recognizing feelings, 168–169. See
    also Affect management
Recollect and Reexperience
    the Deceased and the
    Relationship, 215–217
Recreation, survivors and, 58–59
Reenactment stories, 71
Reinvestment, 225–226
Relational therapy, 33, 234–235
Religion. See Meaning and
    spirituality; Spirituality
Religious community, survivors and,
    59–60
Religious struggle, 95
Relinquishing the Old Attachments
    to the Deceased and the Old
    Assumptive World, 217–218

Remarriage, 101
Resistance, 232
Resource building
    bereavement-specific issues,
        177–182
    clinical integration, 165, 188–189
    coping skills, 170–172
    importance of, 34, 189–190
    meaning and spirituality, 182–185
    overview, 10–13
    self capacities, 165–170
    social support, 172–177
    in structured sessions, 156, 159
    See also Ego resources
Restoration-oriented coping, 116–117
Responses to sudden, traumatic
    death
    behavioral, 42–43
    physical, 42–43
    psychological, 42–43
    social, 42–43
Revenge fantasies, 46, 71
Reviewing and remembering
    realistically, 215, 216
Revising the assumptive world,
    218–220
Reviving and reexperiencing feelings,
    215, 216–217
Risk factors
    characteristics of the death
        confrontation with the deaths of
            others, 74–75
        human-induced events, 72–73
        multiple deaths, 74
        perpetrator's behavior, 76
        physical or emotional suffering
            before death, 71–72
        randomness, 73–74
        threat to one's own life, 74–75
        unnaturalness, 70
        untimeliness, 75–76
        viewing or identifying the body,
            76–77
        violence, 70–71
    defined, 69
    importance of therapeutic attention
        to, 69, 89–90
    modes of death
        accidents, 79–80
        acute natural death, 78
        disasters, 80–82
        homicide, 84–86
        impact on parents, 77–78
        military combat, 82–84
        suicide, 86–89
    recent focus on in research, 114
Risking Connection trauma training
    curriculum (Saakvitne et al.,
    2000), 146, 166, 170, 253,
    256–257
Role-playing, 181
"R" processes, 13
    in the accommodation phase,
        24–25
    in the avoidance phase, 22–23
    challenges of, 234

client assessment of progression
    through, 137–138
clinical integration, 208, 226–227
in the confrontation phase, 23–24
importance to traumatic
    bereavement treatment, 34
interrelatedness of, 209
mourning and, 22, 23, 227–228
multiple deaths and, 74
overview, 113, 208
React to the Separation, 211–215
Readjust to Move Adaptively into the
    New World without Forgetting
    the Old, 218–225
Recognize the Loss, 209–211
Recollect and Reexperience
    the Deceased and the
    Relationship, 215–217
Reinvestment, 225–226
Relinquish the Old Attachments to
    the Deceased and the Old
    Assumptive World, 217–218
in structured sessions, 156, 159

Safety, 243
Same-sex couples, 53
Sample Automatic Thought Record
    Handout, 292
Schemas, 26, 28–29
Second Account of the Death
    Handout, 306
Secondary losses
    discussion of, 19–20
    following disasters, 81
    identifying and mourning, 212,
        214–215
Secondary Losses Handout, 215,
    299–302
Secure attachment style, 101, 102
Self, disrupted domains of, 26–30
Self capacities
    assessment of, 140
    challenges of developing, 232–233
    as a component of the treatment
        approach, 10, 11
    defined, 26, 27
    developing, 166–170
    handouts for, 154, 303, 304–305
    importance to traumatic
        bereavement treatment, 11,
        27, 33–34
    regulation of internal states, 165–166
    strengthening approach in the
        treatment of PTSD, 125–126
    See also Feelings skills
Self-care, in coping with vicarious
    traumatization, 257–258
Self-Care Handout, 277
Self-esteem, adjustment after loss
    and, 98
Self-isolation, 62–63
Self worth
    defined, 11
    developing, 168
    inner stability and, 166, 167–168
    See also Self capacities

Separation distress, 121
Sexual intimacy, 53
Shared trauma, 251–252
Sibling deaths, 53, 55, 99–100, 322
  clinical integration, 135
Six "R" Processes of Mourning
  Handout, 279
Skills training in affect and
  interpersonal regulation
  (STAIR), 125–126
Social, responses to sudden, traumatic
  death, *42–43*
Social ineptitude, 63–64
Social networking bereavement sites,
  176–177
Social support
  assessment of, *140*
  defined, 172
  developing, 172–174
  handouts for, *154, 303, 304–305*
  homicide survivors and, 86
  importance to clients in treatment,
    11, 172
  problems and failures for survivors,
    62–64
  suicide survivors and, 89
Spiritual community, 59–60
Spirituality
  coping with traumatic death and,
    94–98
  defined, 184, 254–255, 259–260
  disrupted spirituality and vicarious
    traumatization, 254–255,
    259–260
  exploring, 184–185
  traumatic bereavement treatment
    and, 266
  See also Meaning and spirituality
Spirituality Handout, 331
Spouse death
  gender differences in grief and
    coping, 92
  impact of attachment style on the
    survivor's reactions to,
    101–103
  impact on the survivor in
    conflictual or ambivalent
    relationships, 100–101
Stage models of grief, 13, 109–111,
  113
Stillbirths, 100
Stimulus-cued precipitants, 178–179
Stress and coping model of mourning,
  13, 113–114
Structured interviews, 242
Structured session format
  challenges of, 234–235
  core treatment components, *156,*
    159
  introduction to the session, *156,*
    157–159
  overview, 156–157
  wrap-up, *156,* 159–161
Subjective assessment, 114
Subjective Units of Distress Scale
  (SUDS), 202–203, 204

Subsequent temporary upsurge of
  grief (STUG) reactions
  addressing in therapy, 179–182
  defined, 177
  impact of, 179
  triggers for, 178–179
Sudden, traumatic death
  characteristics affecting traumatic
    bereavement
    confrontation with the deaths of
      others, 74–75
    human-induced events, 72–73
    multiple deaths, 74
    perpetrator's behavior, 76
    physical or emotional suffering
      before death, 71–72
    randomness, 73–74
    threat to one's own life, 74–75
    unnaturalness, 70
    untimeliness, 75–76
    viewing or identifying the body,
      76–77
    violence, 70–71
  countertransference responses to,
    249, 250
  defined, 4, 18
  examples of, 3, 4
  handouts for, *154, 303, 304–305*
  modes of death. *See* Modes of death
  persistent and pervasive effects of, 7–9
  prevalence, 4
  psychological consequences of, 4–7
Sudden, Traumatic Death and
  Traumatic Bereavement
  Handout, 215, 269–272
Sudden, traumatic loss, 18
Sudden infant death syndrome
  (SIDS), 78
Suffering
  physical or emotional suffering
    before death, 71–72
  preoccupation with the deceased's
    suffering, 48
Suicide
  clinical vignette, 3, 69
  military suicides, 83
  traumatic bereavement and, 73,
    86–89
Suicide notes, 88
Suicide survivors
  blaming others, 87
  disguising the cause of death, 87
  family dynamics and, 88
  feelings of guilt, 47, 87, 88
  social support and, 89
  studies of, 86–87
  suicide notes and, 88
  unanswered questions and, 87–88
Support groups, 174, 175
Survivors
  bereavement overload and psychic
    numbing, 74
  domains of life affected
    extended family, 55–56
    nuclear family, 51–55
    overview, 50–51

grappling with meaning, 44–45
guilt feelings, 47–48, 87, 88
impact of trauma symptoms, 6
problems and failures of social
  support, 62–64
reenactment stories, 71
risk factors for traumatic
  bereavement
  characteristics of the death,
    70–77
  importance of therapeutic
    attention to, 69, 89–90
  mode of death, 77–89
  See also Person-related risk
    factors; Risk factors
structures of daily life affected by
  traumatic death
  faith communities, 59–60
  leisure and recreation, 58–59
  overview, 56–57
  work, 57–58
symptoms and adaptations to
  traumatic death, 39–40, *42–43*
violation of the assumptive world,
  40–41, 44–48
withdrawal, 62–63
Symbolic bonds, 115
Symptoms. *See* Trauma symptoms

Task approach to mourning, 113
Television watching, 59
Termination
  challenges of the focus on,
    235–236
  of therapy, 150–152
Terrorist attacks, 81. *See also*
  Community violence
Thanatology, 3
Therapeutic relationship
  cultivating self capacities in,
    166–167
  importance in treatment, 14,
    145–146
  termination, 150–152, 235–236
Therapeutic window, 138, 153
Therapists
  building weaker suits, 244
  challenges of traumatic
    bereavement therapy. *See*
    Treatment challenges
  clinical consultation and, 260,
    262–263
  countertransference and, 249–254
  effects of the treatment on,
    248–249, 264–266
  identifying stronger and weaker
    suits, 243–244
  peer support groups, 263–264
  rewards of traumatic bereavement
    work, 264
  training and continuing education,
    260
  vicarious traumatization, 254–260
Therapy frame, 146–148
"Thinking–feeling–doing" continuum,
  169–170